Nanotechnology in Skin, Soft Tissue, and Bone Infections

Mahendra Rai

Editor

Nanotechnology in Skin, Soft Tissue, and Bone Infections

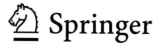 Springer

Editor
Mahendra Rai
Nanobiotechnology Laboratory
Department of Biotechnology
Amravati, Maharashtra, India

ISBN 978-3-030-35149-6   ISBN 978-3-030-35147-2   (eBook)
https://doi.org/10.1007/978-3-030-35147-2

This Springer imprint is published by the registered company Springer Nature Switzerland AG
The registered company address is: Gewerbestrasse 11, 6330 Cham, Switzerland

Preface

Skin, soft tissue, and bone infections are increasing due to the invasion of a wide variety of microorganisms, including bacteria, fungi, viruses, and protozoa. Usually, these infections are mild but they are sometimes fatal to human beings. Such infections can be cutaneous, subcutaneous, or deep-seated in tissues. Among these, bacterial infections occur commonly throughout the world and have created the problem of resistance to drugs. There are alarming reports of methicillin-resistant *Staphylococcus aureus* (MRSA), which accounts for the major part of community-acquired skin infections. Streptococci are also responsible for such infections. These infections are more common in immunocompromised patients. Unfortunately, the rate of development of antibiotics is very slow, and the problem of multidrug-resistance is quickly increasing. These infections are booming in hospitals and mostly community-acquired. Considering these facts, there is a greater need to search for newer antibiotics or potential alternatives to tackle the problem.

In this context, nanotechnology is emerging as a potential tool to fight against multidrug-resistant microbes. It has demonstrated huge potential for the treatment of bone infections through the application of antibacterial nanomaterials. Many nano-biomaterials have been studied for scaffold reinforcement to improve their micro-mechanical and biocompatible properties. For example, calcium phosphate (CaP) bioceramics are commonly used as local delivery agents (nanocarriers) for the treatment of bone infections and can be substituted with antibacterial nanoparticles that possess broad-spectrum activity even against multidrug-resistant bacteria. Metal nanoparticles such as silver nanoparticles and other antimicrobial nanomaterials can be used for coating of implants. This self-assembly at the nanolevel at body temperature may, in the future, be used by way of side chains to direct bone growth or possibly to combat osteomyelitis. Silver nanoparticles are yet another nanostructured material that is attracting increasing attention as an effective antimicrobial agent. Wound dressings impregnated with silver nanoparticles have already proven their remarkable potential against Gram-positive and Gram-negative bacteria.

The present book covers the role of nanotechnology in skin infections such as atopic dermatitis and acne vulgaris, as well as the role of metal nanoparticles as antibacterial and antifungal. It additionally elaborates on the management of wound and bone infections using different nanoparticles. Finally, this book discusses toxicity issues concerning the use of nanoparticles.

This book will be useful for master and postgraduate students, researchers, and teachers dealing with medical microbiology, dermatology, osteology, nanotechnology, nanobiotechnology, pharmacology, microbiology, and biotechnology.

Amravati, Maharashtra, India   Mahendra Rai

Contents

Contributors

Mehran Alavi Laboratory of Nanobiotechnology, Department of Biology, Faculty of Science, Razi University, Kermanshah, Iran

Venâncio Alves Amaral Laboratory of Biomaterials and Nanotechnology, University of Sorocaba, Sorocaba, São Paulo, Brazil

Farnoush Asghari-Paskiabi Department of Mycology, Pasteur Institute of Iran, Tehran, Iran

Fernando Batain Laboratory of Biomaterials and Nanotechnology, University of Sorocaba, Sorocaba, São Paulo, Brazil

Debalina Bhattacharya Department of Microbiology, Maulana Azad College, Kolkata, West Bengal, India

Marco Vinicius Chaud Laboratory of Biomaterials and Nanotechnology, University of Sorocaba, Sorocaba, São Paulo, Brazil

Kessi Marie Moura Crescencio Laboratory of Biomaterials and Nanotechnology, University of Sorocaba, Sorocaba, São Paulo, Brazil

Hanna Dahm Department of Microbiology, Nicolaus Copernicus University, Torun, Poland

Larissa Ciappina de Camargo Department of Microbiology, Biological Sciences Center, Universidade Estadual de Londrina, Londrina, Paraná, Brazil

Parneet Kaur Deol Department of Pharmaceutics, G.H.G. Khalsa College of Pharmacy, Gurusar Sadhar, Ludhiana, Punjab, India

Carolina Alves dos Santos College of Pharmacy, University of Sorocaba, Sorocaba, São Paulo, Brazil

Amoljit Singh Gill Department of Mechanical Engineering, Punjab Technical University, Kapurthala, Punjab, India

Marcelly Chue Gonçalves Department of Microbiology, Biological Sciences Center, Universidade Estadual de Londrina, Londrina, Paraná, Brazil

Avinash P. Ingle Department of Biotechnology, Engineering School of Lorena, University of Sao Paulo, Lorena, SP, Brazil

Zahra Jahanshiri Department of Mycology, Pasteur Institute of Iran, Tehran, Iran

Aswathy Jayakumar School of Biosciences, Mahatma Gandhi University, Kottayam, Kerala, India

Vandita Kakkar Department of Pharmaceutical Sciences, University Institute of Pharmaceutical Sciences, Panjab University, Chandigarh, India

Indu Pal Kaur Department of Pharmaceutics, University Institute of Pharmaceutical Sciences, Panjab University, Chandigarh, India

Renata Katsuko Takayama Kobayashi Department of Microbiology, Biological Sciences Center, Universidade Estadual de Londrina, Londrina, Paraná, Brazil

Parina Kumari Department of Pharmaceutical Sciences, University Institute of Pharmaceutical Sciences, Panjab University, Chandigarh, India

Audrey Alesandra Stinghen Garcia Lonni Department of Pharmaceutical Sciences, Health Sciences Center, Universidade Estadual de Londrina, Londrina, Paraná, Brazil

Milena Menegazzo Miranda-Sapla Department of Pathological Sciences, Biological Sciences Center, Universidade Estadual de Londrina, Londrina, Paraná, Brazil

Fabio Franceschini Mitri Department of Human Anatomy, Biomedical Sciences Institute, Federal University of Uberlandia, Uberlandia, MG, Brazil

Mainak Mukhopadhyay Department of Biotechnology, JIS University, Kolkata, West Bengal, India

Gerson Nakazato Department of Microbiology, Biological Sciences Center, Universidade Estadual de Londrina, Londrina, Paraná, Brazil

Priyanka Narula Department of Pharmaceutical Sciences, University Institute of Pharmaceutical Sciences, Panjab University, Chandigarh, India

Luciano Aparecido Panagio Department of Microbiology, Biological Sciences Center, Universidade Estadual de Londrina, Londrina, Paraná, Brazil

Anita K. Patlolla CSET, Department of Biology, Jackson State University, Jackson, MS, USA

Joana C. Pieretti Center for Natural and Human Sciences (CCNH), Federal University of ABC (UFABC), Santo André, SP, Brazil

Sushant Prajapati Department of Biotechnology and Medical Engineering, NIT, Rourkela, India

E. K. Radhakrishnan School of Biosciences, Mahatma Gandhi University, Kottayam, Kerala, India

Mahendra Rai Nanobiotechnology Laboratory, Department of Biotechnology, Amravati, Maharashtra, India

Thais Cruz Ramalho Laboratory of Pharmaceutical Nanosystems—NANOSFAR, Postgraduate Program in Pharmaceutical Sciences, Federal University of Piauí, Teresina, Piauí, Brazil

Mehdi Razzaghi-Abyaneh Department of Mycology, Pasteur Institute of Iran, Tehran, Iran

Márcia Araújo Rebelo College of Pharmacy, Max Planck University Center, Indaiatuba, São Paulo, Brazil

Guilherme Fonseca Reis Department of Microbiology, Biological Sciences Center, Universidade Estadual de Londrina, Londrina, Paraná, Brazil

Hercília Maria Lins Rolim Laboratory of Pharmaceutical Nanosystems—NANOSFAR, Postgraduate Program in Pharmaceutical Sciences, Federal University of Piauí, Teresina, Piauí, Brazil

Rituparna Saha Department of Biotechnology, JIS University, Kolkata, West Bengal, India

Amaresh Kumar Sahoo Department of Applied Sciences, Indian Institute of Information Technology, Allahabad, India

Amedea B. Seabra Center for Natural and Human Sciences (CCNH), Federal University of ABC (UFABC), Santo André, SP, Brazil

Masoomeh Shams-Ghahfarokhi Department of Mycology, Faculty of Medical Sciences, Tarbiat Modares University, Tehran, Iran

Vishal Singh Department of Applied Sciences, Indian Institute of Information Technology, Allahabad, India

Victória Soares Soeiro Laboratory of Biomaterials and Nanotechnology, University of Sorocaba, Sorocaba, São Paulo, Brazil

Paul B. Tchounwou CSET, Department of Biology, Jackson State University, Jackson, MS, USA

Fernanda Tomiotto-Pellissier Carlos Chagas Institute (ICC), Fiocruz, Curitiba, Paraná, Brazil

Arushi Verma Department of Applied Sciences, Indian Institute of Information Technology, Allahabad, India

Alka Yadav Department of Biotechnology, Sant Gadge Baba Amravati University, Amravati, Maharashtra, India

Mohd Yaseen Department of Pharmaceutical Sciences, University Institute of Pharmaceutical Sciences, Panjab University, Chandigarh, India

Part I
Skin Infections

Chapter 1
Nitric Oxide-Releasing Nanomaterials and Skin Infections

Joana C. Pieretti and Amedea B. Seabra

Abstract The free radical nitric oxide (NO) is an important endogenous molecule that controls several biological processes, ranging from the promotion of vasodilatation to the acceleration of wound repair process and potent antimicrobial effects. NO is synthesized in human skin through the action of three isoforms of nitric oxide synthase (NOS), with an important role in dermal vasodilatation, wound healing process, tissue repair, and skin defense against pathogens. During the past few years, interest has increased in the development of biologically friendly and versatile NO-releasing materials for biomedical applications, in particular, for topical/dermatological applications. Recently, the combination of NO donors/generations with nanomaterials has been emerging as a suitable strategy to carry and deliver therapeutic amounts of NO directly to the target site of application, including human skin, as discussed in this chapter. Thus, NO-releasing nanomaterials present great potential to treat skin diseases, highlighting skin infections caused by pathogens, because of the broad spectrum of antimicrobial activity of NO. In this sense, NO donors/generators have been incorporated in nanoparticles, leading to a sustained and localized delivery of NO. This chapter presents and discusses the recent advantages on the design and applications of NO-releasing nanomaterials for dermatological applications, mainly in promoting wound healing and in combating resistant pathogens.

Keywords Antimicrobial · Nanomaterials · Nanoparticles · Nitric oxide · Nitric oxide donors · Skin infections

J. C. Pieretti · A. B. Seabra (✉)
Center for Natural and Human Sciences (CCNH), Federal University of ABC (UFABC), Santo André, SP, Brazil
e-mail: amedea.seabra@ufabc.edu.br

© Springer Nature Switzerland AG 2020
M. Rai (ed.), *Nanotechnology in Skin, Soft Tissue, and Bone Infections*,
https://doi.org/10.1007/978-3-030-35147-2_1

3

Nomenclature

AgNPs   Silver nanoparticles
AuNPs   Gold nanoparticles
eNOS   Endothelial nitric oxide synthase
GSNO   *S*-Nitroso glutathione
iNOS   Inducible nitric oxide synthase
MRSA   Methicillin-resistant *Staphylococcus aureus*
MSSA   Methicillin-sensitive *Staphylococcus aureus*
nNOS   Neuronal nitric oxide synthase
NO   Nitric oxide
NO_2^- Nitrite
NO_3^- Nitrate
NOS   Nitric oxide synthase
O_2 Oxygen
$RONO_2$ NO-releasing organic nitrates
RSNO   *S*-Nitroso molecules
UV   Ultraviolet radiation
UVA   Ultraviolet A radiation

1.1   Introduction

More than two decades ago, nitric oxide (NO) was only known by its significant role in atmosphere phenomena and pollution, contributing to ozone removal from high levels of the atmosphere. In 1992, NO was considered the molecule of the year by Science (Koshland 1992). In 1998, the Nobel Prize of Medicine and Physiology was awarded to Robert F. Furchgott, Louis J. Ignarro, and Ferid Murad for their path-breaking discoveries regarding the effects of NO on the cardiovascular system (Ignarro 1999; Seabra 2017; Stuehr and Haque 2018). NO is not only a key molecule in the cardiovascular system, but it also controls various fundamental physiological processes, such as cell communication (Eileen et al. 2016), blood pressure control and vasodilatation (Seabra et al. 2015), antitumor and antimicrobial activities (Mollick et al. 2015), and promotion and acceleration of wound healing and tissue repair processes, among others (Seabra 2017).

NO is a small, diatomic molecule, found in the gaseous state, and is a free radical because it has an unpaired electron at the π∗ orbital. Because of its relative lipophilicity, NO freely diffuses within cell membranes, allowing important cell communication (Aktan 2004). In vivo, NO is synthesized by the action of the enzyme nitric oxide synthase (NOS), which catalyzes the oxidation of *L*-arginine to *L*-citrulline, producing NO (Aktan 2004; Seabra and Durán 2018). NOS presents as three isoforms:

1. Endothelial (eNOS), which is able to produce NO in picomolar to nanomolar concentrations in a calcium- dependent manner.
2. Neuronal (nNOS), which is able to produce NO in picomolar to nanomolar range in calcium- dependent manner.
3. Inducible (iNOS), which produces considerably higher amounts of NO for longer periods of time, in the micromolar to millimolar range, in a calcium -independent manner. iNOS is induced by immuno stimuli, and NO produced by iNOS is a potent antimicrobial agent.

After the discovery of key functions of NO in the biological system, several studies have established NO as a fascinating versatile molecule regulating key functions in many organs, including the human skin (Ignarro 2000). NO has been intensively studied for the past 20 years. Advances in the knowledge of NO biological mechanisms, the design of targeted NO delivery systems, and sustained exogenous NO release in different therapies have been successfully achieved for several biomedical applications (Stuehr and Haque 2018). Figure 1.1 indicates a continuous increase in scientific papers with the key words "nitric oxide" in the heading, according to Web of Science from 1990 until now. It is notable that there has been a great increase in the number of scientific publications in the first decade after the Nobel Prize was awarded to Robert F. Furchgott, Louis J. Ignarro, and Ferid Murad, which has followed a linear increase during the past years, reaching an average number of publications of 10,000 scientific papers per year. The scientific journal *Nitric Oxide*, the official journal of the Nitric Oxide Society, also indicates the importance of studies based on the chemistry and biology of this molecule, with an increasing impact

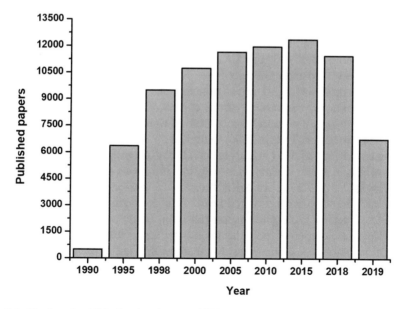

Fig. 1.1 Number of published papers, between 1990 and 2019, with the keyword "nitric oxide" in the heading obtained via Web of Science

factor of 3.45 in 2010 to 4.37 at the present time (www.journals.elsevier.com/nitric-oxide).

NO, which is one of the most studied biological molecules, is a key regulator in many organs, including the human skin. The functions of NO in human skin cover such diverse topics as (1) dermal vasodilatation, (2) inflammation, (3) infection, (4) wound healing, (5) tissue repair, and (6) skin cancer (Cals-Grierson and Ormerod 2004; Seabra et al. 2004; Amadeu et al. 2007; Seabra 2017).

In this direction, this chapter focuses in the roles of NO in human skin, particularly in the combat of skin infections, highlighting the promising use of exogenous NO donors allied to nanomaterials to combat skin infections.

1.2   NO and Human Skin

Skin is the largest organ of the body and provides important functions such as protection, thermoregulation, somatosensory and antioxidant activity, and antibacterial and immunological actions (Stancic et al. 2019). NO and other reactive species are expressed in the skin and contribute to the regulation of physiological and pathophysiological conditions in skin diseases (Jankovic et al. 2016), highlighting the promotion of the wound healing process and the control of infection and inflammation processes (Heuer et al. 2015).

In the skin, NO is produced from all three isoforms of NOS: eNOS, nNOS, and iNOS (Holliman et al. 2017), and it is mostly distributed in keratinocytes, fibroblasts, melanocytes, and endothelial cells (Stancic et al. 2019). eNOS and nNOs are expressed in the epidermis and dermis layers, in melanocytes and keratinocytes, and iNOS was detected in almost all types of cells in skin after cytokine stimulation (Yarlagadda et al. 2017). Figure 1.2 represents the schematic production of NO from NOS in the skin and its activity.

Low concentrations of NO (pico- to nanomolar range), synthesized by eNOs/nNOs in the skin, are responsible for the control of physiological functions in the skin, such as the promotion and acceleration of wound healing, skin pigmentation, and dermal circulation (Ignarro 2000; Georgii et al. 2011; Seabra 2011). In contrast, high concentrations of NO (micro- to milli molar range) produced by iNOS have cytotoxic effects acting in skin defense against infections and skin cancer (Ignarro 2000; Englander and Friedman 2010; Seabra 2011, 2017).

The antimicrobial activity of NO involves its mediation in cytotoxic events in host defense against pathogenic agents (bacteria, fungi, parasites) (Schairer et al. 2012). Upon stimulation of tumor necrosis factor and cytokines, NO is synthesized by iNOS in pathological conditions by macrophages and other cell types (Lyons 1995). NO produced by iNOS has viricidal, antibacterial, antiparasitic, and tumoricidal activity (Halpenny and Mascharak 2010.). The antimicrobial activity of NO involves diverse mechanisms, including (1) impairment of the replication of pathogen DNA, (2) inhibition of mitochondrial respiration by interfering in the electron transport chain in pathogen key enzymes, (3) promotion of S-nitrosation reactions

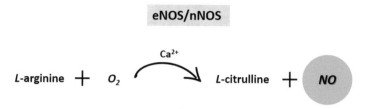

NO pmol L^{-1} - nmol L^{-1} → wound healing, skin pigmentation and dermal circulation

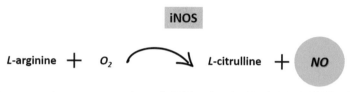

NO μmol L^{-1} – mmol L^{-1} → skin infections, skin disease and skin cancer

Fig. 1.2 Endogenous synthesis of nitric oxide (NO) via nitric oxide synthase (NOS) and its activity in human skin

of cysteine residues of important pathogen enzymes, and (4) generation of other oxygen and nitrogen reactive species (NO$_x$) (Seabra et al. 2016). For reasons of its lipophilicity, NO can easily diffuse through the membranes of pathogens. Once internalized, NO reacts with intracellular targets, leading to toxic effects. NO rapidly and efficiently reacts with superoxide anion radical (O$_2$·$^-$), a product of bacteria cellular respiration, leading to the formation of the highly toxic and oxidant peroxynitrite (ONOO$^-$) (Eq. 1.1).

$$NO^{\bullet} + O_2^{\bullet-} \rightarrow ONOO^-. \tag{1.1}$$

Once produced, peroxynitrite causes severe and irreversible biological damage to the pathogens, including formation of nitrosyl moieties through the attack of metabolic heme-containing enzymes, DNA damage, and peroxidation of the lipid membrane, yielding impairment of the metabolism of skin pathogens (Fang 1997). Therefore, NO is directly involved in host defense against many skin diseases caused by bacteria, fungi, and protozoa.

Recently, it has been reported that human skin is able to store the free radical NO in more stable species (NO$_x$) (Mowbray et al. 2009; Liu et al. 2014; Weller 2016). The main NO$_x$ species that are stored in human skin are nitrite (NO$_2^-$), nitrate (NO$_3^-$), and S-nitrosothiols (RSNOs). In human skin, these NO$_x$ species can release free NO from the skin to the bloodstream upon irradiation with ultraviolet (UV) light (Mowbray et al. 2009; Weller 2016; Pelegrino et al. 2017). UV light-targeted exposure can activate and increase the expression of NOS, resulting in the growth of iNOS in skin after 8–10 h of exposure (Kuhn et al. 1998). In this sense, NO can

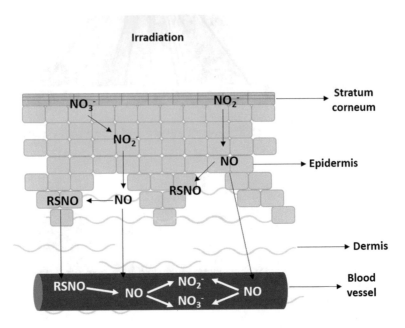

Fig. 1.3 Schematic representation of NO_x species present in human skin: nitrites, nitrates, and *S*-nitroso molecules (RSNOs), which can produce free NO triggered by UV irradiation

also be obtained by a nonenzymatic route, specially by NO_3^- and NO_2^- reduction, and from decomposition of *S*-nitroso molecules (RSNO), such as *S*-nitrosoalbumin, *S*-nitrosoglutathione, and *S*-nitrosocysteine, so- called photolabile compounds that can be triggered by blue light or ultraviolet A (UVA) radiation exposure (Opländer et al. 2013). Under UV irradiation, *S*-nitroso molecules photodecompose, releasing NO, while NO_3^- is reduced to NO_2^-, which is further reduced to NO (Opländer and Suschek 2013). The radiation induces the decomposition of the related NO_x species present in the stratum corneum and epidermis, generating free NO in human skin. NO can permeate skin layers and diffuse from the skin into blood vessels, where it will be further oxidized to nitrite or nitrate, whereas RSNOs can enter the blood system and release free NO, acting as a vasoactive agent (Opländer and Suschek 2013). The role of NO_2^-, NO_3^-, and RSNO in skin is schematically represented in Fig. 1.3.

1.3 Delivering NO to Human Skin

The involvement of NO in many physiological and pathophysiological responses in human skin has led to increasing interest in the development of NO-releasing bio-materials for dermatological purposes, mainly to treat skin infections (Seabra 2011). In this direction, exogenous delivery of NO/NO donors in topical applications presents great potential to enhance the bioavailability of this molecule in skin and, depending on the dosage, a targeted application can be achieved, leading to wound healing (low concentrations) or to combat skin infections (high concentrations of NO, micro- to milli molar range) (Gutiérrez et al. 2016).

As a free radical, NO has a short half-life of 1–5 s in the human; it can rapidly react with different radical species such as molecular oxygen (O_2), leading to the formation of oxidized species including NO_2^- and NO_3^- (Yang et al. 2015). In addition, NO can react with oxyhemoglobin, leading to the formation of methemoglobin and nitrate; this process leads to the inactivation of NO (Doyle and Hoekstra 1981). Therefore, there is increasing interest in the design of strategies to deliver therapeutic amounts of NO in dermatological applications to treat skin infections.

In this sense, NO donors are molecules that present NO in their structure and that are able spontaneously and continuously release NO in situ, for longer periods ranging from hours to days (Wang et al. 2002). There are several classes of NO donors , such as organic nitrates ($RONO_2$), the oldest class of NO donors that have been clinically applied, S-nitrosothiols, also naturally present in skin, which are able to photorelease NO, metal–NO complexes, and hydroxylamines, among others.

Although NO donors are able to increase NO half-life, the combination of NO donors with biomaterials/nanomaterials might significantly enhance the sustained release of therapeutic amounts of NO directly to the target site of application, for instance, in the skin (Friedman et al. 2008). Recently, the combination of NO donors and nanomaterials has been emerging as a suitable strategy to improve the pharmacokinetic, biodisponibility, and targeted release of NO in the treatment of skin infections (Quinn et al. 2015).

1.4 Nanoparticles for Dermatological Applications

Regarding topical applications, it is important to remember that skin is a protective organ that is designed to avoid the penetration of external materials, and thus it is a challenge to develop formulations able to interact and penetrate the skin barrier (Hamblin et al. 2016). The use of nanoparticles for dermatological applications might overcome this challenge, because, depending on the features of the nanomaterial, it can permeate skin, delivering the active drug directly to the skin (Basnet and Skalko-Basnet 2013). Nanomaterials are able to permeate skin barriers through the following routes:

1. Follicular route: nanoparticles are transported through the skin via a follicular penetration happening via sweat ducts, hair follicles, and sebaceous glands that can extend as much as 2 µm into the skin, enabling a controlled and localized release of molecules such as NO (Fang et al. 2014).
2. Intracellular lipidic route: nanoparticle permeation occurs between the corneocytes, diffusing through the intracellular lipid bilayer (Carter et al. 2019).

3. Transcellular route: nanoparticles must traverse through alternate lipophilic and hydrophilic regions through the corneocytes (intracellularly), this being mostly an unfavorable route (Chevalier and Bolzinger 2015).

It is important to highlight that nanoparticle diffusion through the skin is intrinsically dependent on various physicochemical aspects of the nanomaterial such as size, shape, weight, surface charge, and pH (Carter et al. 2019). In this regard, evaluation of the ability of different nanoparticles to act as a drug delivery system in dermatological applications is of fundamental importance to obtain a successful therapy (Parani et al. 2016). The incorporation of NO donors into nanomaterials has been recently explored for dermatological applications to combat skin infections, because high concentrations of NO have potent antimicrobial activity. Nanoparticles have the ability to load high NO concentrations, which is suitable for antimicrobial activity (Carpenter et al. 2012). Different types of nanomaterials that can be used for dermatological applications are described below.

1.4.1 Liposomes

Liposomes are nanoscale lipid vesicles, formed by one or multiple bilayers composed of phospholipids and cholesterol. These nanoparticles are biodegradable and nontoxic, despite being able to load hydrophilic or hydrophobic molecules (Bozzuto and Molinari 2015). Liposomes easily penetrate the epidermal barrier when compared to other classes of nanoparticles because these are similar to the lipid composition of the epidermis. For this reason, studies focusing on liposomes composed of different types of phospholipids are a hot spot to enhance the skin penetration (Sakdiset et al. 2018).

1.4.2 Polymeric Nanoparticles

Polymeric nanoparticles stand out when it comes to skin application mostly because drug degradation can be reduced by adjusting the nanoparticle physicochemical features, providing a controlled drug release (Hamblin et al. 2016). For this application, natural polymer-based nanoparticles mostly are investigated, highlighting chitosan nanoparticles that present controlled drug release for days and antiinflammatory and antibacterial properties in itself (Zou et al. 2016). In addition, chitosan has mucoadhesive properties (Basha et al. 2018). Synthetic polymers such as polyalkylcyanoacrylates and polylactides are common because of their biocompatibility (Grumezescu 2016).

1.4.3 Metallic Nanoparticles

Besides lipid and polymeric nanoparticles, metallic nanoparticles have also been investigated in dermatological applications for their unique properties controlled by choosing the composition of the material, size, and tunable surface characteristics (Goyal et al. 2016). Among various nanoparticles, silver nanoparticles (AgNPs) and gold nanoparticles (AuNPs) have been the most investigated in the field of topical applications (Carter et al. 2019). AgNPs presents great antibacterial and antiinflammatory properties, and their surface can be modified to release drugs and increase diffusion into the skin (Kraeling et al. 2018). AuNPs also present great potential to be functionalized and are notable because their size control enables diffusion even through intact skin (Huang et al. 2010).

Thus, different classes of nanoparticles present great potential in skin treatment applications because most of them can permeate through skin, depending on their design during the synthesis. Furthermore, these nanoparticles can be loaded or functionalized with specific antimicrobial molecules, such as NO, enabling the development of NO-releasing nanoparticles that may enhance NO efficiency in skin application. Thus, the next section presents and discusses the combination of NO/NO donors with nanomaterials for the treatment of skin infections.

1.5 NO-Releasing Nanomaterials for Biomedical Purposes

In biological media, NO donors present low stability, which leads to a noncontrolled and fast release of NO, limiting potential applications (Nguyen et al. 2016). A solution for this problem is the functionalization or encapsulation of NO donors in inorganic or polymeric nanoparticles, which have been studied by various research groups (Barraud et al. 2012; Duong et al. 2014; Seabra and Durán 2017a, b). NO-releasing nanoparticles may enhance NO stability as well as increasing the local concentration and solubility (Sun et al. 2014).

Among various platforms for NO-releasing, polymeric nanoparticles stand out for encapsulating NO, acting as a barrier promoting a slow release. Nguyen et al. (2016) encapsulated NO donors in a polymeric nanoparticle based on oligo(ethylene glycol) methyl ether methacrylate. In this study, the prepared polymeric nanoparticles were able to load the NO donor N-diazeniumdiolate (NONOate) using high-pressure NO gas for 48 h. After encapsulation, NO release was verified by amperometric measurements, at 37 °C, pH 7.4, which instantaneously measures NO released. In this system, NO was quickly released in the first 10 min, achieving 10 % of release; maximum release was 80%, after 17 h of monitoring. NO-releasing polymeric nanoparticles allied to gentamicin, a clinically used antibacterial drug, promoted the dispersal of *Pseudomonas aeruginosa* biofilms into an antibiotic-susceptible planktonic form. Figure 1.4 shows representative images obtained by

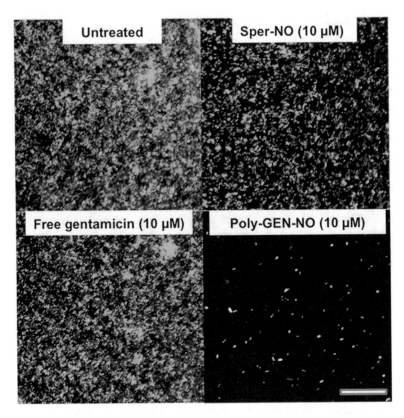

Fig. 1.4 Representative confocal images of *Pseudomonas aeruginosa* biofilms stained with a LIVE/DEAD kit. Biofilms were grown for 6 h and then treated with NO donor spermine NONOate (Sper-NO), free gentamicin, or GEN-NO nanoparticles (NO-releasing nanoparticles), or left untreated for a further 1 h before staining. Viable and nonviable bacteria appear green and red, as well as those stained both green and red, respectively. *Bar* 50 μm. *Note:* Concentration is based on GEN: one mole of GEN-NO nanoparticles is equivalent to one mole of Sper-NO and gentamicin. (Reproduced from Nguyen et al. 2016 under a Creative Commons Attribution 3.0 Unported Licence. Published by The Royal Society of Chemistry)

confocal microscopy of opportunistic pathogen *Pseudomonas aeruginosa* biofilms treated with free NO donor (Sper-NO, at concentration of 10 μM), free gentamicin (at 10 μM), and NO-releasing nanoparticles (Poly-GEN-NO, at 10 μM), compared to untreated *Pseudomonas aeruginosa* biofilm (Nguyen et al. 2016). The biofilms were stained with live/dead dyes: green color indicates live cells, and red color indicates dead cells. It can be clearly observed that biofilm treatment with NO-releasing nanoparticles (GEN-NO nanoparticles at 10 μM) significantly decreased biofilm volume, leading to a greater number of dead cells, in comparison with those treated with free NO donor, gentamicin alone, or the untreated group (Fig. 1.4).

Taken together, NO-releasing nanoparticles were able to release NO, which was made available to biofilms, and consequently induced dispersal of biofilm cells. Therefore, the nanoparticle is able to enhance the stability of the encapsulated NO donor from minutes to almost a day, facilitating potential biomedical applications (Keefer 2011).

When it comes to topical application, polymeric nanoparticles usually are present in larger sizes, compared to metallic nanoparticles, which may hamper skin penetration. Chitosan nanoparticles are a hot topic, mostly for the possibility of loading several different classes of hydrophilic molecules, such as low molecular weight NO donors, and for reasons of their relatively small-sized nanoparticles (i.e., 40 nm), which are able to penetrate skin layers and deliver NO in the targeted location (Zhang et al. 2013). In this sense, Pelegrino and coworkers evaluated the potential dermatological applications of NO-releasing chitosan nanoparticles (Pelegrino et al. 2017). The NO donor S-nitrosoglutathione (GSNO), which belongs to the class of S-nitrosothiols, was encapsulated into chitosan nanoparticles. Topical applications of NO-releasing chitosan nanoparticles directly on human skin allowed an efficiently transdermal NO permeation along the skin layers (Pelegrino et al. 2017). First, chitosan nanoparticles were obtained by a cross-link reaction with the polyanion tripolyphosphate, followed by the encapsulation of the NO donor via electrostatic interactions. The kinetics of NO release from chitosan nanoparticles was monitored, indicating a sustainable diffusion of the encapsulated NO donor. Regarding skin applications, after treating ex vivo human skin slices with NO-releasing chitosan nanoparticles, it was possible to verify a significant increase in the levels of NO in treated skin, compared to nontreated skin, indicating that dermatological application of chitosan nanoparticles containing NO donors is able to promote NO diffusion through skin layers (Pelegrino et al. 2017).

In addition to polymeric nanoparticles, inorganic nanoparticles have been extensively studied for drug transport and biomedical applications. Gold nanoparticles (AuNPs) are one of the most popular nanoparticles studied and have great potential in topical application in the treatment of skin diseases (Huang et al. 2010). Duong et al. (2014) prepared a 10- nm AuNP, coated with poly(oligoethylene glycol methyl ether methacrylate)-b-poly(vinyl benzyl chloride), in which amine groups were further converted to N-diazeniumdiolate NO donor, by exposure to NO gas at high pressure. NO release was monitored by the Griess method. In comparison to the free NO donor, encapsulated NO presented a slow release with no burst and a sustained release up to 6 days. Thus, this material is suitable for topical applications. Topical application of AuNPs has great potential because they penetrate the skin epidermis. The Yang research group demonstrated that small AuNPs (1–10 nm) can create channels through the skin barrier allowing loaded molecules to migrate in the epidermis and dermis. The authors demonstrated a high accumulation of AuNPs in epidermis and dermis (Duong et al. 2014). Thus, functionalization of AuNPs with NO donors is a suitable strategy regarding topical applications, enhancing sustainable NO release and penetration into the skin.

1.5.1 NO-Releasing Nanoparticles in the Management of Skin Infection

Skin infection can be caused by a variety of microorganisms, such as bacteria, virus, fungi, and parasites, affecting high numbers in worldwide populations (Percival et al. 2012). One of the most common skin infections is caused by *Staphylococcus aureus* and its methicillin- resistant form, but other microorganisms are also commonly related to skin infections, including *Pseudomonas aeruginosa*, *Escherichia coli*, *Staphylococcus epidermidis*, *Candida albicans*, and *Leishmania* spp. (Percival et al. 2012).

At low concentrations, NO can stimulate and reinforce the host immune system, whereas at higher concentrations, in the range of micro- to millimolar, NO acts as an antimicrobial agent against the pathogen. For this reason, NO donors have been used in the treatment of dermatological diseases (Seabra et al. 2015). NO donors can be incorporated into gels, creams, or nanoparticles for dermatological applications (Pelegrino et al. 2018). Some NO donors might be stable under ambient conditions, some of them present a long history of use with well- known side effects, and some are easily produced; however, they have some negative points such as limited antibacterial properties and lack of stability for topical uses (Adler and Friedman 2015). The incorporation of the NO donor into a gel, cream matrix, or nanoparticle represents an attractive strategy for allowing the dermatological administration of NO donors. This strategy is easily applied. NO-releasing nanoparticles are suitable for dermatological applications, with a broad spectrum of toxicity against numerous microorganisms, increasing NO stability in localized applications (Adler and Friedman 2015). The next sections present and discuss selective examples of NO-releasing nanomaterials in the management of skin infections caused by different microorganisms.

1.5.1.1 Bacterial Infections

One of the most common skin infections is caused by *Staphylococcus aureus*, leading to superficial and invasive infections, usually developed in the hospital environment (Clebak and Malone 2018). Looking forward to new therapeutics because of bacterial resistance, Martinez and coworkers developed a NO-releasing hydrogel/ glass nanoparticle, encapsulating sodium nitrite ($NaNO_2$), and verified the potential of NO-generating nanoparticles against *Staphylococcus aureus* skin infections (Martinez et al. 2009). First, an in vitro evaluation was conducted with methicillin-resistant *Staphylococcus aureus* (MRSA) and methicillin-sensitive *Staphylococcus aureus* (MSSA), indicating the NO-releasing nanoparticle toxicity against both forms caused cell wall destruction followed by cell lysis. In a further step, in vivo experiments in infected mice were carried out to evaluate the potential of NO-releasing nanoparticles to treat skin infection. The authors observed that NO-releasing nanoparticles exerted antimicrobial activity against MRSA in a

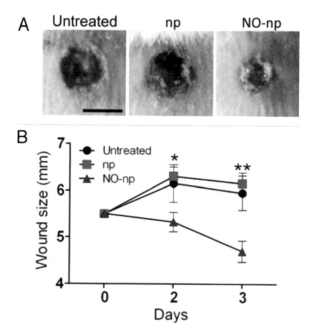

Fig. 1.5 Dermatological application of NO-releasing nanoparticles (NO-NP) accelerated wound healing process in mice. (**a**) Wounds of Balb/c mice untreated and Ab-infected, np-treated and Ab-infected, or Ab-infected NO-np-treated, 3 days post infection. *Bar* 5 mm. (**b**) Wound size analysis of Balb/c mice skin lesions. Time points are the averages of the results for five measurements, and error bars denote standard deviations. ∗$p < 0.05$, ∗∗$p < 0.001$ in comparing the NO-np-treated group with untreated and np-treated groups. (Reproduced from Mihu et al. (2010) under a Creative Commons Attribution 3.0 Unported Licence)

murine wound model, as evidenced by acceleration of infected wound closure in animals treated with dermatological applications of NO-releasing nanoparticles, compared with control groups. Moreover, histology evaluation of the infected wounds showed that treatment with NO-releasing nanoparticles decreased suppurative inflammation, minimized bacterial burden, and decreased collagen degradation, allowing potential mechanisms for biological activity (Martinez et al. 2009).

NO-releasing chitosan nanoparticles were also applied in wound infections caused by *Acinetobacter baumannii* as described by Mihu et al. (2010). This treatment presented great results from the microbicidal activity of NO-releasing nanoparticles, able to reduce bacterial growth after 12 h. Figures 1.5a, b and 1.6 shows the rates of infected wounds of NO-releasing nanoparticles (NO-NP), empty nanoparticles (NP), and untreated wounds (untreated). As indicated, Fig. 1.5 shows that dermatological application of NO-releasing nanoparticles significantly increases the wound healing process, as evidenced by wound closure. In addition, collagen amount and wound healing rate also stood out compared to a control group and pure nanoparticle treatment. According to the authors, this result indicates a great advance in the treatment of skin infections caused by resistant bacteria, especially

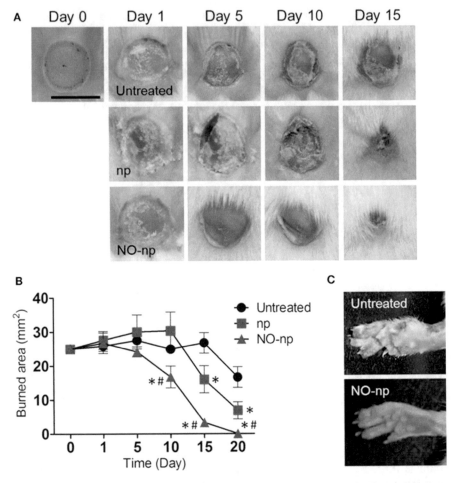

Fig. 1.6 Healing effectiveness of nitric oxide-releasing nanoparticles (NO-np) in *Candida albicans*-induced burn infections. (**a**) Burn injuries of Balb/c mice untreated, treated with np, and treated with NO-np, day 0, 1, 5, 10, and 15. Bar = 5 mm. (**b**) Closure of the burn area of skin lesions of Balb/c mice relative to the initial 5-mm wound. Time points are the averages of the results of the measurements of six different wounds, and error bars denote SDs. ∗$P < 0.001$ in the comparison of the np- (empty nanoparticle) or NO-np-treated group with untreated group. #$P < 0.001$ in the comparison of the np-treated group with the NO-np-treated group. These experiments were performed twice with similar results. (**c**) NO-np prevents cutaneous spread of candidiasis in mice. (Reproduced from Macherla et al. (2012) under the terms of the Creative Commons Attribution Non-Commercial License)

the ease of the treatment and the ability to load high concentration of NO donors into the nanoparticles (Mihu et al. 2010).

Bacterially infected wounds might also lead to severe conditions when biofilm is formed on skin and ducts (Brandwein et al. 2016). When compared to free plank-tonic bacteria, biofilms can be 10,000 times more resistant, leading to common consequences such as difficulty in controlling bacterial infection with a high micro-bial charge, skin ulcers, chronic infections, and a high mortality, because biofilms deposited on skin wounds are in direct contact with the patient's bloodstream (Kon and Rai 2016; Sonesson et al. 2017). NO-releasing nanoparticles also present great potential in combating bacterial biofilm, including MRSA, the most frequent patho-gen in skin infections, as reported by Mihu et al. (2017). Similar to Martinez et al. (2009), a hydrogel/glass nanoparticle with sodium nitrite was developed and anti-microbial activity against *S. aureus* biofilm was evaluated. Results indicated an anti-microbial activity of NO-releasing nanoparticle reducing and preventing biofilm formation, with advantage of minimum resistance development even after frequent exposure to NO.

Other published papers also indicated the potent antibacterial activity of poly-meric and inorganic NO-releasing nanoparticles against *Pseudomonas aeruginosa* and *Staphylococcus aureus* biofilms, indicating minimal bacterial resistance, long-term biofilm prevention, and thus a suitable alternative strategy to combat biofilm-infected wounds in dermatological applications (Slomberg et al. 2013; Hasan et al. 2017; Mihu et al. 2017).

1.5.1.2 Fungal Infections

Fungal infections also present potential risk in skin wounds. *Candida albicans* is one of the causes of deaths after a severe skin burn, and new therapeutics in which fungi are likely to develop resistance are needed (Lakshminarayanan et al. 2018). The Martinez research group developed a NO-releasing silane hydrogel nanoparti-cle and sodium nitrite was encapsulated as the NO generator (Macherla et al. 2012). As NO-releasing nanoparticles demonstrated potent in vitro antifungal potential after only 2 h incubation, in vivo studies in infected burn wound healing were con-ducted. The treatment showed potent results, because topical application of NO-releasing nanoparticles significantly reduced microbial load in the infected wound bed. In addition, NO-releasing nanoparticles prevented fungi penetration into different tissues, as occurred with the control group (untreated group) and ani-mals treated with empty nanoparticles. The curative process was also accelerated upon treating fungi- infected wounds with NO-releasing nanoparticles, leading to complete healing after 20 days of treatment. The curative process progressed rap-idly in animals treated with NO-releasing nanoparticles, with complete healing in all treated mice within 20 days following burn injury and infection. In contrast, a delay in the healing process of animals treated with empty nanoparticles or untreated animals was observed. The authors reported that complete wound closure was not observed within the 20 days following injury. Animals in the control groups experi-enced fungal transmission from the burn site to their paws, possibly by scratching of the infected injury. This result agrees with the observation of superior fungal burdens and prolonged infection (Macherla et al. 2012) (Fig. 1.6).

Friedman's research group also reported a therapy against dermal antifungal infection based on NO-releasing nanoparticles (Mordorski et al. 2017). *Trichophyton rubrum* is a causal agent of dermatophytosis, involving not only the epidermis, but also invading the dermis and subcutaneous tissues, requiring an efficient and secure drug delivery system. Common drugs possess low tissue penetration to reach a targeted location, besides presenting many side effects and antimicrobial resistance (Mordorski et al. 2017). Thus, the use of nanoparticles represents a promising alternative, because NO-releasing nanoparticles are able to penetrate skin tissue, delivering NO directly to the infected tissue, which has already been reported as an efficient antimicrobial agent with low side effects and low probability of causing resistance in the microorganisms (Cabrales et al. 2010; Mordorski et al. 2017).

NO-releasing hydrogel/glass nanoparticles showed low minimum inhibitory concentration values against *Trichophyton rubrum*, and fungal burden was notably decreased after 7 days of treatment; also, after this period fungal growth was not observed (Mordorski et al. 2017). Another work from Friedman's group also demonstrated promising results treating skin infection caused by *Trichophyton mentagrophytes* showing outstanding healing efficacy when compared to a control group after 7 days treatment. Burden decrease was also verified, demonstrating significant results when compared to nontreated skin. NO-releasing nanoparticles enhance skin penetration efficiency, indicating successful penetration of NO through the epidermis, mostly via hair follicles, confirming the potential of NO delivery in dermatological applications (Landriscina et al. 2015).

Fungal- infected wounds can present resistance by the presence of biofilms, as can bacterial infections. Fungal biofilms (i.e., *Candida albicans*) occur in recurrent and persistent infections, presenting a remarkable 2000-fold resistance increase (Nusbaum et al. 2012). NO-releasing nanoparticles have already been reported for their enhanced activity against bacterial biofilm and, regarding fungal biofilms, an intermediary activity was demonstrated (Hetrick et al. 2009; Privett et al. 2010). In this scenario, the development of nanomaterials able to carry and to release NO might lead to an enhanced efficacy against fungal biofilms. This is a promising research topic to be further explored.

1.5.1.3 Parasitic Infections

Parasitic skin diseases are caused by parasites or "cutaneous larvae" and can be classified as epidermis skin infection, related to interactions restricted to the upper layer of skin, or infections in which the parasite is able to penetrate the epidermis and reach deeper skin levels . Some common epidermal diseases are pediculosis and scabies, and leishmaniasis and onchocerciasis represent known deep skin infections (Feldmeier and Heukelbach 2009). All listed diseases are classified as neglected diseases, including, mostly, poor people in low-income countries, with lack of basic sanitation and suffering limited medical care (Seabra and Durán 2017a, b). Despite infecting millions of people, neglected diseases are listed neither nationally nor internationally as a priority, and are not receiving much attention from public or private markets (Engelman et al. 2016).

For parasitic infections, NO should be released in a high sustained concentration, directly to the target site of application, and be able to kill protozoa, without affecting patient tissues (Seabra and Durán 2017a, b). Although studies in this field are scarce, NO potential has been already evaluated in cutaneous leishmaniasis. López-Jaramillo and coworkers evaluated a NO patch against *Leishmania panamensis,* and despite results indicating a potential effect of NO, issues reported concerned an improved sustained and high concentration of released NO and efficient skin diffusion (López-Jaramillo et al. 2010), which clearly indicates the great potential for NO-releasing nanoparticles.

In addition, unloaded nanoparticles (i.e., AgNPs) have already been studied and demonstrated great potential against parasitic infections (Moreno et al. 2014). In this sense, there is still much potential to be explored by combining nanoparticles to NO donors to enhance and target the application to neglected cutaneous diseases, representing not only a technological, but also a social, advance.

1.6 Conclusions

NO is a small molecule with various potential biomedical applications that can be enhanced by loading or functionalize different nanoparticles, leading to a sustained and targeted treatment. Regarding topical applications, loaded NO nanoparticles also represent a promising strategy to enhance NO penetration into the skin barrier. Even though some reports have already indicated an improved result using NO-releasing nanoparticles in the treatment of skin infections, there is still much to be explored, such as nanoparticles of different compositions and diverse NO donors, to find the most appropriate combination for each treatment, and new applications, highlighting neglected diseases in which only a few have already been studied and reported. Therefore, this chapter intended to highlight the promising applications of NO-releasing nanoparticles applied to skin infections, showing an outstanding potential of this platform. We expect that it might encourage new research and development in this area.

Acknowledgments We appreciate the support from CNPq (404815/2018-9) and FAPESP (2018/08194-2, 2018/02832-7).

References

Adler BL, Friedman AJ (2015) Nitric oxide therapy for dermatologic disease. Future Sci OA 1:FSO37
Aktan F (2004) iNOS-mediated nitric oxide production and its regulation. Life Sci 75:639–653
Amadeu TP, Seabra AB, de Oliveira MG, Costa AMA (2007) *S*-Nitrosoglutathione containing hydrogel accelerates rat cutaneous wound repair. J Eur Acad Dermatol Venereol 21:629–637

Barraud N, Kardak BG, Yepuri NR, Howlin RP, Webb JS, Faust SN, Kjelleberg S, Rice SA, Kelso MJ (2012) Cephalosporin-3'-diazeniumdiolates: targeted NO-donor prodrugs for dispersing bacterial biofilms. Angew Chem Int Ed Engl 51:9057–9060

Basha M, Abou Samra MM, Awad GA, Mansy SS (2018) A potential antibacterial wound dressing of cefadroxil chitosan nanoparticles in situ gel: fabrication, in vitro optimization and in vivo evaluation. Int J Pharm 544:129–140

Basnet P, Skalko-Basnet N (2013) Nanodelivery systems for improved topical antimicrobial therapy. Curr Pharm Des 19:7237–7243

Bozzuto G, Molinari A (2015) Liposomes as nanomedical devices. Int J Nanomedicine 10:975–999

Brandwein M, Steinberg D, Meshner S (2016) Microbial biofilms and the human skin microbiome. NPJ Biofilms Microbiomes 2:3

Cabrales P, Han G, Roche C, Nacharaju P, Friedman AJ, Friedman JM (2010) Sustained release nitric oxide from long-lived circulating nanoparticles. Free Radic Biol Med 49:530–538

Cals-Grierson MM, Ormerod AD (2004) Nitric oxide function in the skin. Biol Chem 10:179–193

Carpenter AW, Worley BV, Slomberg DL, Schoenfisch MH (2012) Dual action antimicrobials: nitric oxide release from quaternary ammonium-functionalized silica nanoparticles. Biomacromolecules 13:3334–3342

Carter P, Narasimhan B, Wang Q (2019) Biocompatible nanoparticles and vesicular systems in transdermal drug delivery for various skin diseases. Int J Pharm 555:49–62

Chevalier Y, Bolzinger M (2015) Percutaneous penetration enhancers chemical methods in penetration enhancement, 1st edn. Springer, Berlin

Clebak K, Malone M (2018) Skin infections. Prim Care 45:433–454

Doyle MP, Hoekstra JW (1981) Oxidation of nitrogen oxides by bound dioxygen in hemoproteins. J Inorg Biochem 14:351–358

Duong HTT, Adnan NNM, Barraud N, Basuki JS, Kutty SK, Kenward J, Kumar N, Davis TP, Boyer C (2014) Functional gold nanoparticles for the storage and controlled release of nitric oxide: applications in biofilm dispersal and intracellular delivery. J Mater Chem B 2:5003–5011

Eileen O, Marika VD, Eoin S, Andrew H (2016) Novel targets in the glutamate and nitric oxide neurotransmitter systems for the treatment of depression. In: Systems neuroscience in depression. Academic Press, Cambridge, pp 81–113

Engelman D, Fuller LC, Solomon AW (2016) Opportunities for integrated control of neglected tropical diseases that affect the skin. Trends Parasitol 32:843–854

Englander L, Friedman A (2010) Nitric oxide nanoparticle technology: a novel antimicrobial agent in the context of current treatment of skin and soft tissue infection. J Clin Aesthet Dermatol 3:45–50

Fang FC (1997) Mechanisms of nitric oxide-related antimicrobial activity. J Clin Invest 99:2818–2825

Fang CL, Aljuffali IA, Li YC, Fang JY (2014) Delivery and targeting of nanoparticles into hair follicles. Ther Deliv 5:991–1006

Feldmeier H, Heukelbach J (2009) Epidermal parasitic skin diseases: a neglected category of poverty-associated plagues. Bull World Health Organ 87:152–159

Friedman AJ, Han G, Navati MS, Chacko M, Gunther L, Alfieri A, Friedman JM (2008) Sustained release nitric oxide releasing nanoparticles: characterization of a novel delivery platform based on nitrite containing hydrogel/glass composites. Nitric Oxide 19:12–20

Georgii JL, Amadeu TP, Seabra AB, de Oliveira MG, Monte-Alto-Costa A (2011) Topical S-nitrosoglutathione-releasing hydrogel improves healing of rat ischaemic wounds. J Tissue Eng Regen Med 5:612–619

Goyal R, Macri LK, Kaplan HM, Kohn J (2016) Nanoparticles and nanofibers for topical drug delivery. J Control Release 240:77–92

Grumezescu AM (2016) Nanobiomaterials in galenic formulations and cosmetics applications, 1st edn. William Andrew, Elsevier, Amsterdam

Gutiérrez V, Seabra AB, Reguera RM et al (2016) New approaches from nanomedicine for treating leishmaniasis. Chem Soc Rev 45:152–168

Halpenny GM, Mascharak PK (2010) Emerging antimicrobial applications of nitric oxide (NO) and NO-releasing materials. Antiinfect Agents Med Chem 9:187–197

Hamblin MR, Avci P, Prow TW (2016) Nanoscience in dermatology, 1st edn. Academic Press, Cambridge

Hasan S, Thomas N, Thierry B, Prestidge CA (2017) Biodegradable nitric oxide precursor-loaded micro- and nanoparticles for the treatment of *Staphylococcus aureus* biofilms. J Mater Chem B 5:1005–1014

Hetrick EM, Shin JH, Paul HS, Schoenfisch MH (2009) Anti-biofilm efficacy of nitric oxide-releasing silica nanoparticles. Biomaterials 30:2782–2789

Heuer K, Hoffmanns MA, Demir E, Baldus S, Christine MV, Röhle M, Fuchs PC, Awakowicz P, Suschek CV, Opländer C (2015) The topical use of non-thermal dielectric barrier discharge (DBD): nitric oxide related effects on human skin. Nitric Oxide 44:52–60

Holliman G, Lowe D, Cohen H, Felton H, Felton S, Raj K (2017) Ultraviolet radiation-induced production of nitric oxide: a multi-cell and multi-donor analysis. Sci Rep 7:1–11

Huang Y, Yu F, Park YS, Wang J, Shin MC, Chung HS, Yang VC (2010) Co-administration of protein drugs with gold nanoparticles to enable percutaneous delivery. Biomaterials 31:9086–9091

Ignarro LJ (1999) Nitric oxide: a unique endogenous signaling molecule in vascular biology (Nobel lecture). Angew Chem Int Ed 38:1882–1892

Ignarro LJ (2000) Nitric oxide, biology and pathobiology, 3rd edn. Academic Press, Cambridge

Jankovic A, Ferreri C, Filipovic M, Ivanovic-Burmazovic I, Stancic A, Otasevic V, Korac A, Buzadzic B, Korac B (2016) Targeting the superoxide/nitric oxide ratio by *L*-arginine and SOD mimic in diabetic rat skin. Free Radic Res 50:S51–S63

Keefer LK (2011) Fifty years of diazeniumdiolate research: from laboratory curiosity to broad-spectrum biomedical advances. ACS Chem Biol 6:1147–1155

Kon K, Rai M (2016) Antibiotic resistance: mechanisms and new antimicrobial approaches, 1st edn. Academic Press, Cambridge

Koshland DE Jr (1992) The molecule of the year. Science 258:186

Kraeling MEK, Topping VD, Keltner ZM, Belgrave KR, Bailey KD, Gao X, Yourick JJ (2018) *In vitro* percutaneous penetration of silver nanoparticles in pig and human skin. Regul Toxicol Pharmacol 95:314–322

Kuhn A, Fehsel K, Lehmann P, Krutmann J, Ruzicka T, Kolb-Bachofen V (1998) Aberrant timing in epidermal expression of inducible nitric oxide synthase after UV irradiation in cutaneous lupus derythematosus. J Invest Dermatol 111:149–153

Lakshminarayanan R, Ye E, Young DJ, Li Z, Loh XJ (2018) Recent advances in the development of antimicrobial nanoparticles for combating resistant pathogens. Adv Healthc Mater 7:1–13

Landriscina A, Rosen J, Blecher-Paz K, Long L, Ghannoum MA, Nosanchuk JD, Friedman AJ (2015) Nitric oxide-releasing nanoparticles as a treatment for cutaneous dermatophyte infections. Sci Lett J 4:193–198

Liu D, Fernandez BO, Hamilton A, Lang NN, Gallagher JMC, Newby DE, Feelisch M, Weller RB (2014) UVA irradiation of human skin vasodilates arterial vasculature and lowers blood pressure independently of nitric oxide synthase. J Invest Dermatol 134:1839–1846

López-Jaramillo P, Rincón MY, García RG, Silva SY, Smith E, Kamoeerapappun P, García C, Smith DJ, López M, Vélez ID (2010) A controlled, randomized-blinded clinical trial to assess the efficacy of a nitric oxide releasing patch in the treatment of cutaneous leishmaniasis by *Leishmania* (V.) *panamensis*. Am J Trop Med Hyg 83:97–101

Lyons CR (1995) The role of nitric oxide in inflammation. Adv Immunol 60:323–371

Macherla C, Sanchez DA, Ahmadi MS, Vellozzi EM, Friedman AJ, Nosanchuk JD, Martinez LR (2012) Nitric oxide releasing nanoparticles for treatment of *Candida albicans* burn infections. Front Microbiol 3:1–9

Martinez LR, Han G, Chacko M, Mihu MR, Jacobson M, Gialanella P, Friedman AJ, Nosanchuk JD, Friedman JM (2009) Antimicrobial and healing efficacy of sustained release nitric oxide nanoparticles against *Staphylococcus aureus* skin infection. J Invest Dermatol 129:2463–2469

Mihu MR, Sandkovsky U, Han G, Friedman JM, Nosanchuk JD, Martinez LR (2010) Nitric oxide releasing nanoparticles are therapeutic for *Acinetobacter baumannii* wound infections. Virulence 1:62–67

Mihu MR, Cabral V, Pattabhi R, Tar MT, Davies KP, Friedman AJ, Martinez LR, Nosanchuk JD (2017) Sustained nitric oxide-releasing nanoparticles interfere with methicillin-resistant *Staphylococcus aureus* adhesion and biofilm formation in a rat central venous catheter model. Antimicrob Agents Chemother 61:1–11

Mollick MMR, Rana D, Dash SK, Chattopadhyay S, Bhowmick B, Maity D, Mondal D, Pattanayak S, Roy S, Chakraborty M, Chattopadhyay D (2015) Studies on green synthesized silver nanoparticles using *Abelmoschus esculentus* (L.) pulp extract having anticancer (in vitro) and antimicrobial applications. Arab J Chem 2015:1–13

Mordorski B, Costa-Orlandi CB, Baltazar LM, Carreño LJ, Landriscina A, Rosen J, Navati M, Mendes-Giannini MJS, Friedman JM, Nosanchuk JD, Friedman AJ (2017) Topical nitric oxide releasing nanoparticles are effective in a murine model of dermal *Trichophyton rubrum* dermatophytosis. Nanomedicine 13:2267–2270

Moreno E, Schwartz J, Fernández C et al (2014) Nanoparticles as multifunctional devices for the topical treatment of cutaneous leishmaniasis. Expert Opin Drug Deliv 11:579–597

Mowbray M, McLintock S, Weerakoon R, Lomatschinsky N, Jones S, Rossi AG, Weller RB (2009) Enzyme-independent NO stores in human skin: quantification and influence of UV radiation. J Invest Dermatol 129:834–842

Nguyen TK, Selvanayagam R, Ho KKK, Chen R, Kutty SK, Rice SA, Kumar N, Barraud N, Doung HTT, Boyer C (2016) Co-delivery of nitric oxide and antibiotic using polymeric nanoparticles. Chem Sci 7:1016–1027

Nusbaum AG, Kirsner RS, Charles CA (2012) Biofilms in dermatology. Skin Therapy Lett 17(7):1–5

Opländer C, Suschek CV (2013) The role of photolabile dermal nitric oxide derivates in ultraviolet radiation (UVR)-induced cell death. Int J Mol Sci 14:191–204

Opländer C, Deck A, Volkmar CM, Kirsch M, Liebmann J, Born M, van Abeelen F, van Faassen EE, Kröncke KD, Windolf J, Suschek CV (2013) Mechanism and biological relevance of blue-light (420–453 nm)-induced nonenzymatic nitric oxide generation from photolabile nitric oxide derivates in human skin *in vitro* and *in vivo*. Free Radic Biol Med 65:1363–1377

Parani M, Lokhande G, Singh A, Gaharwar AK (2016) Engineered nanomaterials for infection control and healing acute and chronic wounds. Appl Mater Interfaces 8:10049–10069

Pelegrino MT, Weller RB, Chen X, Bernardes JS, Seabra AB (2017) Chitosan nanoparticles for nitric oxide delivery in human skin. Med Chem Commun 8:713–719

Pelegrino MT, de Araújo DR, Seabra AB (2018) *S*-Nitrosoglutathione-containing chitosan nanoparticles dispersed in Pluronic F-127 hydrogel: potential uses in topical applications. J Drug Delivery Sci Technol 43:211–220

Percival SL, Emanuel C, Cutting KF, Williams DW (2012) Microbiology of the skin and the role of biofilms in infection. Int Wound J 9:14–32

Privett BJ, Nutz ST, Schoenfisch MH (2010) Efficacy of surface-generated nitric oxide against *Candida albicans* adhesion and biofilm formation. Biofouling 26:973–983

Quinn JF, Whittaker MR, Davis TP (2015) Delivering nitric oxide with nanoparticles. J Control Release 205:190–205

Sakdiset P, Okada A, Todo H, Sugibayashi K (2018) Selection of phospholipids to design liposome preparations with high skin penetration-enhancing effects. J Drug Delivery Sci Technol 44:58–64

Schairer DO, Chouake JS, Nosanchuk JD, Friedman AJ (2012) The potential of nitric oxide releasing therapies as antimicrobial agents. Virulence 3:271–279

Seabra AB (2011) Nitric oxide-releasing nanomaterials and skin care. In: Beck R, Pohlmann A, Guterres S (eds) Nanocosmetics and nanomedicines, 1st edn. Springer, New York, pp 253–268

Seabra AB (2017) Nitric oxide donors: novel biomedical applications and perspectives, 1st edn. Elsevier, New York

Seabra AB, Durán N (2017a) Nanoparticulated nitric oxide donors and their biomedical applications. Mini Rev Med Chem 17(3):216–223

Seabra AB, Durán N (2017b) Nitric oxide donors for treating neglected diseases. In: Nitric oxide donors: novel biomedical applications and perspectives, 1st edn. Elsevier, Amsterdam, pp 25–54

Seabra AB, Durán N (2018) Nitric oxide donors for prostate and bladder cancers: current state and challenges. Eur J Pharmacol 826:158–168

Seabra AB, Fitzpatrick A, Paul J, De Oliveira MG, Weller R (2004) Topically applied S-nitrosothiol-containing hydrogels as experimental and pharmacological nitric oxide donors in human skin. Br J Dermatol 151:977–983

Seabra AB, Justo GZ, Haddad PS (2015) State of the art, challenges and perspectives in the design of nitric oxide-releasing polymeric nanomaterials for biomedical applications. Biotechnol Adv 33:1370–1379

Seabra AB, Pelegrino MT, Haddad PS (2016) Can nitric oxide overcome bacterial resitance to antibiotics? In: Antibiotic resistance: mechanisms and new antimicrobial approaches, 1st edn. Elsevier, Amsterdam, pp 187–204

Slomberg DL, Lu Y, Broadnax AD, Hunter RA, Carpenter AW, Schoenfisch MH (2013) Role of size and shape on biofilm eradication for nitric oxide-releasing silica nanoparticles. ACS Appl Mater Interfaces 5:9322–9329

Sonesson A, Przybyszewska K, Eriksson S, Mörgelin M, Kjellström K, Davies J, Potempa J, Schmidtchen A (2017) Identification of bacterial biofilm and the *Staphylococcus aureus* derived protease, staphopain, on the skin surface of patients with atopic dermatitis. Sci Rep 7:1–12

Stancic A, Jankovic A, Koracb A et al (2019) The role of nitric oxide in diabetic skin (patho)physiology. Mech Ageing Dev 172:21–29

Stuehr DJ, Haque MM (2018) Nitric oxide synthase enzymology in the twenty years after the Nobel prize. Br J Pharmacol 176(2):177–188

Sun T, Zhang YS, Pang B, Hyun DC, Yang M, Xia Y (2014) Engineered nanoparticles for drug delivery in cancer therapy. Angew Chem Int Ed 53:12320–12364

Wang PG, Xian M, Tang X, Wu X, Wen Z, Cai T, Janczuk AJ (2002) Nitric oxide donors: chemical activities and biological applications. Chem Rev 102:1091–1134

Weller RB (2016) Sunlight has cardiovascular benefits independently of vitamin D. Blood Purif 41:130–134

Yang Y, Qi PK, Yang ZL, Huang N (2015) Nitric oxide based strategies for applications of biomedical devices. Biosurf Biotribol 1(3):177–201

Yarlagadda K, Hassani J, Foote IP, Markowitz J (2017) The role of nitric oxide in melanoma. Biochim Biophys Acta Rev Cancer 1868:500–509

Zhang Z, Tsai PC, Ramezanli T, Michniak-Kohn BB (2013) Polymeric nanoparticles-based topical delivery systems for the treatment of dermatological diseases. Wiley Interdiscip Rev Nanomed Nanobiotechnol 5(3):205–218

Zou P, Yang X, Wang J, Li Y, Yu H, Zhang Y, Liu G (2016) Advances in characterisation and biological activities of chitosan and chitosan oligosaccharides. Food Chem 190:1174–1181

Chapter 2
Metal Nanoparticle Based Antibacterial Nanocomposites for Skin Infections

Arushi Verma, Vishal Singh, and Amaresh Kumar Sahoo

Abstract There are ample numbers of patients who have been suffering from skin and soft tissue infections (SSTIs) all over the world. Development of SSTIs associates with various symptoms such as inflammatory response, fever and formation of lesions. Conventional antibiotic therapy has been used as routine practice for this kind of medical situation. However, the present scenario becomes more challenging due to the prevalence of antibiotic resistant bacterial infections. Moreover, the delayed wound healing due to certain medical conditions such as diabetes leads to an exaggeration of the complicacy of the skin infections. Therefore, healing bacterial skin infections with conventional antibiotics is not always found to be effective. Moreover, skin infections sometimes result in permanent scarring on infected areas after complete recovery also. This demands new therapeutics for skin infections as well as removal of the scar. In order to address these issues, for last few decades, nanotechnology-based approaches have been attempted by various research groups. These offer significant prospects of developing new therapeutic agents which exhibit heightened bactericidal activity against Gram-positive and Gram-negative bacterial infection. Additionally, the nanoscale materials have been used as an integrated component of several skincare products like gels and creams which assist the removal of the scar and the protection of the skin from potentially toxic UV light and other harmful agents like pollutants too. There have been several nanoscale materials such as metal and metal oxide nanoparticles (NPs), nanospheres, nanocapsules and various other nanocomposites which show huge potential of using these to combat against skin infections due to antibiotic resistant bacteria also.

Keywords Skin infections · Nanoparticles · Nanoformulation · Antibiotic resistant · Bacterial infection

---

Arushi Verma and Vishal Singh contributed equally to this work.

A. Verma · V. Singh · A. K. Sahoo (✉)
Department of Applied Sciences, Indian Institute of Information Technology,
Allahabad, India
e-mail: asahoo@iiita.ac.in

© Springer Nature Switzerland AG 2020
M. Rai (ed.), *Nanotechnology in Skin, Soft Tissue, and Bone Infections*,
https://doi.org/10.1007/978-3-030-35147-2_2

Nomenclature

Ag NPs	Silver nanoparticles
ATP	Adenosine triphosphate
Au NPs	Gold nanoparticles
Cu NPs	Copper nanoparticles
CuO	Copper oxide
DNA	Deoxyribonucleic acid
ECM	Extracellular matrix
FDA	Food and Drug Administration
Fe_3O_4	Iron oxide
MDR	Multidrug resistant
MgO	Magnesium oxide
NPs	Nanoparticles
RNA	Ribonucleic acid
ROS	Reactive oxygen species
SPION	Super-paramagnetic iron oxide
SSTIs	Skin and soft tissue infections
TiO_2	Titanium dioxide
UV	Ultraviolet
XDR	Extensive drug resistant
ZnO	Zinc oxide

2.1 Introduction

Bacterial skin infections have always been a major concern globally due to its potential impact on human health. A dermatological or skin infection often begins as small, red bumps which cause itching, pain, tenderness and several other side effects. While the skin infection invades into the nearby tissues, it is called as skin and soft tissue infections (SSTIs). Essentially, complete SSTIs formations depend on the three steps, first bacterial adherence to skin cells of the host, then invasion of bacterial strain into deeper layer of tissue, followed by formation of toxins. Most commonly, these are treated with conventional antibiotics, which have been used as 'gold standard' medicine for all kind of bacterial infections for several decades. While these infections are not treated with utmost care, it may result into visible lesions and are likely to leave scars on the patient's body for a lifetime. Sometimes, chronic skin infections also cause a potential death threat to the patients without proper medication. This is very often seen in case of post medical surgery. Moreover, increasing cases of bacterial infections due to multidrug resistant (MDR) and extensive drug resistant (XDR) strains have also raised a concern, and this demands an alternative of conventional antibiotics (Gupta et al. 2013; Niska et al. 2018). Thereby, researchers are looking forward to overcome these challenges by developing nanotechnology-based antimicrobial substances that are having superior physicochemical properties suitable for skincare. Nanoscale materials—manmade engineered materials and structures—offer great deal of opportunities to use it as novel nanotherapeutics owing to its unique dimensionality that offers better therapeutic indexes than conventional agents. This is an emerging area of research which is gaining huge attention from the scientific communities for last few decades in order to develop various novel therapeutic agents particularly suitable for the bacterial skin infections (Beyth et al. 2015).

Nanoscale materials are very small, usually in the size range of 1–100 nm (1 nm = 10^{-9} m). Actually, nanoscale materials are approximately 10^3 times smaller than the diameter of human hair. In this size realm, the material shows unique properties such as high surface area to volume ratio, high conductivity of heat and electricity, super magnetism and high catalytic activity which are distinctly different from its bulk counterpart (Gupta et al. 2013; Beyth et al. 2015). However, synthesis of nanoscale materials with desired size and physicochemical properties greatly relies on its precursors and synthesis methods. There are various physical and chemical methods available which are found to be quite promising and suitable for the synthesis of 'desired' nanoscale materials. Moreover, experts from various fields like physics, chemistry and biology sciences have been striving their common interest in the field of nanotechnology that lead to develop methods of generation of user-defined nanoscale materials with atomic precision. This also provides the development of nanoscale materials with various sizes, shapes and physicochemical properties that are considered to be valuable in various fields starting from optoelectronics to healthcare. It would be mentioned here that the easy surface modifications, favourable mechanical properties and tuneable surface charge distribution allow these nanoscale materials to easily penetrate through cell membranes and other biological barriers. This aspires various researchers to test the efficacy of the nanomaterials in dermatological and dermocosmetological purposes also. Skin being the largest organ of the body and maximally exposed to the external environment is at maximum risk to radiations and infections. Even small damage or cut (e.g. surgery) in the skin causes a skin infection which subsequently leads to colonization and proliferation of microbial flora (Niska et al. 2018; Rajendran et al. 2018). Amongst various types of skin infections, bacterial infections are predominant due to versatile adaptation nature of the bacteria which leads to proliferate this at even very harsh environment also. It is worth mentioning that the detailed mechanism of interaction of bacterial cells with the human skin cells, which influences the growth of the bacterial cells and successive colonization into various layers of the skin, is not fully explored yet. This lack of understanding of physicochemical interactions and microarchitecture of the colonization are one of the major hurdles for development of the novel therapeutics against various kinds of bacterial skin infections. This is very important as conventional antibiotic therapy has been found to be futile against several bacterial skin infections whose number is increasing day-by-day all over the world. To address these issues, nanotechnology-based products for treatments of dermatological infections are considered to be more effective as they can interact at sub-atomic level with the skin tissues owing to their unique dimensional properties (Beyth et al. 2015). Nanomaterials can also be used as drug delivery agents and in formulations of creams and gels which can facilitate faster healing process and also suppress scar visibility (Kuotsu et al. 2010). Importantly, the establishment of the Nanodermatology Society established in 2010 is a major step towards increasing the inclination of researchers in favour of using nanoparticles (NPs) for treating skin infections. Amongst several available options, metal and metal oxide NPs have proved their potential candidature due to their exceptional antimicrobial activities such as antibacterial, antifungal and antiviral, in the treatment of dermatological infections (Gupta et al. 2013). In this chapter, we are going to highlight some of the recent research outcomes and prospects of nanotechnology-based approaches in order to address the issue of bacterial skin infections.

2.2   Anatomy and Physicochemical Properties of Skin

Human skin is the outermost continuous protective layer of the body; however, thickness of skin is not uniform throughout the body. Thickness of the skin depends on the exposer and use of the specific area of the body. For example, skin of palm is thicker as compared to skin of face. Apart from the protection from the invasion of the pathogens, it is responsible for many vital functions such as thermoregulation, sensation to stimuli (touch/heat/cold), synthesis of Vitamin D, secretion of sweat and many more. The cross section of skin can broadly be divided into three layers namely epidermis, dermis and hypodermis (Prost-Squarcioni 2006; Proksch et al. 2008; Kolarsick et al. 2011) that are summarized in Fig. 2.1.

Basically, epidermis is a thin, avascular, continuous and outermost covering of the skin. The epidermis further can be divided into five sub-layers (Kanitakis 2002; McGrath and Uitto 2010; Ng and Lau 2015).

1. *Stratum Corneum*: Uppermost layer of epidermis. This layer mainly consists of 15–30 mono layers of cells. Cells of these layers are replaced in every 15–30 days. Cells from the lower layer like granulosum or lucidum help in replacing the dead cells of corneum layer.
2. *Stratum Lucidum*: This layer is present just below stratum corneum and is smooth and translucent. It generally acts as a water barrier.
3. *Stratum Granulosum*: It is located just below the stratum lucidum. The grainy behaviour of this layer is due to the presence of keratin and keratohyalin.
4. *Stratum Spinosum*: It is the intermediate layer of epidermis and it also generates keratin protein.
5. *Stratum Basale*: This layer separates epidermis from dermis through basal lamina. This layer is made up of collagen and proteins.

Also, epidermis layer of skin contains various vital cell lines like melanocytes, keratinocytes, Langerhans' cells and Merkel's cells. Melanocyte cells synthesize pigment called as melanin which is responsible for skin colour and also protects skin

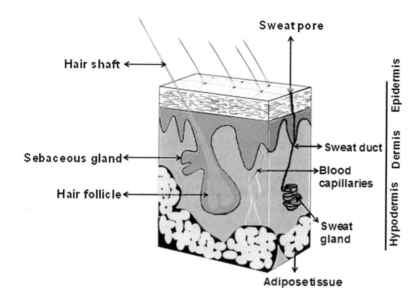

Fig. 2.1 Cross-sectional view of human skin showing the presence of various layers, i.e. dermis, epidermis and hypodermis. Dermis is outermost layer of the skin which mainly acts as a barrier preventing entry of any external substance. The innermost areas comprises of blood vessels and adipose tissues

from radiation. Keratinocyte cells usually originate in stratum basale which produces keratin protein. Keratin proteins provide strength to the skin and also act as an important component for water barrier. Langerhans' cells which are tissue-resident macrophage of the skin that constitute 2–8% of the total epidermal cells are derived from bone marrow. These cells may also behave as dendritic and antigen presenting cell, and also express MHC II.

Dermis is the second layer of skin which is comparatively thicker than epidermis. It is further divided into two sub-layers called as papillary layer and reticular layer. Papillary layer is thin and superficial layer of dermis which is composed of loosely bound connective tissue and that contains collagen and elastin. This layer also constitutes of adipocytes, phagocytes, nerve cells and meissner corpuscles. Reticular layer is present beneath papillary layer which is composed of dense connective tissue and nerve cells. Elastin provides elasticity and collagen contribute strength to this layer.

Hypodermis is the deepest layer of skin which is also called as subcutaneous layer. This layer play a very important role in connecting skin with muscle and bone. This layer contains well-developed vascularization, loose connective tissue and lots of adipocytes.

2.3   Type of Bacterial Infections in Skin

In 1998, the US Food and Drug Administration (FDA) proposed classification methods of SSTIs. Based upon the characteristics of the infections, SSTIs can be broadly classified into two categories, i.e. (1) Uncomplicated—this is superficial infection which may be cured by conventional antimicrobial therapy or surgical incision alone, and (2) Complicated—this includes deeper tissue infections where surgery is essential as only conventional antimicrobial agents could not resolve the issues of infections. Importantly, both of them show different symptoms based on the type of infections which are summarized below. Depending on the specific body parts of skin, specific bacterial colonization is observed. Apart from this anatomical feature, various other factors such as genetics, age, sex, nutrition and hygienic conditions also determine the type and behaviour of bacterial flora (Nizet et al. 2001).

- *Cellulitis*: This is a small breakage in the skin and/or cut results in entering of the bacteria and spreading cellulitis. The common symptoms of this type of bacterial infection are that infected part will be red in colour and usually warm. This also causes huge pain and swelling of the infected area. It may appear in any part of the body; however, leg and face are most vulnerable for this type of infections. Several types of bacteria cause these types of infections; however, more predominantly *β-haemolytic streptococci,* or *S. aureus* bacteria strains are found to be responsible for this type of infections.
- *Folliculitis*: It is another type of bacterial infection that is mainly seen in case of infections of the hair follicles which appears like red bumps. This causes itching, constant scratching and hair loss also. This may be caused due to various reasons such as unhygienic bath and shavings, which may harvest bacteria that cause folliculitis.
- *Impetigo*: It is very transmissible bacterial skin infection which commonly affects the face of young children and infants, but person of any age may be affected by this. Its onset is characterized by appearance of tiny blisters which become bigger with time. *Staphylococcus aureus* and/or *Streptococcus pyogenes* are the foremost cause of this type of infection. Quite often this infection enters into the deeper layer of skin, which is commonly termed as ecthyma.
- *Boils*: This type of deep skin infections start as a red lump and with the progress of time it appears as red and tender bumps.

2.4   Emergence of Various Types of Metal Nanoparticles (MNPs) and Its Composites

With the advancement of nanotechnology-based research works, nanoparticles (NPs) are becoming an essential component of conventional therapeutics. The market of cosmetics is flooded with extensive usage of NPs as an integral part of the formulations. Some of the most common NPs manufactured for use in treatment of skin infections include silver nanoparticles (Ag NPs), titanium oxide NPs (TiO$_2$ NPs), zinc oxide NPs (ZnO NPs), copper oxide NPs (CuO NPs) and so on (Thakur et al. 2018). The major advantages of nanoscale materials are that they show strong antimicrobial activity. Additionally, protection from the exposure of the UV radiation is one of the essential aspects of any skincare products, in this regard, NPs-based product showed remarkable results. Several nanoscale materials block the ultraviolet radiations very efficiently and thus offer the scope of using it as vital component of numerous cosmetic products. Furthermore, the NPs can be functionalized to form a composite to perform targeted drug delivery in case of skin cancer or melanoma as well (Hashim et al. 2019).

Skin is basically a barrier formed by the body towards external environment. It is impermeable to drugs due to the occurrence of stratum corneum lipids and cellular cohesion. However, due to high patient compliance topically applicable formulations are most preferred methods of treatment. Thus, for any skincare materials, the first and foremost property which needs to attend priority basis is its permeation through skin that needs to be enhanced. In this aspect, nanotechnology comes into play a very pivotal role as size and tuneable physicochemical properties of the NPs allow it to permeate more efficiently through various layers of skin. Additionally, metal NPs and its composites can be mixed with conventional drugs that essentially enhance its permeability and penetration through skin. NPs of a suitable size can easily cross the skin barriers and enter in the body as well as enable other drug components to be carried along with it, thereby proving its potency as a nanocarrier. There are plenty of NPs which itself possess antibacterial properties in in vivo model and thus enhance the scope of using it as drug. These also produced effective results against antibiotic resistant infections where antibiotics utterly fail to produce effective outcomes, hence, these nanoscale materials offer a huge scope of filling up the gap in skin treatment particularly in case of bacterial skin infections. They are even helpful in fighting against multidrug resistant (MDR) and biofilm infections. Moreover, the formulations involving metal and metal oxide NPs reduce the need of chemical enhancers (organic solvents/surfactants) which are generally used to deliver therapeutic agents topically. It is well-proven fact that extensive use of chemical enhancers hampers the proper functioning of the skin and also is responsible for allergic reactions and damaging of skin (Gupta et al. 2013; Beyth et al. 2015; Rajendran et al. 2018; Niska et al. 2018). Recent experimental evidences support that several metal NPs have the potential to kill both Gram positive and Gram negative bacterial strains.

Proposed Mechanism of Antibacterial Activity of MNPs
- Metal NPs interact with bacterial cells depending upon the surface properties; however, strong interactions of NPs cause damage to bacterial cell wall which is commonly known as direct 'particle effects'. This leads to mechanical damage to the cell wall that releases intracellular component outside to the cells due to osmotic imbalance.

- Disruption of the bacterial cell wall alters the membrane potential followed by membrane depolarization and loss of membrane integrity. This creates a discrepancy in the electron transport chain, influences cellular respiration and interrupts energy transduction that leads to bacterial cell death.
- Some studies suggested that release of the metal ions from metal NPs causes the ionic disproportions within the cells. This also results in incongruity in several cellular pathways which ultimately causes cell death.
- Bacterial cell death is mediated due to generation of high levels of reactive oxygen species (ROS) or free radicals of oxygen. The elevated amount of ROS leads to lipid peroxidation, protein alteration, enzyme inhibition and disruption/mutation of genetic material which finally causes cell death.

From the above, it was clear that metal and its oxide NPs would be ideal choices to control the bacterial skin infection as these target several pathways simultaneously to kill bacterial cells. Moreover, bacteria are not able to develop resistance against NPs. Therefore, several research groups have been engaged in order to develop novel NPs and its composites suitable for bacterial skin infections. Essentially, these nanoparticles and nanocomposites open up several new avenues and prospects in order to develop next-generation skincare products, some of that are already available in the market and many more are in the pipeline, these will be marketed in the near future.

2.5 Essences of New Class of Nanoscale Materials Suitable Against Skin Infections

Besides metal NPs and their composites, there are several new classes of nanoscale materials which are also being used in skin infection such as nanospheres, nanocapsules, nanoemulsions, niosomes and so on (Thakur et al. 2018). Most commonly used nanostructures are nanospheres which are generally polymeric matrices of size approximately 100 nm. These are formed by using a controlled polymerization process (e.g. alkyl cyanoacrylates or its derivatives) while the active compounds or drugs are adsorbed, dispersed or dissolved into them. Nanospheres usually increase the stability of the active substances and improve the biocompatibility of the pharmaceutical products. Similarly, nanocapsules are the modified form of nanospheres, which have the capability to captivating the active substances within itself and providing a controlled release of it at desired time. However, the size of the nanocapsules is considerable bigger than nanospheres. Both these types of nanostructures are essential as they help the active ingredients to penetrate deeper into the dermis of the skin (Guterres et al. 2007). They also help in protecting the active compounds from the external environment.

Another very popular nanoformulation is nanoemulsions, which are colloidal particulates contained in oil-in-water/water-in-oil/bi-continuous emulsion. They are of size ranging from 10 to 1000 nm based of the synthesis methods and reactants.

With a lipophilic and amorphous surface, these form solid spherical drug carriers having a negative charge. They are highly stable thermally and have high viscosity, fluidity and solubility, and this enables them to effortlessly integrate biologically active substances or drugs into it. However, there are several drawbacks associated with it such as its accumulation of the substances in layers of the skin unable to penetrate into deeper layers of the skin (Jaiswal et al. 2015).

Niosomes are nanocarriers similar to liposomes and are composed of synthetic, non-ionic surfactants formed by self-assembly and have vesicular structure. These are moulded by mingling non-ionic surfactant of alkyl or dialkyl polyglycerol ether with cholesterol. A bilayer vesicular structure is formed by these surfactants in aqueous media because of its amphiphilic nature. The structures are composed of hydrophilic heads and hydrophobic tails which make it suitable to encapsulate a wide range of drug molecules of varied solubility. They are also equipped with specific chemical receptors for targeted drug delivery. In dermatology, they are used in the transfer of hyaluronic acid, antioxidants, vitamins and other peptides to deeper layers of skin (Kuotsu et al. 2010).

Similarly, various other types of nanomaterials are also being employed for treatment of skin infections in a more specific and targeted manner. However, here in this chapter, we would discuss only about the role of metal and metal oxide NPs in the treatment of skin infections.

2.6 Nanoscale Materials as Antibacterial Skincare Agents

2.6.1 Metal Nanoparticles

Contribution of nanotechnology is rapidly increasing in several areas to find out the innovative solutions including skin infections and dermatological treatments that have the immense potential to improve the quality of life of patients. Various nanotechnology-based products already proved their mettle by being a component of numerous beauty products and modern anti-ageing formulations. It is to be deemed that NP-based products would essentially overcome plenty of drawbacks associated with the conventional skincare products. Therefore, this is one of the faster growing areas of research suitable for personal care industry and its use has risen substantially over last few decades (Table 2.1). Amongst various nanoparticle-based products, metal NPs are in forefront, which is considered one of the most vital nanotherapeutic agents in order to control the skin infections. This exhibits bactericidal activity against wide range of Gram-positive, Gram-negative bacteria and even antibiotic resistant bacterial species. Modern nanotechnology offers the scope of synthesis of metal NPs with precise number of atoms in its metal core. Additionally, the suitable ligands play a crucial role in the transportation of the NPs through various layer of the skin and could be easily tagged with the NPs. These programmed metal NPs provided the opportunities of developing various new materials which

Table 2.1 Types of commercialized products containing nanoparticles used to prevent skin infections or diseases

Commercial product	Nanoparticles	Properties
Sunscreen	Zinc and titanium oxide NPs	Protection of skin from UVA (400–320 nm) and UVB (320–290 nm)
Anti-aging cream	Gold and silver based NPs	Skin tissue regeneration
Facial cleanser	Gold and silver NPs, zinc and titanium dioxide NPs	Antibacterial, anti-inflammatory, restoring skin texture
Bandage fabric	Zinc oxide and silver NPs	Antibacterial, treatment of infected wounds, retains wettability in bandage
Soaps	Silver NPs	Antimicrobial
Shaving creams	Titanium dioxide NPs	Antibacterial, protection of skin from UVA (400–320 nm) and UVB (320–290 nm)
Shampoos	Silver and titanium dioxide NPs	Antibacterial, antifungal and anti-inflammatory
Deodorant	Zinc and titanium dioxide NPs	Antimicrobial

have better performance and are economical, biocompatible and more stable in the ambient conditions.

Important Properties of Metal NPs Suitable for Skin Infections
- Metal NPs can be formulated easily of desirable size (nm to μm) and shape which can easily infiltrate through various layers of skin, thus suitable for treatment of deep tissue infections.
- Surface of the metal NPs can be functionalized with wide range of chemical molecules in order to monitor the surface characteristics of the NPs (hydrophilic/ hydrophobic).
- Transition metal NPs (e.g. Au NPs, Ag NPs, etc.) exhibit size and shape dependent exquisite optical properties in the visible to near infrared regions which help in tracking the nanoparticle trajectories inside the cells and organs.
- There are several metal NPs (e.g. Au NPs and Cu NPs) which are biocompatible and raise less chances of immunogenic responses.

2.6.1.1 Silver Nanoparticles (Ag NPs)

Silver NPs (Ag NPs) have a long history of using it as effective antimicrobial agents. Owing to its intense antibacterial, antifungal and antiviral abilities, it is the most appreciated metal NP in medicinal industry. Since ancient times, silver is being used as an antimicrobial agent. Silver nitrate was used in World War I as disinfecting agent. In skin treatment, silver (Ag) is being looked upon for treating wounds, burns and other infectious or prone to infection diseases. The increasing rate of antibiotic resistance has led to a demand of agents that do not allow resistance to be developed against them (Tian et al. 2007; Niska et al. 2018); in this regard, silver NPs based product offers very promising outcomes. The best part of Ag NPs is that it is equally effective against both Gram-positive and Gram-negative bacteria.

With the onset of the era of nanomaterial, Ag NPs were synthesized and they have proved to be more effective against treating infections and healing wounds by various research groups. The Ag NPs show better biological activities than conventional silver nitrate based products that have been used for a long time. As per a report by Tian et al., in 2007 Ag NPs augmented the process of wound healing by decreasing the bacterial activity as well as reducing the inflammation. Wound healing involves a process in which keratinocyte cells migrate and then divides in the epidermal layer of skin which is known as re-epithelialization. It was found that Ag NPs based agents showed significant improvement in the re-epithelialization process; however, the exact mechanism of action of Ag NPs is not yet known. On the other hand, mechanism of antibacterial activity is more validated for Ag NPs. It was established that Ag NPs created holes in the cell wall that increases the membrane permeability and causing failure of the respiratory chain (Qing et al. 2018). Another report stated that Ag NPs bind to thiol group and disrupt protein structure (Dakal et al. 2016). However, higher dose of Ag NPs is toxic to the human body, although the toxicity varies based on size, surface charge and shape of the NPs (Zhang et al. 2016). Szmyd et al. (2013) in their study claimed that human epidermal keratinocytes upon exposure to 15 nm Ag NPs decreased its cell viability and metabolic activities. Additionally, the study found that prolonged exposure of it also induced DNA damage.

2.6.1.2   Gold Nanoparticles (Au NPs)

Gold nanoparticles (Au NPs) are extensively used in wound healing, drug delivery and tissue regeneration due to their suitable physicochemical properties. They are biocompatible and offer antimicrobial activity also. However, unlike silver it cannot be used individually as an antimicrobial agent and thus must be incorporated with other antibacterial macromolecules for effective results. While Au NPs are integrated or cross-linked with collagen, gelatin, chitosan or amphiphilic molecules, these become more biocompatible and biodegradable at the same time potent bactericidal too, thereby hastening the wound healing process. Additionally, Au NPs can even be conjugated with other existing conventional drugs to increase their ability to kill bacterial infections. Recently, several studies came up with another very promising applications of Au-based material, whereas it was demonstrated that gold nanorod can be used effectively in photothermal therapies by conjugating with pathogen-specific antibodies. Moreover, it may be used along with photosensitizing agents also for photodynamic therapy in order to kill pathogenic bacterial strains. These methods are very effective for killing of both wild-type and resistant bacterial species.

The modes of bacterial cell death after treatment with Au NPs are not fully understood yet. However, it was proposed that there might be two different pathways which lead to bacterial cell death. (1) NPs after entering into the bacterial cells cause alteration of membrane potential leading to inhibition of enzyme ATP synthase (ATP depletion and finally collapse in energy metabolism) (2) Au NPs also lead to formation of higher amount of intracellular ROS that ultimately kill the bacteria by ROS dependent pathways (Niska et al. 2018).

Apart from this antibacterial activity of gold-based nanoformulation, there are studies which established that these nanoformulations help in the tissue regeneration and wound healing too. Moreover, Au NPs enhance healing by reducing inflammation via cytokine regulation and increasing angiogenesis. For example, Naraginti et al. (2016) applied Au NPs topically on cutaneous wounds of rat and to their surprise a higher rate of re-epithelialization, granular tissue formation and extracellular matrix (ECM) deposition was observed. These all led to a faster rate of wound healing process which is a very important aspect of Au-based nanoformulations. They also compared the wound healing process using Au NPs and Ag NPs. The comparative studies of Au NPs and Ag NPs showed that Au NPs revealed better free radical scavengers' activities and thus enhanced wound healing process at faster rate as compared to Ag NPs. Hence, it would be inferred that Au NPs hold great potential to be used as effective nanotherapeutics in treating skin infections.

2.6.2 Metal Oxide NPs

2.6.2.1 Titanium Dioxide Nanoparticles

Titanium dioxide (TiO_2) has been known since ancient times for its antibacterial properties against both Gram-positive and Gram-negative bacteria (Wei et al. 1994). They have even emerged as strong antiviral and antiparasitic agents according to some recent studies (Zan et al. 2007; Allahverdiyev et al. 2013; Amin et al. 2014). Their mode of action is very similar to that of Au NPs, i.e. their toxicity might be induced by visible light, near UV or UV light causing excessive ROS generation. Study showed that TiO_2 NPs were effective against spores of *Bacillus* also, which is one of the most resistant pathogens (Hamal et al. 2010). Reports have also shown that nanocomposite of TiO_2 NPs with other nanomaterial, for instance, Ag NPs, demonstrated enhanced antibacterial activity (Pratap Reddy et al. 2007).

Owing to their high photostability TiO_2 NPs are used to combat photoallergy as an active ingredient of topical formulations and sunscreens. However, studies revealed that these NPs may have adverse effects on human dermal fibroblasts (Pan et al. 2009). It was observed that it damaged the cells in multiple ways such as by decreasing cell proliferation, mobility and fibroblast area. Eventually, when these same NPs were functionalized with certain hydrophobic polymer the adverse effects were much more reduced and the cells were protected from damage. Also the rutile form of TiO_2 showed lesser phototoxicity than its anatase form (Gomathi Devi and Nagaraj 2014).

2.6.2.2 Zinc Oxide Nanoparticles

Zinc oxide nanoparticles (ZnO NPs) are also an active ingredient of the sunscreens due to their ability of absorbing radiations. They prevent photoageing and photoallergy of skin as well as formation of cancerous skin lesions due to broad ultraviolet A (UVA) spectrum by absorbing them. It is also an efficient antibacterial agent depending upon its concentration being used and size of particles. They are also known to be effective against various drug resistant bacterial strains. It showed antibacterial activities against methicillin resistant *S. aureus*, methicillin sensitive *S. aureus* and methicillin resistant *S. epidermidis* (Ansari et al. 2012; Malka et al. 2013). They also prevent biofilm formation. They act upon bacteria by either disrupting the cell membrane, altering its membrane potential or by inducing high level of ROS generation (Huang et al. 2008; Jin et al. 2009; Liu et al. 2009).

However, ZnO NPs may exhibit toxic effects on human skin by disturbing the mitochondrial function in epidermal keratinocytes causing leakage of lactate dehydrogenase (LDH). It also induces ROS generation causing damage to cell organelles. Its phototoxicity study on skin revealed the production of hydroxyl radicals, leakage of LDH and 8-hydroxy-2′-deoxyguanosine generation. These are known to be the byproducts of oxidative DNA damage and used as a biomarker of oxidative stress and carcinoma (Tran and Salmon 2011; Wang et al. 2013; Pati et al. 2014). Therefore, it could be stated that prior to using this NPs for in vivo treatment of skin infections its adverse effects need to be taken care.

2.6.2.3 Copper Oxide Nanoparticles

Copper oxide NPs (CuO NPs) also recently are being explored as antibacterial and antifungal agents. However, its antibacterial property is slightly less than both of Ag NPs and ZnO. It is preferably used as an enhancer of antibacterial activity in form of nanocomposites. The studies showed that Ag NPs were found to be more effective against *E. coli* and *S. aureus*, while CuO NPs were more toxic towards *B. subtilis* and *B. anthracis* possibly due to its better interaction with amine and carboxyl group on pathogen's cell surface (Ruparelia et al. 2008; Ren et al. 2009; Pandey et al. 2014).

2.6.2.4 Other Metal Oxide Nanoparticles

Several other NPs are also being explored in order to treat dermatological infections because some of the above-mentioned NPs cause certain adverse effects. Magnesium oxide nanoparticles (MgO NPs) are also known to possess antibacterial properties against both Gram-positive and Gram-negative bacteria as well as spores and viruses. The MgO NPs have the potential to directly inhibit essential enzymes of the bacteria and also induce generation of ROS (Kuotsu et al. 2010). It also inhibits the biofilm formation mainly occurred by *E. coli* and *S. aureus* (Lellouche et al. 2009, 2012; Blecher et al. 2011).

Another class of nanoparticle, which has been drawn significant attention, is iron oxide (Fe_3O_4) which possesses almost negligible antibacterial properties in its bulk form. However, their nanoscale formed possesses bactericidal activity while stabilized with suitable agents. More commonly, Fe_3O_4 NPs were seen to reduce growth of both Gram-positive and Gram-negative bacterial colonies (Anghel et al. 2014). Similarly, use of super-paramagnetic iron oxide (SPION) is a completely new approach in this field. The concept behind it is to use magnetic nanoparticles to cause local magnetic-hyperthermia in presence of oscillating magnetic field, which kills the bacteria by controlled and local heating. These are also very effective in disruption of the bacterial biofilm infections, for example, usually SPIONs are tagged with other NPs (e.g. Ag NP) and/or drugs as bactericidal agents and then the magnetic property is utilized to penetrate inside and destroy the bacterial biofilm (Taylor et al. 2012; Durmus et al. 2013; Vasanth and Kurian 2017). It should be mentioned here that biofilms are communities of microorganisms that are often formed on solid surfaces and are organized to protect the individual cells from the harsh environment. Very often, it is noticed that the biofilm-associated microorganisms exhibit an extreme resistance to antibiotics. One of the important reasons for low susceptibility of biofilm to antimicrobial agents is the failure of antibiotics to penetrate the full depth of the biofilm. In this regard, NPs exhibit significant results.

2.6.3 Nanocomposites

Metal and metal oxide NPs show strong bactericidal property against both Gram-positive and Gram-negative bacteria. However, these are failed to produce expected outcomes in the in vivo model owing to its cytotoxicity and issues of biocompatibility (Soenen et al. 2011; Takamiya et al. 2016; Vasanth and Kurian 2017). Very often these NPs also suffer from the challenges of the clearance from the human body by normal sequester mechanisms. Moreover, issues of stabilization of these NPs in the biological interface raise several concerns in the real-life applications for the newly developed NPs. On the other hand, organic nanostructures are comparatively more stable in the biological interface and mechanically more flexible than inorganic nanoparticles (i.e. metal and metal oxide NPs). They are also known to produce lesser side effects than the latter one. The issue of inflammation due to administration of certain metal and metal oxide NPs on skin can be surpassed by usage of organic NPs. But since organic NPs possess weaker bactericidal property, the researchers have been working upon combining the two of them to form nanocomposites. These nanocomposites resolve the issues of cytotoxicity without compromising the bactericidal properties of the nanocomposites.

One of the extensively used organic nanostructures is collagen which is naturally available, thus economical and biocompatible. There are several studies which showed that it can be combined with various metal NPs to suppress the adverse effects caused by it and make it more biocompatible. Interestingly, these collagen-based nanocomposites exhibited synergistic antibacterial activity (Grigore et al. 2017). For example, Cardoso et al. (2014) synthesized nanocomposite of Ag NPs by taking collagen as stabilizing agent of NPs. Surprisingly, their results established that the nanocomposite provided minimum toxic effects and enhanced antibacterial activity in case of *S. aureus* and *E. coli* bacteria. Subsequent studies revealed the effect of nanocomposite of TiO_2-Ag encapsulated with collagen matrix upon skin cells. It was observed that although collagen did not increase the antibacterial property of the composite, it enhanced the biocompatibility and fastened skin regeneration (Patrascu et al. 2015; Spoiala et al. 2015). Similar studies are also carried out by Ren et al. 2009 by developing nanocomposite of collagen-CuO NP that also demonstrated greater effectiveness than CuO NP alone as antibacterial agent.

Another biopolymer which has been used extensively for last few decades in various biomedical applications is chitosan. The chitosan-based nanocomposites are also implied effectively to combat bacterial infections. Various types of nanocomposite such as chitosan-Ag NPs, chitosan-Au NPs, chitosan-Cu NPs, chitosan-ZnO NPs, and chitosan-TiO_2 NPs based nanocomposites are being highly explored in this context. It was reported that chitosan-Ag NP nanocomposite showed 1.5 times better antimicrobial activity against *P. aeruginosa*, *S. aureus* and *E. coli,* when compared to conventionally available wound dressing agents containing only Ag NPs. In case of manufacturing sponge dressing, nanocomposites are formed of chitosan-Ag NPs and hyaluronic acid, which found to be excellent bactericidal agent against *P. aeruginosa, S. aureus, MRSA* and *K. pneumonia* strains of bacteria. (Mohandas et al. 2018). Sandri et al. in 2019 published their work on development of electrospun scaffolds loaded with silver nanoparticles (Ag NPs) to augment cutaneous healing and inhibiting wound infections. Various other inorganic NPs bound with chitosan also demonstrated better bactericidal properties and increased the biocompatibility of it, thus proving it to be an essence in treating skin infections effectively with reduced side effects.

2.7 Proposed Mathematical Models of Penetration of NPs Through Skin

There are several mathematical models that tried to explore the basic understanding of structural organization and physicochemical behaviour of the skin (Table 2.2). Mathematical model of skin can be classified into three classes: (1) Structural models of skin, (2) Phenomenological models of skin and (3) Structurally based phenomenological models (Limbert 2017; Anissimov 2014). Each model has its assumptions and limitations. For any model to mimic the physiochemical behaviour of skin, it is significant for the model to consider all the features of skin like biomechanical, biochemical, interaction between the components of skin, stress condition, etc. The phenomenological model assumes the general behaviour of skin

Table 2.2 Some of the functional models being used these days (Limbert 2017)

Type of model	Characteristic mathematical approaches
Structural model	Image-based microstructural finite-element model (Leyva-Mendivil et al. 2015)
Nonlinear elastic models of the skin	1. Lanir's model 2. Bischoff–Arruda–Grosh's formulation 3. Limbert–Middleton's/Itskov–Aksel's formulation 4. Gasser–Ogden–Holzapfel's anisotropic hyperelastic formulation 5. Flynn–Rubin–Nielsen's formulation 6. Limbert's formulation 7. Weiss's transversely isotropic hyperelastic formulation
Nonlinear viscoelastic models of skin	1. Quasi-linear viscoelasticity model 2. Explicit rate-dependent model

tissue. This model considers the overall phenomena of tissue, and it does not consider the individual nature of components of skin. The drawback of this model is that the resulting parameters/factors often have no physical explanation and thus more or less it acts as 'black box' (Limbert 2017).

Structural model considers skin as assembly or arrangement of different constituent components of tissue in the matrix like keratin and collagen fibres. The model considers only the biophysical property (mechanical and physicochemical properties) of building block of the tissue. In order to make this model more realistic, more features like geometrical arrangement, interspatial arrangement and how they interact with each other under different physiological conditions will have to incorporate. Structural and phenomenological model both have several limitations. So, to overcome these limitations a third model has been framed combining the features of above-mentioned model. The combined model can be named as structurally based phenomenological models (Limbert 2017). This model has more efficiency to mimic the real skin as it includes various features like mechanical properties, chemical properties, interspatial arrangement, geometrical arrangements and many more.

2.8 Diffusion of NPs Through Skin

Diffusion of nanoparticles/drug through skin depends on various factors like size of NPs, its surface charge and the pathways NPs follow for the penetration through skin. Selection of pathway is not random or fixed; it depends on physiochemical properties of NPs and nature of formulation of the nanoparticles.

The pathways for absorption of any materials by skin can be divided into two categories: (1) Epidermal route and (2) Transappendageal route/trans-follicular route/shunt pathways. Epidermal route can be again subdivided into two subclasses called as intracellular (across cells) and other is intercellular (between cells). Drug that follows intracellular route passes through the cell membrane (Schneider et al. 2009; Boer et al. 2016; Herskovitz et al. 2016). The processes like endocytosis, transcytosis and diffusion of small and polar molecule through membrane generally follow this route passively. But due to lipid layer in stratum corneum, the permeability of drug is very less. It was established that permeability of NPs/drug is inversely proportional to size and its hydrophilicity (Bhowmick et al. 2013). Several small molecules like penetration enhancer can be used to enhance the permeability. However, intercellular route is comparatively faster and predominantly used route for transportation of NPs. In this mode of transportation, the molecules travel between the cells. Actually, molecules travel very long distance as compared to the thickness of stratum corneum (~20 nm); still this mode of transportation is faster and preferred. Shunt pathways is another important route of penetration through skin. The molecules find a route to penetrate stratum corneum through hair follicles and its sebaceous glands, through apocrine sweat gland (Fig. 2.2). Numerous researches have been done which supports the fact that nanoparticles are better drug candidate for permeability and specific drug delivery (Couto et al. 2014).

Recently few researchers have tried to explore the penetration of the Au NPs through human skin (Filon et al. 2011). The study was done by considering Franz diffusion method in biological skin cells. The outer surface of skin was considered to be the donor phase, whereas inner surface was the receiver (physiological solution). Varying amount of Au NPs of concentration 100 mg L^{-1} was applied over the

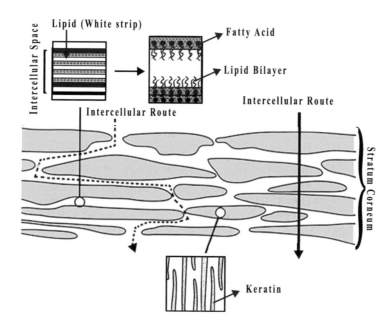

Fig. 2.2 Various routes of transportation of the materials through skin. Mainly two types of pathways are available: (1) Intracellular and (2) Intercellular route of transportation of the substance through skin

Table 2.3 Diffusion of nanoparticles through skin

Type of NPs	Total conc. used	Conc. diffused	Rate of diffusion	References
Ag NP (rat skin)	1 mL (280 μg mL^{-1})	0.2 μg cm^{-2}	–	Dhar et al. (2012)
Au NP	0.5 mL (100 mg L^{-1})	0.214 μg cm^{-2}	7.8 ± 2 ng cm^{-2} h^{-1}	Filon et al. (2011)
TiO$_2$ NP	2.5 mL (1 g L^{-1})	0.47 ± 0.33 μg cm^{-2}	–	Crosera et al. (2015)

donor phase and the results were observed for 24 h. Mean gold content found in the receiver solution depended upon the dosage given at the donor phase. Intact skin showed 214.0 ± 43.7 ng cm^{-2} and damaged skin showed 187.7 ± 50.2 ng cm^{-2} mean gold content. Gold permeation flux for 24 h was found to be 7.8 ± 2.0 ng cm^{-2} h^{-1} and 7.1 ± 2.5 ng cm^{-2} h^{-1} for intact and damaged skin, respectively. Similarly experiments on diffusion of Ag NPs through rat skin were conducted by Dhar et al. in 2012 which included exposing the skin with 1 mL Ag NPs of concentration 280 μg mL^{-1} for 24 h. When exposed in form of dispersions 0.2 μg cm^{-2} of Ag was identified in the receptor section. Though the penetration was found to be low, the study indicated size dependent permeation of Ag NPs and its localization upon skin surface (Table 2.3).

2.8.1 Mathematical Model for Diffusion Through Skin

Diffusion of particles through skin barrier is well-studied topic and depends on various factors like physicochemical properties, size, concentration of particles and pathways of diffusion. Considering all these features, mathematical model for diffusion has been formulated. This model is based on Fick's equation. However, there are some limitations in this model. So, there are various other diffusion models that have been developed assuming different mathematical assumptions like Fick's first law, Fick's second law, Laplace transform, homogeneous membrane model and scaled particle theory (Couto et al. 2014). According to Fick's laws, diffusion of particle takes place from higher concentration to lower concentration.

While any substances (e.g. drugs/NPs/creams/ointment) apply on the skin, these pass through it via normal passive diffusion, by following appropriate laws of mass transfer. Most commonly used equation which governs the mass transfer rate through biological skin is Fick's laws (first and the second law of Fick), which are based on a pure mathematical model suitable for the study of diffusional behaviour of various solutes. However, diffusion in skin is a complex process which associates several other factors like the architecture of the stratum corneum, the number of hair follicles and sebaceous glands, and all these intrinsic parameters of skin determine the feasibility of the outcomes of the models. Therefore, several other models are also proposed such as the scaled particle theory, the homogeneous membrane model or hybrid approach (uses both first and the second law of Fick). Use of proper boundary conditions which are the physical attributes in the mathematical model provides the rational solutions of the equations.

Let us consider M as the amount of material that is flowing in a small time interval of t through a surface area of A and thickness L (stratum corneum (SC)) due to the concentration gradient of ∇C between outer and inner SC layers. It would be mentioned here that mathematical modelling of mass transfer through skin mainly includes the modelling of mass transfer through SC only as it is the main barrier to any kind of solute permeation through skin. Initially the diffusion through the SC is time dependent and is described by the diffusion equation. With time, rate of diffusion will reach at a steady state. The relationship between ∇C and M would be according to the Fick's first law that describes the skin transportation under steady-state conditions. We can write the following equation:

$$M = D\frac{A}{L}t\nabla C$$

$$J_{ss} = \frac{M}{At} = \frac{D}{L}\nabla C$$

where D is the diffusion constant and J_{ss} is steady-state flux of solute passing through skin.

Experimentally, it is established that due to easy and faster rate of clearance of the solutes in the dermis, the concentration in the inner layer of the SC generally is much less than in the outer layer. So, the following assumption may be incorporated in the above equation.

$$\Delta C \approx C = K_{sc}C_v$$

$$J_{ss} = \frac{DP}{L}C_v$$

$$J_{ss} = kC_v$$

where $k = \dfrac{DP}{L}$ is the permeability coefficient of the SC, C_v is drug concentration within vesicles (i.e. nanospheres/nanocarriers, etc.) and P is the partition coefficient between skin and vesicle.

This is the Fick's first law of diffusion which can be applied to explain the skin transportation under steady-state conditions.

2.8.2   Metal and Metal Oxide NPs Diffusion Through Skin

Numerous researches have been done which supports the fact that nanoparticles are better drug candidates for permeability and specific drug delivery (Couto et al. 2014). In recent past, lots of research has been done to see how and how much nanoparticles penetrate the skin barrier (stratum corneum) (Larese et al. 2009; DeLouise 2012; Gupta et al. 2013). Researchers are trying to establish the relationship between size, concentration, time and absorption of NPs in systemic circulation of the body through dermal penetration. A series of work are being done these days to investigate the qualitative and quantitative study of many type of nanoparticles like TiO_2, ZnO, Au NPs and quantum dots (DeLouise 2012). Reports suggested that Au NPs (5 nm) have showed high rate of penetration through mouse skin barrier (Huang et al. 2010). Diffusion of Au NPs of different sizes (15, 102 and 198 nm) was investigated to see the extent of penetration (Sonavane et al. 2008). The authors observed that the penetration of Au NPs depends upon the size, whereas the extent of penetration decreases with increase in size of nanoparticles. Maximum penetration was observed in case of 15 nm and comparatively lesser penetration in case of 102 nm and least in case of 198 nm. In another study, TiO_2 and ZnO NPs enriched sunscreen were applied to pigs to observe the penetration through stratum corneum (Monteiro-Riviere et al. 2011) which showed better permeation of the sunscreen through skin due to presence of NPs. In contrast, another research group reported that penetration of topically applied TiO_2 NPs was negligible through the skin (Filipe et al. 2009).

2.9   Conclusion

Skin being the essential first line of barrier against microbial invasion constantly interacts with a wide range of microbial flora and prevents their entry into the host. However, any discrepancy in its functions due to skin damage or cut may help in colonization of bacterial strains. Various nanocomposites have been explored and showed significant outcomes in in - vitro as well as in - vivo studies that offer the scope of using it as an alternative of antibacterial agents. However, proper evaluation of toxicity of these newly developed nanoscale materials on human need to be carried out in much more comprehensive ways prior to any clinical applications. Fortunately, many nanocomposites are in the process of clinical trials. Several metallic and organic NPs have already found valuable and beneficial in medicinal and cosmetic products. Moreover, their ability to combat with antibiotic resistant bacterial strains has created a new ray of hope in treatment of patients suffering from resistant strains. However, there are few demerits still associated with these like sequester mechanism and risks of long-term use associated with these nanocomposites are not explored extensively in many cases. Research is being carried out to develop several new strategies to address these issues throughout the world to overcome the challenges associated with the use of nanoformulations in therapeutics and their success is also being reported. Thus, we are anticipating that in near future nanoformulations would become an essential component for various skincare and wound healing materials.

References

Allahverdiyev AM, Abamor ES, Bagirova M, Baydar SY, Ates SC, Kaya F, Kaya C, Rafailovich M (2013) Investigation of antileishmanial activities of Tio2@Ag nanoparticles on biological properties of L. tropica and L. infantum parasites, in vitro. Exp Parasitol 135:55–63

Amin MT, Alazba AA, Manzoor U (2014) A review of removal of pollutants from water/wastewater using different types of nanomaterials. Adv Mater Sci Eng 2014:1–24

Anghel AG, Grumezescu AM, Chirea M, Grumezescu V, Socol G, Iordache F, Oprea AE, Anghel I, Holban AM (2014) MAPLE fabricated Fe3O4@Cinnamomum verum antimicrobial surfaces for improved gastrostomy tubes. Molecules 19:8981–8994

Anissimov YG (2014) Mathematical models for skin toxicology. Expert Opin Drug Metab Toxicol 10:551–560

Ansari MA, Khan HM, Khan AA, Sultan A, Azam A (2012) Characterization of clinical strains of MSSA, MRSA and MRSE isolated from skin and soft tissue infections and the antibacterial activity of ZnO nanoparticles. World J Microbiol Biotechnol 28:1605–1613

Beyth N, Houri-Haddad Y, Domb A, Khan W, Hazan R (2015) Alternative antimicrobial approach: nano-antimicrobial materials. Evid Based Complement Alternat Med 2015:246012

Bhowmick P, Pancsa R, Guharoy M, Tompa P (2013) Functional diversity and structural disorder in the human ubiquitination pathway. PLoS One 8:e65443

Blecher K, Nasir A, Friedman A (2011) The growing role of nanotechnology in combating infectious disease. Virulence 2:395–401

Boer M, Duchnik E, Maleszka R, Marchlewicz M (2016) Structural and biophysical characteristics of human skin in maintaining proper epidermal barrier function. Adv Dermatol Allergol XXXIII(1):1–5

Cardoso VS, Quelemes PV, Amorin A, Primo FL, Gobo GG, Tedesco AC, Mafud AC, Mascarenhas YP, Corrêa JR, Kuckelhaus SA, Eiras C, Leite JRS, Silva D, dos Santos Júnior JR (2014) Collagen-based silver nanoparticles for biological applications: synthesis and characterization. J Nanobiotechnol 12:36

Couto A, Fernandes R, Cordeiro MNS, Reis SS, Ribeiro RT, Pessoa AM (2014) Dermic diffusion and stratum corneum: A state of the art review of mathematical models. J Control Release 177:74–83

Crosera M, Prodi A, Mauro M, Pelin M, Florio C, Bellomo F, Adami G, Apostoli P, De Palma G, Bovenzi M, Campanini M, Filon F (2015) Titanium dioxide nanoparticle penetration into the skin and effects on HaCaT cells. Int J Environ Res Public Health 12:9282–9297

Dakal TC, Kumar A, Majumdar RS, Yadav V (2016) Mechanistic basis of antimicrobial actions of silver nanoparticles. Front Microbiol 7:1831

DeLouise LA (2012) Applications of nanotechnology in dermatology. J Invest Dermatol 132:964–975

Dhar S, Murawala P, Shiras A, Pokharkar V, Prasad BLV (2012) Gellan gum capped silver nanoparticle dispersions and hydrogels: cytotoxicity and in vitro diffusion studies. Nanoscale 4:563–567

Durmus NG, Taylor EN, Kummer KM, Webster TJ (2013) Enhanced efficacy of superparamagnetic iron oxide nanoparticles against antibiotic-resistant biofilms in the presence of metabolites. Adv Mater 25:5706–5713

Filipe P, Silva JN, Silva R, Cirne de Castro JL, Marques Gomes M, Alves LC, Santus R, Pinheiro
     T (2009) Stratum corneum is an effective barrier to TiO2 and ZnO nanoparticle percutaneous
     absorption. Skin Pharmacol Physiol 22:266–275
Filon FL, Crosera M, Adami G, Bovenzi M, Rossi F, Maina G (2011) Human skin penetration of
     gold nanoparticles through intact and damaged skin. Nanotoxicology 5:493–501
Gomathi Devi L, Nagaraj B (2014) Disinfection of Escherichia Coli gram negative Bacteria using
     surface modified TiO2: optimization of Ag metallization and depiction of charge transfer
     mechanism. Photochem Photobiol 90(5):1089–1098
Grigore M, Grumezescu A, Holban A, Mogoşanu G, Andronescu E (2017) Collagen-nanoparticles
     composites for wound healing and infection control. Metals 7:516
Gupta S, Gupta S, Jindal N, Jindal A, Bansal R (2013) Nanocarriers and nanoparticles for skin care
     and dermatological treatments. Indian Dermatol Online J 4:267
Guterres SS, Alves MP, Pohlmann AR (2007) Polymeric nanoparticles, nanospheres and nanocap-
     sules, for cutaneous applications. Drug Target Insights 2:147–157
Hamal DB, Haggstrom JA, Marchin GL, Ikenberry MA, Hohn K, Klabunde KJ (2010) A multi-
     functional biocide/sporocide and photocatalyst based on titanium dioxide (TiO$_2$) Codoped with
     silver, carbon, and sulfur. Langmuir 26:2805–2810
Hashim PW, Nia JK, Han G, Ratner D (2019) Nanoparticles in dermatologic surgery. J Am Acad
     Dermatol S0190-9622(19)30606-1
Herskovitz I, Macquhae F, Fox JD, Kirsner RS (2016) Skin movement, wound repair and develop-
     ment of engineered skin. Exp Dermatol 25:99–100
Huang Z, Zheng X, Yan D, Yin G, Liao X, Kang Y, Yao Y, Huang D, Hao B (2008) Toxicological
     effect of ZnO nanoparticles based on Bacteria. Langmuir 24:4140–4144
Huang Y, Yu F, Park Y-S, Wang J, Shin M-C, Chung HS, Yang VC (2010) Co-administration of pro-
     tein drugs with gold nanoparticles to enable percutaneous delivery. Biomaterials 31:9086–9091
Jaiswal M, Dudhe R, Sharma PK (2015) Nanoemulsion: an advanced mode of drug delivery sys-
     tem. 3 Biotech 5:123–127
Jin T, Sun D, Su JY, Zhang H, Sue H-J (2009) Antimicrobial efficacy of zinc oxide quantum dots
     against Listeria monocytogenes, Salmonella Enteritidis, and Escherichia coli O157:H7. J Food
     Sci 74:M46–M52
Kanitakis J (2002) Anatomy, histology and immunohistochemistry of normal human skin. Eur
     J Dermatol 12:390–399; quiz 400–401
Kolarsick PAJ, Kolarsick MA, Goodwin C (2011) Anatomy and physiology of the skin. J Dermatol
     Nurs Assoc 3:203–213
Kuotsu K, Karim K, Mandal A, Biswas N, Guha A, Chatterjee S, Behera M (2010) Niosome: a
     future of targeted drug delivery systems. J Adv Pharm Technol Res 1:374
Larese FF, D'Agostin F, Crosera M, Adami G, Renzi N, Bovenzi M, Maina G (2009) Human skin
     penetration of silver nanoparticles through intact and damaged skin. Toxicology 255:33–37
Lellouche J, Kahana E, Elias S, Gedanken A, Banin E (2009) Antibiofilm activity of nanosized
     magnesium fluoride. Biomaterials 30:5969–5978
Lellouche J, Friedman A, Lahmi R, Gedanken A, Banin E (2012) Antibiofilm surface function-
     alization of catheters by magnesium fluoride nanoparticles. Int J Nanomedicine 7:1175–1188
Leyva-Mendivil MF, Page A, Bressloff NW, Limbert G (2015) A mechanistic insight into the
     mechanical role of the stratum corneum during stretching and compression of the skin. J Mech
     Behav Biomed Mater 49:197–219
Limbert G (2017) Mathematical and computational modelling of skin biophysics: a review. Proc
     Math Phys Eng Sci 473:20170257
Liu Y, He L, Mustapha A, Li H, Hu ZQ, Lin M (2009) Antibacterial activities of zinc oxide
     nanoparticles against Escherichia coli O157:H7: antibacterial ZnO nanoparticles. J Appl
     Microbiol 107:1193–1201
Malka E, Perelshtein I, Lipovsky A, Shalom Y, Naparstek L, Perkas N, Patick T, Lubart R, Nitzan Y,
     Banin E, Gedanken A (2013) Eradication of multi-drug resistant bacteria by a novel Zn-doped
     CuO nanocomposite. Small 9:4069–4076

McGrath JA, Uitto J (2010) Anatomy and organization of human skin. In: Burns T, Breathnach S, Cox N, Griffiths C (eds) Rook's textbook of dermatology. Wiley-Blackwell, Oxford, pp 1–53

Mohandas A, Deepthi S, Biswas R, Jayakumar R (2018) Chitosan based metallic nanocomposite scaffolds as antimicrobial wound dressings. Bioact Mater 3:267–277

Monteiro-Riviere NA, Wiench K, Landsiedel R, Schulte S, Inman AO, Riviere JE (2011) Safety evaluation of sunscreen formulations containing titanium dioxide and zinc oxide nanoparticles in UVB sunburned skin: an in vitro and in vivo study. Toxicol Sci 123:264–280

Naraginti S, Kumari PL, Das RK, Sivakumar A, Patil SH, Andhalkar VV (2016) Amelioration of excision wounds by topical application of green synthesized, formulated silver and gold nanoparticles in albino Wistar rats. Mater Sci Eng C 62:293–300

Ng KW, Lau WM (2015) Skin deep: the basics of human skin structure and drug penetration. In: Dragicevic N, Maibach HI (eds) Percutaneous penetration enhancers chemical methods in penetration enhancement. Springer, Berlin, pp 3–11

Niska K, Zielinska E, Radomski MW, Inkielewicz-Stepniak I (2018) Metal nanoparticles in dermatology and cosmetology: interactions with human skin cells. Chem Biol Interact 295:38–51

Nizet V, Ohtake T, Lauth X, Trowbridge J, Rudisill J, Dorschner RA, Pestonjamasp V, Piraino J, Huttner K, Gallo RL (2001) Innate antimicrobial peptide protects the skin from invasive bacterial infection. Nature 414:454–457

Pan Z, Lee W, Slutsky L, Clark RAF, Pernodet N, Rafailovich MH (2009) Adverse effects of titanium dioxide nanoparticles on human dermal fibroblasts and how to protect cells. Small 5:511–520

Pandey P, Packiyaraj MS, Nigam H, Agarwal GS, Singh B, Patra MK (2014) Antimicrobial properties of CuO nanorods and multi-armed nanoparticles against B. anthracis vegetative cells and endospores. Beilstein J Nanotechnol 5:789–800

Pati R, Mehta RK, Mohanty S, Padhi A, Sengupta M, Vaseeharan B, Goswami C, Sonawane A (2014) Topical application of zinc oxide nanoparticles reduces bacterial skin infection in mice and exhibits antibacterial activity by inducing oxidative stress response and cell membrane disintegration in macrophages. Nanomedicine 10:1195–1208

Patrascu JM, Nedelcu IA, Sonmez M, Ficai D, Ficai A, Vasile BS, Ungureanu C, Albu MG, Andor B, Andronescu E, Rusu LC (2015) Composite scaffolds based on silver nanoparticles for biomedical applications. J Nanomater 2015:1–8

Pratap Reddy M, Venugopal A, Subrahmanyam M (2007) Hydroxyapatite-supported Ag–TiO2 as Escherichia coli disinfection photocatalyst. Water Res 41:379–386

Proksch E, Brandner JM, Jensen J-M (2008) The skin: an indispensable barrier. Exp Dermatol 17:1063–1072

Prost-Squarcioni C (2006) [Histology of skin and hair follicle]. Med Sci (Paris) 22:131–137

Qing Y, Cheng L, Li R, Liu G, Zhang Y, Tang X, Wang J, Liu H, Qin Y (2018) Potential antibacterial mechanism of silver nanoparticles and the optimization of orthopedic implants by advanced modification technologies. Int J Nanomedicine 13:3311–3327

Rajendran NK, Kumar SSD, Houreld NN, Abrahamse H (2018) A review on nanoparticle based treatment for wound healing. J Drug Delivery Sci Technol 44:421–430

Ren G, Hu D, Cheng EWC, Vargas-Reus MA, Reip P, Allaker RP (2009) Characterisation of copper oxide nanoparticles for antimicrobial applications. Int J Antimicrob Agents 33:587–590

Ruparelia JP, Chatterjee AK, Duttagupta SP, Mukherji S (2008) Strain specificity in antimicrobial activity of silver and copper nanoparticles. Acta Biomater 4:707–716

Sandri G, Miele D, Faccendini A, Bonferoni MC, Rossi S, Grisoli P, Taglietti A, Ruggeri M, Bruni G, Vigani B, Ferrari F (2019) Chitosan/glycosaminoglycan scaffolds: the role of silver nanoparticles to control microbial infections in wound healing. Polymers 11:1207

Schneider M, Stracke F, Hansen S, Schaefer UF (2009) Nanoparticles and their interactions with the dermal barrier. Dermatoendocrinol 1:197–206

Soenen SJ, Rivera-Gil P, Montenegro J-M, Parak WJ, De Smedt SC, Braeckmans K (2011) Cellular toxicity of inorganic nanoparticles: common aspects and guidelines for improved nanotoxicity evaluation. Nano Today 6:446–465

Sonavane G, Tomoda K, Makino K (2008) Biodistribution of colloidal gold nanoparticles after intravenous administration: effect of particle size. Colloids Surf B Biointerfaces 66:274–280

Spoiala A, Voicu G, Ficai D, Ungureanu C, Albu MG, Vasile BS, Ficai A, Andronescu E (2015) Collagen/TiO2-Ag composite nanomaterials for antimicrobial applications. UPB Sci Bull Ser B 77:275–290

Szmyd R, Goralczyk AG, Skalniak L, Cierniak A, Lipert B, Filon FL, Crosera M, Borowczyk J, Laczna E, Drukala J, Klein A, Jura J (2013) Effect of silver nanoparticles on human primary keratinocytes. Biol Chem 394:113

Takamiya AS, Monteiro DR, Bernabé DG, Gorup LF, Camargo ER, Gomes-Filho JE, Oliveira SHP, Barbosa DB (2016) In vitro and in vivo toxicity evaluation of colloidal silver nanoparticles used in endodontic treatments. J Endod 42:953–960

Taylor EN, Kummer KM, Durmus NG, Leuba K, Tarquinio KM, Webster TJ (2012) Superparamagnetic iron oxide nanoparticles (SPION) for the treatment of antibiotic-resistant biofilms. Small 8:3016–3027

Thakur K, Sharma G, Singh B, Chhibber S, Katare OP (2018) Current state of nanomedicines in the treatment of topical infectious disorders. Recent Pat Antiinfect Drug Discov 13:127–150

Tian J, Wong KKY, Ho C-M, Lok C-N, Yu W-Y, Che C-M, Chiu J-F, Tam PKH (2007) Topical delivery of silver nanoparticles promotes wound healing. ChemMedChem 2:129–136

Tran DT, Salmon R (2011) Potential photocarcinogenic effects of nanoparticle sunscreens: Photocarcinogenic and NP sunscreens. Australas J Dermatol 52:1–6

Vasanth SB, Kurian GA (2017) Toxicity evaluation of silver nanoparticles synthesized by chemical and green route in different experimental models. Artif Cells Nanomed Biotechnol 45:1721–1727

Wang C-C, Wang S, Xia Q, He W, Yin J-J, Fu PP, Li J-H (2013) Phototoxicity of zinc oxide nanoparticles in HaCaT keratinocytes-generation of oxidative DNA damage during UVA and visible light irradiation. J Nanosci Nanotechnol 13:3880–3888

Wei C, Lin WY, Zainal Z, Williams NE, Zhu K, Kruzic AP, Smith RL, Rajeshwar K (1994) Bactericidal activity of TiO2 photocatalyst in aqueous media: toward a solar-assisted water disinfection system. Environ Sci Technol 28:934–938

Zan L, Fa W, Peng T, Gong Z (2007) Photocatalysis effect of nanometer TiO2 and TiO2-coated ceramic plate on hepatitis B virus. J Photochem Photobiol B Biol 86:165–169

Zhang XF, Shen W, Gurunathan S (2016) Silver nanoparticle-mediated cellular responses in various cell lines: an in vitro model. Int J Mol Sci 17

Chapter 3
Combination Therapy Using Metal Nanoparticles for Skin Infections

Debalina Bhattacharya, Rituparna Saha, and Mainak Mukhopadhyay

Abstract Nowadays skin infections have emerged as a serious health problem worldwide. Over the years research has been conducted to develop new therapeutic agents for the treatment and prevention of various skin infections. Frequent use of conventional antibiotics and drugs increases multi-drug resistance. Therefore, it requires a continuous need for newer and more effective therapies. Nanotechnology is the most promising and novel area in the field of medicine for safe and targeted drug delivery to combat various skin infections. Nanomaterials especially metallic nanoparticles are increasingly utilized in dermatology and cosmetology due to their unique properties such as small size, shape, and high surface-area-to-volume ratio. Metallic nanoparticles have the ability to interact with the cell membrane and cell wall of the pathogens and can easily penetrate into the skin. Therefore, metal-based nanoparticles can effectively combine with conventional drugs to develop successful combination therapies. The aim of this chapter is to describe the combination therapy of metallic nanoparticles for the treatment of various skin infections.

Keywords Combination therapy · Dermatology · Nanomaterials · Metal nanoparticles · Skin infections

Nomenclature

AuNPs	Gold nanoparticles
BCCs	Basal cell carcinomas
CFU	Colony-forming unit
CL	Cutaneous leishmaniasis
CuO NPs	Copper oxide nanoparticles
EPR	Permeability and retention effect

D. Bhattacharya (✉)
Department of Microbiology, Maulana Azad College, Kolkata, West Bengal, India

R. Saha · M. Mukhopadhyay
Department of Biotechnology, JIS University, Kolkata, West Bengal, India

© Springer Nature Switzerland AG 2020
M. Rai (ed.), *Nanotechnology in Skin, Soft Tissue, and Bone Infections*,
https://doi.org/10.1007/978-3-030-35147-2_3

EPSD   Epidermal parasitic skin diseases
HSV   Herpes simplex virus
IDs   Infectious diseases
MDR   Multi-drug resistance
NMSC   Non-melanocytic skin cancer
NPs   Nanoparticles
NRs   Nanorod
ROS   Reactive oxygen species
SC   Stratum corneum
SPIONs   Superparamagnetic iron oxide nanoparticles
SSTIs   Skin structure infections
TiO$_2$ Titanium dioxide

3.1 Introduction

Infectious diseases (IDs) are caused by various types of microorganisms. It is one of the prime therapeutic challenges of this era because of the appearance of numerous new IDs and the revival of several old ones (Jones et al. 2008). In developing countries due to the resource-restricted conditions like poverty and subordinate livelihood, the right to use primary health care facilities has to put up with a burden of skin infections. The treatment of skin infectious diseases is hampered by drug resistance, indicating a serious need to develop a new approach for therapy which can overcome drug resistance. Nanotechnology has gained attention for the treatment of various IDs. Among all the nanoparticles, metal-based nanoparticles are the most promising agent to control IDs due to their unique physicochemical properties such as size, shape, solubility, and high surface-area-to-volume ratio (Kamaruzzaman et al. 2019). Due to their small size and shape, metal-based nanoparticles offer many advantages for pathogen detection and identification. Over the time metallic nanoparticles like silver, gold, zinc oxide, and titanium dioxide are gaining importance in antimicrobial formulations and dressings due to the production of reactive oxygen species (ROS) (Allaker and Ren 2008). The best part of using the metallic nanoparticles is that the microbes cannot produce resistance against them or they find it difficult to develop resistance against them without multiple mutations in their genetic materials (Betts et al. 2018). Therefore, to win the fight against multiple drug-resistant microbial species, the metallic nanoparticles are a huge helping hand and a very powerful tool to combat skin infections. The most common mechanisms through which metallic nanoparticles exhibit their microbiocidal activity involve (1) disruption of cell membrane (Xi and Bothun 2014), (2) perturbation of the metabolism such as purine metabolism (Sirelkhatim et al. 2015), (3) denaturation of microbial protein and DNA damage (Zhou et al. 2013), (4) disruption of respiratory chain (Choi et al. 2008), (5) induction of oxidative stress and free radical formation

(Pati et al. 2014), (6) mutations (Ahmad et al. 2012), and (7) inhibition of DNA replication by binding to DNA (Zhou et al. 2013). Through surface modification metal-based nanoparticles can be tailored with microbial surface markers, antibodies, toxins, nucleic acids, peptides, and enzymes for targeted drug delivery and better efficacy of the drugs over conventional formulations. Conjugation of drugs, antibodies and proteins onto metal nanoparticles allows sustained release of the drug, protects them against the body's immune system, and reduces the drug-induced side effects and drug adhesivity to the skin. Today nanotechnology combines with both standard and developing detection techniques, which gives us faster, more sensitive, and more economical diagnostic assays for the various skin infectious diseases.

Therefore, the aim of this chapter is to provide an in-depth look into the therapeutic uses of metallic nanoparticles with respect to skin infections. The various types and occurrence of skin infections are also discussed. Additionally, an outlook into the diverse range of metallic nanoparticles which plays a role against a wide range of microorganisms is also mentioned.

3.2 Skin Infections

Skin is known to be the chief protecting layer as well as the most exposed organ of the human body. It is composed of mainly three layers, i.e., epidermis, dermis, and hypodermis with many appendages, such as hair follicles, sweat glands, and sebaceous glands. The epidermis layer, mainly the stratum corneum (SC) acts as a barrier to protect our body from infections. Skin infections are a reason for concern due to their increasing number of cases all over the world. There are many factors involved with skin infections such as environmental conditions, the host's immune system, the type of the pathogens and its pathogenicity, etc. The skin acts as a host for various types of microflora and they can be categorized into two groups, resident flora and transient flora. Resident floras securely adhere to the skin. They are present in stable numbers and are able to tolerate an acidic environment. Transient floras are the opportunistic pathogens which come from the environment and only attach if the skin is damaged or broken (Fredricks 2001). The most common transient bacteria on the skin that causes infection are *Group A Streptococcus* (GAS, *Streptococcus pyogenes*) and *Staphylococcus aureus* (Chiller et al. 2001). Skin structure infections (SSTIs) are also referred to as skin and soft tissue infections, which indicate a group of infections that are different in their clinical symptoms and degree of severity; and are broadly classified into two categories: purulent infections (e.g., furuncles, carbuncles, abscesses) and nonpurulent infections (e.g., erysipelas, cellulitis, necrotizing fasciitis). Symptoms of these infections can vary from mild to serious; mild infections may be treatable with counter medications and home remedies, whereas moderate to severe infections may require medical attention and sometimes it may be life-threatening. The host's immune system also has a crucial role in skin infections. If the host has low immunity conditions, then there are clinical signs of deeper infection, or infection that fails to improve with incision and drainage (I&D) and oral antibiotics are also administered in severe cases. Antimicrobial treatments are often designed based on host characteristics, most likely pathogens, and local susceptibility patterns and if the causative organisms are isolated, microbiology culture and sensitivity is also studied (Stevens et al. 2014).

3.3 Types of Skin Infections

Skin infections are caused by an array of microorganisms such as bacteria, fungi, viruses, parasites, etc. The four types of skin infections which occur in our body are summarized below.

3.3.1 Bacterial Skin Infections

Our skin acts as a host of both pathogenic and symbiotic (non-pathogenic) bacteria. Pathogenic bacteria try to invade the skin, whereas the commensal bacteria work for the defense of the host skin from other pathogenic bacteria. Most common Gram-positive microflora on the skin includes *Staphylococcus*, *Micrococcus*, and *Corynebacterium* sp., but severe skin infections are caused by *S. aureus* and *S. pyogenes*. These pathogenic bacteria possess adherence property as well as some virulence genes. Their ability to adhere to host cells results in their colonization, and the development of various molecular strategies enhances their adhesion to the host cells (Abeylath and Turos 2008). Nowadays, bacterial infections can be treated very simply with a variety of antibiotics, whereas some of the bacteria are resistant to many drugs resulting in a worldwide public health threat. The major bacterial skin infections caused by *S. aureus* or a variant of *Streptococcus* (the same bacteria responsible for strep throat) are as follows:

1. Epidermal infections: impetigo and ecthyma
2. Dermal infections: erysipelas, cellulitis, and necrotizing fasciitis
3. Follicular infections (boils): folliculitis, furunculosis, and carbunculosis

Furthermore, the bacterial toxins can also evoke the super antigen response, which causes mass production of cytokines. The super antigens trigger toxic shocks, staphylococcal scalded skin syndrome, and scarlet fever. Reports indicate that Gram-negative bacteria such as *Acinetobacter* sp., *Pseudomonas aeruginosa*, *Pasteurella multocida*, *Capnocytophaga canimorsus*, *Bartonella* sp., *Klebsiella rhinoscleromatis*, and *Vibrio vulnificus* may also cause skin infections (Bassetti et al. 2019).

3.3.2 Fungal Skin Infections

Like bacteria, there are some fungi that live naturally within the body. When some harmful fungi also invade the human body, then fungal (cutaneous or superficial mycoses) infections or mycoses occur (Valderrama-Beltrán et al. 2019). These types of skin infections are most likely to develop in moist areas of the body such as the feet or armpit. Some fungal infections are not contagious and non-life-threatening. These fungi harbor on SC and do not penetrate deeply but sometimes harmful fungi are difficult to kill as they can survive in the environment and re-infect the person. These recurrent infections are very hard to handle for the immune system of the human body. Different types of fungal infections which occur in our body are as follows:

3.3.2.1 Athlete's Foot or *Tinea pedis*

Athlete's foot is a most common fungal infection caused by a dermatophyte *Trichophyton rubrum*, causes peeling, redness, itching, burning, and sometimes blisters and sores. The fungus will grow in warm and moist environmental conditions such as shoes, socks, swimming pools, sports equipment, the floors of a public toilet, etc. Persons wearing tight shoes or sweaty socks are more susceptible to these infections (Kang and Lipner 2019).

3.3.2.2 Jock Itch or *Tinea cruris*

Tinea cruris, commonly known as jock itch, is another common fungal skin infection caused by a dermatophyte. These fungi also love to grow in moist areas of the body, such as the groin, buttocks, and inner thighs. Jock itch appears on the body as an itchy, red rash that often appears as circular in shape (El-Gohary et al. 2014).

3.3.2.3 Ringworm or *Tinea corporis*

Tinea corporis or ringworm is a superficial fungal infection caused by dermato-phytes. These fungi live on the dead tissues of the skin, scalp (*Tinea capitis*), nails, hand (*Tinea manuum*), and beard areas (*Tinea barbae*). Ringworm is caused by the same fungus that causes both jock itch and athlete's foot. It can appear anywhere in the body and is highly contagious. Any type of itchy or scaly red patch can often turn into a slightly raised, ring-shaped patch of skin very swiftly. The fungus that causes ringworm can linger on surfaces, clothes, towels, in combs and brushes (Khurana et al. 2019).

3.3.2.4   Yeast Infections

Yeast infections of the skin are called cutaneous candidiasis and the causative agent is yeast-like fungi called *Candida*. Although not overtly contagious, they often occur on the skin where yeast grows more actively and leads to a red, scaly and itchy rash. *Candida* can cause diaper rash in infants and in the nail known as *Tinea unguium*. Another form of *Candida* infection is the oral thrush which occurs in the mouth (Kühbacher et al. 2017).

3.3.3   Viral Skin Infections

Viral skin infections mostly generate localized or dispersed lesions and range from mild to severe. Superficial viral infection outbreaks have been reported among athletes (college wrestlers, rugby players) and in daycares or schools. Based on clinical symptoms, the viral infections are classified into several types:

3.3.3.1   Herpes Simplex Virus (HSV)

Herpes simplex viruses are categorized into two types: herpes type 1 (HSV-1, or oral herpes) and herpes type 2 (HSV-2, or genital herpes). Most commonly, HSV-1 causes sores around the mouth and lips (sometimes called fever blisters or cold sores). HSV-2 causes genital herpes, where the infected person may have sores around the genitals or rectum (Whitley and Baines 2018).

3.3.3.2   Chickenpox (Varicella zoster)

Chickenpox or varicella zoster is a very common viral skin infections in childhood caused by the Varicella zoster virus. Symptoms include itchy, red, bumpy rashes throughout the body. The chickenpox virus is a highly infective contagion for those who are not immunized to it.

3.3.3.3   Shingle (Herpes zoster)

Shingle is an infection caused by the Varicella zoster virus, which is the same virus that causes chickenpox in childhood. This infection is highly contagious. A red skin rash that can cause pain and burning characterizes shingle. Shingle usually appear as a stripe of blisters on one side of the body, typically on the torso, neck, or face.

3.3.3.4   Molluscum Contagiosum

It is a skin infection caused by the virus *Molluscum contagiosum*. It produces benign raised bumps or lesions on the upper layers of the skin of children.

3.3.3.5   Measles and Rubella

Measles is a highly infectious illness caused by the rubeola virus in children. German measles, also known as rubella, is a viral skin infection in children that causes a red rash on the body and swollen lymph nodes.

3.3.3.6   Hand-Foot-and-Mouth Disease

Hand-foot-and-mouth disease is a mild and contagious viral infection. It is characterized by fever, sores in the mouth, and a rash on the hands and feet of young children. Hand-foot-and-mouth disease is most commonly caused by coxsackievirus (A and B) (Kimmis et al. 2018).

3.3.3.7   Roseola

Roseola infantum is a viral skin infection of infants or very young children that causes a high fever followed by a pinkish macular rash. It is caused by human herpes simplex 6 viruses.

3.3.3.8   Warts

Warts are benign (not cancerous) skin growths that appear when human papilloma virus (HPV) infects the top layer of the skin. Warts are highly contagious. There are five major types of warts affected on the hand, feet, fingernails, and toes. They are common warts, plantar warts, flat warts, filiform warts, and periungual warts (Clebak and Malone 2018).

3.3.4   Parasitic Infections

These types of skin infections are caused by a parasite in which parasite–host interactions are confined to the upper layer of the skin. So these infections are also known as epidermal parasitic skin diseases (EPSD) (Feldmeier and Heukelbach 2009). The six major EPSD are scabies, pediculosis (capitis, corporis, and pubis), tungiasis (sand flea disease) and hookworm-related cutaneous larva migrans.

3.4   Metal and Metal Oxide Nanoparticles on Skin Infections

Metal-based nanoparticles that have been reported with microbicidal activity against skin infectious diseases include silver, gold, copper, copper oxide, iron oxide, titanium dioxide, and zinc oxide, which are illustrated in Fig. 3.1.

3.4.1   Silver Nanoparticles (AgNPs)

Among metal and metal oxide nanoparticles, silver remains the most extensively studied nanoparticles due to its exhibition of remarkable antimicrobial activity. Silver has gained importance from ancient times due to its strong antimicrobial properties and is used in the treatment of burn wound, food additives, clothing, cosmetics, jewelry, contact lens cases, disinfectants, ointments, dental products, catheters, and antibacterial coatings in the forms of metallic silver, silver nitrate, and silver sulfadiazine (Dibrov et al. 2002). The Ag^+ ions released from textiles and wound dressings can interact with the skin and penetrate into it. Larese and coworkers demonstrated in vitro skin penetration of AgNPs of 25 nm through intact and damaged human skin using static diffusion cells (Larese et al. 2009). TEM (Transmission Electron Microscopy) images confirmed the presence of AgNPs into the stratum corneum (SC), the outermost surface of the epidermis but not inside the dermal layer. These results suggest that a fraction of the NPs were dissolved and

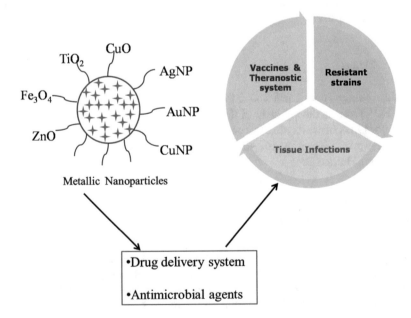

Fig. 3.1 Application of metallic nanoparticles in skin infectious disease

diffused through the skin layers as elemental Ag. Different forms of silver nanoparticles have proven to be effective against different bacteria, viruses, and fungi (Bhattacharya et al. 2012; Kaushik et al. 2010; Marin et al. 2015). Silver nanoparticles have shown antimicrobial property against drug-resistant pathogens such *as Vibrio cholerae* O1, *Shigella flexneri* (IDH00177 and IDH00178) (Bhattacharya et al. 2012), *Klebsiella pneumoniae, erythromycin-resistant Streptococcus pyogenes*, MRSA (Ruparelia et al. 2008), onychomycosis (Ouf et al. 2015), trichophyton (Rezaie and Shahverdi 2011), dermal leishmaniasis (Allahverdiyev et al. 2011), *Proteus vulgaris, Salmonella typhimurium* (Kędziora et al. 2018), etc. The multi-drug-resistant bacteria show sensitivity to silver nanoparticles at concentrations as low as 20 µg/mL (Nakamura et al. 2019).

3.4.2 Gold Nanoparticles (AuNPs)

Gold nanoparticles (AuNPs) have been widely used in recent years for visualization of cells and in many other scientific purposes. Their uses have gained recognition due to their relatively small size and versatile preparation procedures to the good contrasting capability for electron microscope (Azubel et al. 2014). Many experiments are also carried out for studying the dermal penetration of the AuNPs. One study has reported that AuNPs of different sizes (22 nm, 105 nm, and 186 nm) penetrate the thick skin of the hind paw of the rat. The researchers observed that the AuNPs of the smallest size (22 nm) have higher epidermal penetration as compared to the 105 and 186 nm particles. Studies confirm that nanoparticles can circulate in the blood, and histological analysis revealed that AuNPs in epidermal layers just below the SC have no tissue toxicity (Raju et al. 2018). Gold nanoparticles are used as an excellent intracellular targeting vector for the following reasons:

1. They can be readily converted to a suitable size from 0.8 to 200 nm.
2. Their surface can be altered to communicate various functionalities and good biocompatibility.
3. They possess visible light extinction property, which is applied as a nanoparticle tracking system inside the cells. AuNPs allow long-wavelength light directed tumor photothermolysis and may allow deeper targeting of cutaneous tumors (Nasir 2010).

AuNPs are stable in the body (Niidome et al. 2006) and so they have been largely used to study the tissue distribution, following administration through different routes (Cho et al. 2009; Balasubramanian et al. 2010). AuNPs are nontoxic to skin cells, but depending on the size, shape, and coating materials, AuNPs will exert toxicity. In another study, Payne et al. (2016) evaluated the antibacterial activities of kanamycin and AuNP-kanamycin conjugates against the Gram-positive *Staphylococcus epidermidis* and the Gram-negative *Enterobacter aerogenes*, and concluded that the minimum inhibitory concentration of the conjugate was significantly lower than that of free kanamycin (Payne et al. 2016).

3.4.3 Copper Nanoparticles (CuNPs)

Copper has been utilized for decades especially for its antifungal and antibacterial properties, although its antimicrobial activity is less studied. The activity of copper nanoparticles (CuNPs) loaded polymer thin films which uniformly release copper has been demonstrated against *S. cerevisiae*, molds, and bacteria, including *E. coli*, *S. aureus*, and *Listeria monocytogenes*. When tests were conducted, it was seen that copper nanocomposites resulted in lower counts of colony-forming units (CFUs), and this effect was clarified with *S. cerevisiae* because no CFUs were observed. Reports demonstrated that the higher the CuNP loading, the lower the number of CFUs was found, showing a biostatic effect (Cioffi et al. 2005). In another study, Usman et al. demonstrated the antifungal activity of CuNPs against *Candida albicans* (Usman et al. 2013). Additionally, they found that CuNPs inhibited the growth of *methicillin-resistant S. aureus*, *B. subtilis*, *P. aeruginosa*, and *Salmonella choleraesuis*. Due to this research, CuNPs are currently used as additives for medical textiles: cotton fabric in socks, t-shirts, work wear, etc.

3.4.4 Copper Oxide Nanoparticles (CuO NPs)

Copper oxide nanoparticles (CuO NPs) are widely used as an antimicrobial agent and industrial materials. The antimicrobial properties of CuO NPs have been evaluated in many species, including *E. coli*, *B. subtilis*, *P. aeruginosa*, and *S. aureus* (Ahamed et al. 2014; Hu et al. 2009; Das et al. 2013). CuO NPs also show remarkable broad-spectrum antimicrobial activity against pathogenic bacteria. It is believed that the toxicity of CuO NPs is not solely due to the release of Cu^{2+} ions (Wang et al. 2013) but also depends on the size (Gilbertson et al. 2016) and surface coatings (Das et al. 2013). Using green synthesis Sutradhar et al. (2014) synthesized CuO NPs with a size range of 50–100 nm. These nanoparticles have shown antimicrobial activity against pathogens such as *K. pneumoniae*, *S. dysenteriae*, and *V. cholerae*. In another report, it was (Azam et al. 2012) found that small CuO NPs around 20 nm have significantly stronger antibacterial activities against Gram-positive *B. subtilis* and *S. aureus*, and Gram-negative *E. coli* and *P. aeruginosa*. It was also found that CuO nanosheets have better antimicrobial activity against *E. coli* K12 than CuO nanopowders (Gilbertson et al. 2016). Some studies described that the release of Cu^{2+}ions from CuO NPs which generates ROS and DNA damage gives the antimicrobial property (Gilbertson et al. 2016; Azam et al. 2012). But, other studies argue that the amount of Cu^{2+} ions released from CuO NPs is not competent enough and contributes less to the antibacterial activity of the NPs (Applerot et al. 2012). It was further shown that ROS generation was not due to the Cu^{2+} ions but due to its nano form. CuO NPs also bind to $-SH$ groups of proteins causing the modification of proteins or their denaturation and inhibit bacterial enzyme synthesis (Hermida-Montero et al. 2019).

3.4.5 Titanium Oxide Nanoparticles (TiO₂ NPs) and Zinc Oxide Nanoparticles (ZnO NPs)

Titanium dioxide (TiO_2) or zinc oxide (ZnO) NPs are widely used in modern personal care products, particularly in sunscreens and cosmetics due to their high photostability and low photoallergic potentials. It is well reported that TiO_2 and ZnO NPs can easily penetrate from the skin outermost barrier SC to the dermis. TiO_2 undergoes photocatalysis forming active oxygen species when exposed to UV light. The resulting oxygen species, i.e., hydrogen peroxide and hydroxyl radicals, destroy bacterial cell membranes (Gerrity et al. 2008; Kim et al. 2003). The compatibility of ZnO with human skin makes it a suitable additive for textiles and surfaces that come in contact with the human body (Nohynek et al. 2008; Cross et al. 2007). The antibacterial effect of ZnO NPs has been observed on Gram-positive and Gram-negative bacteria as well as the thermostable spores which are resistant to high temperature and high pressure (Jones et al. 2008; Liu et al. 2009). ZnO NPs are normally opaque, greasy and have an elegant feel on the skin when applied (Nasir 2010). Nanometer-sized emulsions are less oily, have a better texture and penetrate skin and hair more deeply when incorporated into emollients and hair conditioners. The shape of the ZnO NPs is also very important in terms of skin penetration. Studies have demonstrated that spherical shaped ZnO NPs were nontoxic to human cells and can be easily applied in sunscreen, antibacterial ointment, and cosmetic industries (Bhattacharya et al. 2014). Multiple layers of nano-ZnO deposited on cotton fabrics act as a good antibacterial agent against *S. aureus* (Ugur et al. 2010). ZnO NPs act through the breakdown of proteins and lipids of the bacterial cell wall that causes cell lysis, ultimately leading to bacterial cell death (Liu et al. 2009; Chandra et al. 2019).

3.5 Human Skin Penetration of Metallic Nanoparticles

The skin is the most exposed part of the external environment; the ill effects of radiation and UV rays (Hadgraft 2001) readily affect it. The systemic treatment for dermatological problems is a cause of concern because it comes with its potential adverse effects. Therefore, topical application is the favored mode due to higher patient acquiescence and satisfaction. The skin is also impermeable to the drugs due to epidermal cell cohesion and stratum corneum lipids. Nanoparticle dimensions are considered as the most important parameter because chemical penetration into the skin can occur through pilosebaceous pores (diameter: 10–70 μm) (Lauer et al. 1996), sweat gland pores (diameter: 60–80 μm) and most commonly through the lipidic matrix that fills a gap of 75 nm, in air-dried conditions (Johnson et al. 1997) between the SC dead corneocytes, cementing them (Fig. 3.2). By comparing the dimensions of skin openings and possible routes of the entrance with nanoparticle sizes, it was hypothesized that individual nanoparticles might be small enough to

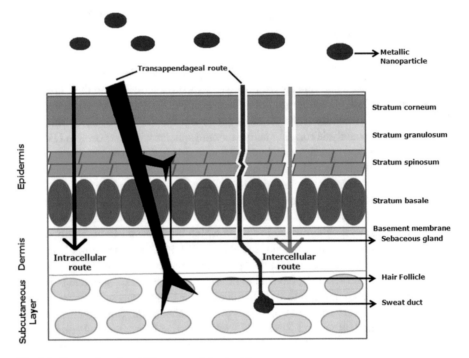

Fig. 3.2 Penetration of metallic nanoparticles in skin

potentially penetrate into the skin. However, the extent of penetration as well as the route of the entrance was considered to depend strongly on all the interactions that could occur between nanoparticles and skin structures. Moreover, the penetration of nanoparticles whose dimensions are compatible with skin absorption routes might be further influenced by their superficial charges.

Nanotechnology plays a promising role to transform the diagnosis and treatment of dermatological conditions because of its interaction at the sub-atomic level with the skin tissue. By controlling the release of active substances and increasing the period of skin permeability, nanotechnology can be used to modify drug permeation/penetration (Hadgraft 2001). Besides ensuring direct contact with the SC and skin appendages (Guterres et al. 2007), metallic nanoparticles protect the drug against chemical or physical instability. Further, the delivery of therapeutic agents without chemical enhancers is required to maintain the normal skin barrier function. Treatment with surfactants and organic solvents which are chemical enhancers causes a reduction in the barrier function of the skin and leads to skin irritation and damage (Lademann et al. 2007; Crissey 1998). Nano-structured carriers are a futuristic option for drug delivery due to their advantages over the typical preparations. The colloidal particulate systems with size ranging from 10 to 1000 nm offer targeted drug delivery, sustained release, protection of labile groups from degradation, less toxic and drug adherences to the skin (Gao and Zhang 2015).

3.6 Combined Therapy of Metallic Nanoparticles in Bacterial Skin Infections

Bacterial skin infections have been a major concern for the medical treatment process. Antibiotic therapy plays an important role in fighting against infections. Nowadays, rising incidents of multi-drug-resistant bacterial strains mediated infections have drawn worldwide attention (Pati et al. 2014). In recent studies, it was reported that metal oxide nanoparticles such as TiO_2 and ZnO NPs are widely used in different fields of textiles and cosmetics and the antibacterial activity of zinc oxide ceramic nanopowder is taken into account (Nair et al. 2008; Hanley et al. 2008; Le Lay et al. 2008; Thevenot et al. 2008). The metal oxide nanoparticles are used widely due to their stable conformations and high safety standards over the organic antimicrobial agents (Anagnostakos et al. 2008). Studies suggest that the production of hydrogen peroxide is responsible for bacterial cell death (Sawai et al. 1996, 1997, 1998), whereas another researcher proposed that the electrostatic force occurring due to the binding of the ZnO NPs to the bacterial cell surface causes the death of the bacteria (Pal et al. 2007). Naturally occurring antibacterial substances, carbon-based nanomaterials, and surfactant-based nanoemulsions are the antibacterial nanoparticles (Niska et al. 2018). The large ratios between the surface area to volume and unique physicochemical attributes of nanomaterials are the reasons for their operative antimicrobial property. In recent studies, it is proposed that the naturally occurring bacterial species are not resistant to the metal nanoparticles (Khan et al. 2016). The mode of action of the metal nanoparticles consists of various processes, which are as follows:

1. Production of ROS by photocatalysis, damaging the cellular components of the pathogens
2. Increases the vulnerability of the bacterial cell wall/membrane
3. Cessation of energy transfer
4. Retardation of enzyme and DNA synthesis

3.7 Combined Therapy of Metallic Nanoparticles in Fungal Skin Infections

Dandruff is a well-known scalp problem caused by the growth of fungus *Malassezia furfur*, potentially cascading into dermal inflammation, itching, and tissue damage. Reports have outlined a detailed analysis into the treatment of scalp infection using silver nanomaterials (Ag NMs) that focuses on the biocidal activity with reference to manipulation of size, shape, and structure (Anwar et al. 2016). Monodisperse silver spherical nanoparticles (NPs) and nanorods (NRs) have also demonstrated an enhanced biocidal activity by showing greater zones of inhibition against the fungus, in comparison to the drugs like itraconazole and ketoconazole that are available in the market. Biosynthesized AgNPs and AuNPs have shown antifungal activity against opportunistic pathogenic yeast and dermatophytes. AgNPs were able to inhibit the growth of several opportunistic *Candida* or *Cryptococcus* sp. and were highly potent against filamentous *Microsporum* and *Trichophyton dermatophytes*, whereas AuNPs exert bactericidal activity only against *Cryptococcus neoformans* (Anwar et al. 2016). Though many antibacterial studies have been carried out on the metal or metal oxide nanoparticles, very limited study about the antifungal properties of the metallic nanoparticles is available. In one study, Sawai et al. demonstrated that ZnO nanopowder shows a very weak antifungal activity against *Candida albicans*. However, the growth inhibition and conductivity changes were observed only at a concentration above 100 mg/mL. As a result, ZnO nanopowder lost authenticity for its influence on fungal population (Sawai et al. 1997). Gomes et al. examined ZnO with calcium hydroxide plus 2% chlorhexidine and treated microbial infections at the external tooth root surface but could not achieve successful results (Gomes et al. 2009). Research has demonstrated the desirable results, where ZnO in a "whisker" form was reported to retard the growth of *C. albicans* (Fang et al. 2006). Due to its antimicrobial properties, ZnO powder has been used for a long time as an active ingredient for dermatological applications in creams, lotions, and ointments (Sawai et al. 1998). In another study, Tiwari et al. has observed that ZnO NPs combined with petal extract of Rosa *indica* L. (rose) have strong antifungal activity against two dermatophytes, namely *Trichophyton mentagrophytes* and *Microsporum canis*, which cause onychomycosis infection (Tiwari et al. 2017).

3.8 Combined Therapy of Metallic Nanoparticles in Viral Skin Infections

Virucidal nanoparticles and drug delivery models have been focused mainly for the fight against human immunodeficiency virus (HIV), hepatitis (type A, B, C, and E), influenza virus, and HSV-1 and -2. The use of nanoparticles for virucidal outcomes is still under investigation and has not been approved for clinical or pre-clinical trials. The ELISA for detecting HIV/AIDS virus with the help of AuNPs is performed most easily by observing the color change of the AuNPs attached to the HIV/AIDS virus sample. Magnetic nanoparticles and colloidal AuNPs are a breakthrough in the detection of HSV. Recent advances in nanotechnology have developed metal oxide nanostructured compounds that have a binding affinity towards viral glycoproteins. Several metal-based nanoparticles have shown antiviral properties such as ZnO (Antoine et al. 2012), tin oxides (SnO) (Trigilio et al. 2012), and AuNPs capped with mercaptoethane sulfonate (Au-MES) (Baram-Pinto et al. 2010). The use of ZnO tetrapods with prophylactic, therapeutic, and virostatic potential has been shown against both HSV-1 (Antoine et al. 2012) and HSV-2 (Mishra et al. 2011). The combined effect of the above metal and metal oxides NPs will initiate improved viral clearance and effective antiviral activity.

3.9 Combined Therapy of Metal Nanoparticles in Parasitic Skin Infections

Scientists use colloidal drug vehicles such as emulsions, liposomes, and nanoparticles for parasitic skin infections because of their polyvalent behavior and alluring benefits. Their different abilities and versatility attract the attention of various researchers and their uses are being revised widely (Niska et al. 2018). The most studied colloidal carrier particle is the liposome. They are microscopic vacuoles containing one or more spheres having a common center of lipid bilayer separated by aqueous or buffer compartments. This spherical colloidal carrier particle can have diameters ranging from 80 to 100 μm (Sharma and Sharma 1997). Cutaneous leishmaniasis (CL) was one of the first studied parasitic infections by objecting the macrophages by liposomes (Owais and Gupta 2005).

3.10 Nanoparticles and Skin Cancers

Skin cancers are the most common malignancy of humans, particularly in the white population with UV being the main contributing factor responsible for skin cancer development. Skin cancers are broadly classified into three types with basal cell carcinomas (BCCs) and squamous cell carcinomas (SCCs) (both referred as non-melanocytic skin cancer—NMSC) and cutaneous malignant melanomas (CMs) (also referred to malignant melanoma of the skin or melanoma). One of the most aggressive skin cancers is multi-drug resistant (MDR) melanoma, which has originated from the malignant transformations of melanocytes, and have a low survival rate and is easy to relapse.

The metallic nanoparticles can be used as a powerful tool for selectively targeting the cancer cells due to the preferred delivery of drugs to tumors enhancing the permeability and retention effect (EPR), minimizing toxicity, increasing the circulation in tissue, etc. The metallic nanoparticles such as Au, Ag, Ni, and TiO_2 are widely used as an anticancer agent. Moreover, TiO_2 and ZnO NPs may be used as skin protectors (Raj et al. 2012). Among all the metallic nanoparticles, AuNPs are widely used for the treatment of cancers. AuNPs conjugated with several molecules including small drugs, proteins, and DNA were found to be effective against more than a few types of tumors including melanoma. Moreover, the metallic nanoparticle conjugated with biodegradable polymer helps in diffusion of hydrophobic drugs by modifying their pharmacological aspects and increases the drug half-life by reducing immunogenicity, improves bioavailability and reduces the metabolic rate of the drug (Hainfeld et al. 2007; Pan et al. 2007). Another metallic nanoparticle used for destroying melanoma cells is super paramagnetic iron oxide nanoparticles (SPIONs). SPIONs can convert the energy supplied by an externally applied alternating magnetic field into heat (Johannsen et al. 2007). This generated heat can be used for the selective destruction of tumor cells, which are more vulnerable to heating than normal body cells (Johannsen et al. 2007; Huang et al. 2011).

3.11 Conclusions and Future Perspectives

Our skin is the main barrier of our body, so it is affected by different kinds of bacterial, fungal, parasitic, and viral infections. The infection critically affects the skin, causes severe damages to it and due to skin invasion, the pathogens enter the bloodstream and affect the whole body. To overcome these infections, mostly antibiotics are used, but due to increased cases of multiple drug resistance, these pathogens are kept unhurt. Therefore, here comes the use of nanotechnology especially metals and metal oxides nanoparticles because the microbes are not able to develop drug resistance against them and it acts as an advantage for the fight against the pathogens. The metallic nanoparticles are small and due to their flexible formulations and stability, they can be widely used for selective drug delivery. In the treatment of cancer, the metallic nanoparticles are used to deliver therapeutic agents in different dosages and they have overcome the barriers of non-solubility of the drugs into the cancerous cells. The imaging and drug delivery are now easier by the use of metallic nanoparticles and they cause less or no harm to the healthy cells. Due to all these potential advantages, the metallic nanoparticles are a noble tool for combating skin infections as well as skin cancer-related difficulties.

The growing interest in studying and developing nanoparticle-enabled drug delivery has resulted in the improvement of several diagnostic and therapeutic functions in disease management. This has proved to be a blessing in disguise for personalized health issues. But the unintended rise in the effects of nanomedicine in the form of particle–particle interactions, allergens, irritants, and toxicity has led to diseases. Extensive studies are required to identify the different safety issues related to the nanomaterials that are released in the market for consumption. Hence, it is critical to evaluate and understand this technology for its constructive use. Therefore, more efficient, target-based as well as cost-effective nanomedicine is necessary for better future disease management.

References

Abeylath SC, Turos E (2008) Drug delivery approaches to overcome bacterial resistance to beta-lactam antibiotics. Expert Opin Drug Deliv 5:931–949

Ahamed M, Alhadlaq HA, Khan M, Karuppiah P, Al-Dhabi NA (2014) Synthesis, characterization, and antimicrobial activity of copper oxide nanoparticles. J Nanomater 2014:637858. https://doi.org/10.1155/2014/637858

Ahmad J, Dwivedi S, Alarifi S, Al-Khedhairy AA, Musarrat J (2012) Use of-galactosidase (lacZ) gene-complementation as a novel approach for assessment of titanium oxide nanoparticles induced mutagenesis. Mutat Res 747:246–252

Allahverdiyev AM, Abamor ES, Bagirova M, Rafailovich M (2011) Antimicrobial effects of TiO(2) and Ag(2)O nanoparticles against drug-resistant bacteria and leishmania parasites. Future Microbiol 6:933–940

Allaker RP, Ren G (2008) Potential impact of nanotechnology on the control of infectious disease. Trans R Soc Trop Med Hyg 102:1–2

Anagnostakos K, Hitzler P, Pape D, Kohn D, Kelm J (2008) Persistence of bacterial growth on antibiotic-loaded beads—is it actually a problem? Acta Orthop 79:302–307

Antoine TE, Mishra YK, Trigilio J, Tiwari V, Adelung R, Shukla DP (2012) Therapeutic and neutralizing effects of zinc oxide tetrapod structures against herpes simplex virus type-2 infection. Antiviral Res 96:363

Anwar MF, Yadav D, Jain S, Kapoor S, Rastogi S, Arora I, Samim M (2016) Size- and shape-dependent clinical and mycological efficacy of silver nanoparticles on dandruff. Int J Nanomedicine 6:147–161

Applerot G, Lellouche J, Lipovsky A, Nitzan Y, Lubart R, Gedanken A, Banin E (2012) Understanding the antibacterial mechanism of CuO nanoparticles: revealing the route of induced oxidative stress. Small 8:3326–3337

Azam A, Ahmed AS, Oves M, Khan MS, Memic A (2012) Size-dependent antimicrobial properties of CuO nanoparticles against Gram positive and -negative bacterial strains. Small 8:3326–3337

Azubel M, Koivisto J, Malola S, Bushnell D, Hura GL, Koh AL, Tsunoyama H, Tsukuda T, Pettersson M, Häkkinen H, Kornberg RD (2014) Electron microscopy of gold nanoparticles at atomic resolution. Science 345:909–912

Balasubramanian SK, Jittiwat J, Manikandan J, Ong CN, Yu LE, Ong WY (2010) Biodistribution of gold nanoparticles and gene expression changes in the liver and spleen after intravenous administration in rats. Biomaterials 31(8):2034–2042

Baram-Pinto D, Shukla S, Gedanken A, Sarid R (2010) Inhibition of HSV-1 attachment, entry, and cell-to-cell spread by functionalized multivalent gold nanoparticles. Small 6:1044

Bassetti M, Castaldo N, Carnelutti A, Peghin M, Giacobbe DR (2019) Tedizolid phosphate for the treatment of acute bacterial skin and skin-structure infections: an evidence-based review of its place in therapy. Core Evid 14:31–40

Betts JW, Hornsey M, La Ragione RM (2018) Novel antibacterials: alternatives to traditional antibiotics. Adv Microb Physiol 73:123–169

Bhattacharya D, Samanta S, Mukherjee A, Santra CR, Ghosh AN, Neyogi SK, Karmakar P (2012) Antibacterial activities of poly ethylene glycol, tween 80 and sodium dodecyl sulphate coated silver nanoparticles in normal and multi-drug resistant bacteria. J Nano Sci Nanotechnol 12:1–9

Bhattacharya D, Santra CR, Ghosh AN, Karmakar P (2014) Differential toxicity of rod and spherical zinc oxide nanoparticles on human peripheral blood mononuclear cells. J Biomed Nanotechnol 10:707–716

Chandra H, Patel D, Kumari P, Jangwan JS, Yadav S (2019) Phyto-mediated synthesis of zinc oxide nanoparticles of Berberisaristata: characterization, antioxidant activity and antibacterial activity with special reference to urinary tract pathogens. Korean J Couns Psychother 102:212–220

Chiller K, Selkin BA, Murakawa GJ (2001) Skin microflora and bacterial infections of the skin. J Investig Dermatol Symp Proc 6:170–174

Cho WS, Cho M, Jeong J, Choi M, Cho HY, Han BS, Kim SH, Kim HO, Lim YT, Chung BH, Jeong J (2009) Acute toxicity and pharmacokinetics of 13 nm-sized PEG-coated gold nanoparticles. Toxicol Appl Pharmacol 236:16–24

Choi O, Deng KK, Kim NJ, Ross L Jr, Surampalli RY, Hu Z (2008) The inhibitory effects of silver nanoparticles, silver ions, and silver chloride colloids on microbial growth. Water Res 42(12):3066–3074

Cioffi N, Torsi L, Ditaranto N, Tantillo G, Ghibelli L, Sabbatini L (2005) Copper nanoparticle/polymer composites with antifungal and bacteriostatic properties. Chem Mater 17:5255–5262

Clebak KT, Malone MA (2018) Skin infections. Prim Care 45:433–454

Crissey JT (1998) Common dermatophyte infections. A simple diagnostic test and current management. Postgrad Med 103:191–202

Cross SE, Innes B, Roberts MS, Tsuzuki T, Robertson TA, McCormick P (2007) Human skin penetration of sunscreen nanoparticles: in-vitro assessment of a novel micronized zinc oxide formulation. Skin Pharmacol Physiol 20:148–154

Das D, Nath BC, Phukon P, Dolui SK (2013) Synthesis and evaluation of antioxidant and antibacterial behavior of CuO nanoparticles. Colloids Surf B Biointerfaces 101:430–433

Dibrov P, Dzioba J, Gosink KK, Häse CC (2002) Chemiosmotic mechanism of antimicrobial activity of Ag+ in Vibrio cholera. Antimicrob Agents Chemother 46:2668–2670

El-Gohary M, van Zuuren EJ, Fedorowicz Z, Burgess H, Doney L, Stuart B, Moore M, Little P (2014) Topical antifungal treatments for tinea cruris and tinea corporis. Cochrane Database Syst Rev 4:CD009992. https://doi.org/10.1002/14651858.CD009992

Fang M, Chen JH, Xu XL, Yang PH, Hildebrand HF (2006) Antibacterial activities of inorganic agents on six bacteria associated with oral infections by two susceptibility tests. Int J Antimicrob Agents 27:513–517

Feldmeier H, Heukelbach J (2009) Epidermal parasitic skin diseases: a neglected category of poverty-associated plagues. Bull World Health Organ 87(2):152–159

Fredricks DN (2001) Microbial ecology of human skin in health and disease. J Investig Dermatol Symp Proc 6:167–169

Gao W, Zhang L (2015) Coating nanoparticles with cell membranes for targeted drug delivery. J Drug Target 23:619–626

Gerrity D, Ryu H, Crittenden J, Abbaszadegan M (2008) Photocatalytic inactivation of viruses using titanium dioxide nanoparticles and low-pressure UV light. J Environ Sci Health Pt A 43:1264–1270

Gilbertson LM, Albalghiti EM, Fishman ZS, Perreault F, Corredor C, Posner JD, Elimelech M, Pfefferle LD, Zimmerman JB (2016) Shape-dependent surface reactivity and antimicrobial activity of nano-cupricoxide. Environ Sci Technol 50:3975–3984

Gomes BP, Montagner F, Berber VB, Zaia AA, Ferraz CC, de Almeida JF, Souza-Filho FJ (2009) Antimicrobial action of intracanal medicaments on the external root surface. J Dent 37:76–81

Guterres SS, Alves MP, Pohlmann AR (2007) Polymeric nanoparticles, nanospheres, and nanocapsules, for cutaneous applications. Drug Target Insights 2:147–157

Hadgraft J (2001) Skin, the final frontier. Int J Pharm 224:1–18

Hainfeld JF, Dilmanian FA, Slatkin DN, Smilowitz HM (2007) Radiotherapy enhancement with gold nanoparticles. J Pharm Pharmacol 60:977–985

Hanley C, Layne J, Punnoose A, Reddy KM, Coombs I, Coombs A, Feris K, Wingett D (2008) Preferential killing of cancer cells and activated human T cells using ZnO nanoparticles. Nanotechnology 19:295103

Hermida-Montero LA, Pariona N, Mtz-Enriquez AI, Carrión G, Paraguay-Delgado F, Rosas-Saito G (2019) Aqueous-phase synthesis of nanoparticles of copper/copper oxides and their antifungal effect against Fusarium oxysporum. J Hazard Mater 380:120850

Hu H, Zheng X, Hu H, Li Y (2009) Chemical compositions and antimicrobial activities of essential oils extracted from Acanthopanaxbrachypus. Arch Pharm Res 32:699–710

Huang H, Barua S, Sharma G, Dey SK, Rege K (2011) Inorganic nanoparticles for cancer imaging and therapy. J Control Release 155(3):344–357

Johannsen M, Gneveckow U, Taymoorian K (2007) Morbidity and quality of life during thermotherapy using magnetic nanoparticles in locally recurrent prostate cancer: results of a prospective phase I trial. Int J Hyperthermia 23:315–323

Johnson ME, Blankschtein D, Langer R (1997) Evaluation of solute permeation through the stratum corneum: lateral bilayer diffusion as the primary transport mechanism. J Pharm Sci 86:1162–1172

Jones KE, Patel NG, Levy MA, Storeygard A, Balk D, Gittleman JL, Daszak P (2008) Global trends in emerging infectious diseases. Nature 451:990–993

Kamaruzzaman NF, Tan LP, Hamdan RH, Choong SS, Wong WK, Gibson AJ, Chivu A, Pina MF (2019) Antimicrobial polymers: the potential replacement of existing antibiotics? Int J Mol Sci 20:2747–2778

Kang R, Lipner S (2019) Consumer preferences of antifungal products for treatment and prevention of tinea pedis. J Dermatolog Treat 24:1–5

Kaushik D, Khokra SL, Kaushik P, Sharma C, Aneja KR (2010) Evaluation of antioxidant and antimicrobial activity of Abutilon indicum. Pharmacologyonline 1:102–108

Kędziora A, Speruda M, Krzyżewska E, Rybka J, Łukowiak A, Bugla-Płoskońska G (2018) Similarities and differences between silver ions and silver in nanoforms as antibacterial agents. Int J Mol Sci 19:444–461

Khan ST, Musarrat J, Al-Khedhairy AA (2016) Countering drug resistance, infectious diseases, and sepsis using metal and metal oxides nanoparticles: current status. Colloids Surf B Biointerfaces 1:70–83

Khurana A, Sardana K, Chowdhary A (2019) Antifungal resistance in dermatophytes: recent trends and therapeutic implications. Fungal Genet Biol 19:103255. https://doi.org/10.1016/j.fgb.2019.103255

Kim SH, Kwak S, Sohn B, Park TH (2003) Design of TiO_2 nanoparticle self-assembled aromatic polyamide thinfilm-composite (TFC) membrane as an approach to solve biofouling problem. J Membr Sci 211:157–165

Kimmis BD, Downing C, Tyring S (2018) Hand-foot-and-mouth disease caused by coxsackievirus A6 on the rise. Cutis 102:353–356

Kühbacher A, Burger-Kentischer A, Rupp S (2017) Interaction of Candida species with the skin. Microorganisms 5:32. https://doi.org/10.3390/microorganisms5020032

Lademann J, Richter H, Teichmann A, Otberg N, Blume Peytavi U, Luengo J (2007) Nanoparticles: an efficient carrier for drug delivery into the hair follicles. Eur J Pharm Biopharm 66:159–164

Larese FF, D'Agostin F, Crosera M, Adami G, Renzi N, Bovenzi M, Maina G (2009) Human skin penetration of silver nanoparticles through intact and damaged skin. Toxicology, 255(1–2), 33–37

Lauer AC, Ramachandran C, Lieb LM, Niemiec S, Weiner ND (1996) Targeted delivery to the pilosebaceous unit via liposomes. Adv Drug Deliv Rev 18:311–324

Le Lay C, Akerey B, Fliss I, Subirade M, Rouabhia M (2008) Nisin Z inhibits the growth of Candida albicans and its transition from blastospore to hyphal form. J Appl Microbiol 105:1630–1639

Liu Y, He L, Mustapha A, Li H, Hu ZQ, Lin M (2009) Antibacterial activities of zinc oxide nanoparticles against Escherichia coli O157:H7. J Appl Microbiol 107:1193–1201

Marin S, Vlasceanu GM, Tiplea RE, Bucur IR, Lemnaru M, Marin MM, Grumezescu AM (2015) Applications and toxicity of silver nanoparticles: a recent review. Curr Top Med Chem 15:1596–1604

Mishra YK, Adelung R, Röhl C, Shukla D, Spors F, Tiwari V (2011) Virostatic potential of micro-nanofilopodia-like ZnO structures against herpes simplex virus-1. Antiviral Res 92:305

Nair S, Sasidharan A, Divya Rani VV, Menon D, Nair S, Manzoor K, Raina S (2008) Role of size scale of ZnO nanoparticles and microparticles on toxicity toward bacteria and osteoblast cancer cells. J Mater Sci Mater Med 20:S235–S241

Nakamura S, Sato M, Sato Y, Ando N, Takayama T, Fujita M, Ishihara M (2019) Synthesis and application of silver nanoparticles (AgNPs) for the prevention of infection in healthcare workers. Int J Mol Sci 20:3620–3638

Nasir A (2010) Nanotechnology and dermatology: part II risks of nanotechnology. Clin Dermatol 28:581–588

Niidome T, Yamagata M, Okamoto Y, Akiyama Y, Takahashi H, Kawano T, Katayama Y, Niidome Y (2006) PEG-modified gold nanorods with a stealth character for in vivo applications. J Control Release 114:343–347

Niska K, Zielinska E, Radomski MW, Inkielewicz-Stepniak I (2018) Metal nanoparticles in dermatology and cosmetology: interactions with human skin cells. Chem Biol Interact 295:38–51

Nohynek GJ, Dufour EK, Roberts MS (2008) Nanotechnology, cosmetics and the skin: is there a health risk? Skin Pharmacol Physiol 21:136–149

Ouf SA, El-Adly AA, Mohamed AH (2015) Inhibitory effect of silver nanoparticles mediated by atmospheric pressure air cold plasma jet against dermatophyte fungi. J Med Microbiol 64:1151–1161

Owais M, Gupta CM (2005) Targeted drug delivery to macrophages in parasitic infections, Curr. Drug Deliv 2:311–318

Pan Y, Neuss S, Leifert A (2007) Size-dependent cytotoxicity of gold nanoparticles. Small 3:1941–1949

Pati R, Mehta RK, Mohanty S, Padhi A, Sengupta M, Vaseeharan B, Goswami C, Sonawane A (2014) Topical application of zinc oxide nanoparticles reduces bacterial skin infection in mice and exhibits antibacterial activity by inducing oxidative stress response and cell membrane disintegration in macrophages. Nanomedicine 10:1195–1208

Payne JN, Waghwani HK, Connor MG, Hamilton W, Tockstein S, Moolani H, Chavda F, Badwaik V et al (2016) Novel synthesis of kanamycin conjugated gold nanoparticles with potent antibacterial activity. Front Microbiol 7:607

Pal S, Tak YK, Song JM (2007) Does the antibacterial activity of silver nanoparticles depend on the shape of the nanoparticle? A study of the gram-negative bacterium Escherichia coli. Appl. Environ. Microbiol. 27, 1712–1720

Raj S, Jose S, Sumod US, Sabitha M (2012) Nanotechnology in cosmetics: opportunities and challenges. J Pharm Bioallied Sci 4:186–193

Raju G, Katiyar N, Vadukumpully S, Shankarappa SA (2018) Penetration of gold nanoparticles across the stratum corneum layer of thick-skin. J Dermatol Sci 89:146–154

Rezaie S, Shahverdi AR (2011) Antifungal effects of silver nanoparticle alone and with combination of antifungal drug on dermatophyte pathogen Trichophyton rubrum. In: 2011 International Conference on Bioscience, Biochemistry and Bioinformatics, vol 5. IACSIT, Singapore

Ruparelia JP, Chatterjee AK, Duttagupta SP, Mukherji S (2008) Strain specificity in antimicrobial activity of silver and copper nanoparticles. Acta Biomater 4:707–716

Sawai J, Kawada E, Kanou F, Igarashi H, Hashimoto A, Kokugan T, Shimizu M (1996) Detection of active oxygen generated from ceramic powders having antibacterial activity. J Chem Eng Jpn 29:627–633

Sawai J, Kojima H, Igarashi H, Hashimoto A, Shoji S, Takehara A, Sawaki T, Kokugan T, Shimizu M (1997) Escherichia coli damage by ceramic powder slurries. J Chem Eng 30:1034–1039

Sawai J, Shoji S, Igarashi H, Hashimoto A, Kokugan T, Shimizu M, Kojima H (1998) Hydrogen peroxide as an antibacterial factor in zinc oxide powder slurry. J Ferment Bioeng 86:521–532

Sharma A, Sharma U (1997) Liposomes in drug delivery: progress and limitations. Int J Pharm 154:123–140

Sirelkhatim A, Mahmud S, Seeni A, Kaus NHM, Ann LC, Bakhori SKM, Hasan H, Mohamad D (2015) Review on zinc oxide nanoparticles: antibacterial activity and toxicity mechanism. Nano Micro Lett 7:219–242

Stevens DL, Bisno AL, Chambers HF, Dellinger EP, Goldstein EJ, Gorbach SL, Hirschmann JV, Kaplan SL, Montoya JG, Wade JC (2014) Practice guidelines for the diagnosis and management of skin and soft tissue infections: update by the Infectious Diseases Society of America. Clin Infect Dis 59:e10–e52

Sutradhar P, Saha M, Maiti D (2014) Microwave synthesis of copper oxide nanoparticles using tea leaf and coffee powder extracts and its antibacterial activity. J. Nanostruct. Chem. 4, 86

Thevenot P, Cho J, Wavhal D, Timmons RB, Tang L (2008) Surface chemistry influences cancer-killing effect of TiO₂ nanoparticles. Nanomedicine 4:226–236

Trigilio J, Antoine TE, Paulowicz I, Mishra YK, Adelung R, Shukla D (2012) Tin oxide nanowires suppress herpes simplex virus-1 entry and cell-to-cell membrane fusion. PLoS One 7:e48147

Tiwari N, Pandit R, Gaikwad S, Gade A, Rai M (2017) Biosynthesis of zinc oxide nanoparticles by petals extract of Rosa indica L., its formulation as nail paint and evaluation of antifungal activity against fungi causing onychomycosis. IET Nanobiotechnology, 11(2), 205–211

Ugur SS, Sarışık M, Aktaş AH, Uçar MC, Erden E (2010) Modifying of cotton fabric surface with nano-ZnO multilayer films by layer-by-layer deposition method. Nanoscale Res Lett 5:1204–1210

Usman MS, El Zowalaty ME, Shameli K, Zainuddin N, Salama M, Ibrahim NA (2013) Synthesis, characterization, and antimicrobial properties of copper nanoparticles. Int J Nanomedicine 8:4467–4479

Valderrama-Beltrán S, Gualtero S, Álvarez-Moreno C, Gil F, Ruiz-Morales Á, Rodríguez JY, Osorio J, Tenorio I, Quintero CG, Mackenzie S, Caro MA, Zhong A, Arias G, Berrio I, Martinez E, Cortés G, De la Hoz A, Arias CA (2019) Risk factors associated with methicillin-resistant Staphylococcus aureus skin and soft tissue infections in hospitalized patients in Colombia. Int J Infect Dis 19:30292–302910

Wang Z, Von Dem Bussche A, Kabadi PK, Kane AB, Hurt RH (**2013**) Biological and environmental transformations of copper-based nanomaterials. ACS Nano 7:8715–8727

Whitley R, Baines J (2018) Clinical management of herpes simplex virus infections: past, present, and future. F1000 Res 7(F1000 Faculty Rev):1726

Xi A, Bothun GD (2014) Centrifugation-based assay for examining nanoparticle–lipid membrane binding and disruption. Analyst 139:973–981

Zhou Z, Wang L, Chi X, Bao J, Yang L, Zhao W, Chen Z, Wang X, Chen X, Gao J (2013) Engineered iron-oxide-based nanoparticles as enhanced T1 contrast agents for efficient tumor imaging. ACS Nano 7:3287–3296

Chapter 4
Applications of Nanometals in Cutaneous Infections

Gerson Nakazato, Audrey Alesandra Stinghen Garcia Lonni, Luciano Aparecido Panagio, Larissa Ciappina de Camargo, Marcelly Chue Gonçalves, Guilherme Fonseca Reis, Milena Menegazzo Miranda-Sapla, Fernanda Tomiotto-Pellissier, and Renata Katsuko Takayama Kobayashi

Abstract Nanoparticles have been largely applied in industrial fields, engineering, and medicine, and are considered as efficient biotechnology tool. Metallic nanoparticles are incorporated into different material with biological properties mainly as antimicrobial. Nanoparticles are the particles with size between 1 and 100 nm being used to different goals due to the beneficial properties. According to the size, NPs can be selected for each function. NPs smaller than 4 nm can usually penetrate and permeate intact skin and reach deeper organs; however, NPs greater than 45 nm cannot penetrate or permeate into the skin. Nanometals have a great potential to different applications in medicine, due to their properties and features. One of these applications is on cutaneous infections, such as acne vulgaris, mycoses, cutaneous leishmaniasis, and wound, which will be discussed here in detail.

Keywords Antimicrobial · AgNP · AuNP · Acne vulgaris · Mycoses · Cutaneous leishmaniasis · Wound

G. Nakazato · L. A. Panagio · L. C. de Camargo · M. C. Gonçalves · G. F. Reis
R. K. T. Kobayashi (✉)
Department of Microbiology, Biological Sciences Center, Universidade Estadual de Londrina, Londrina, Paraná, Brazil
e-mail: kobayashirkt@uel.br

A. A. S. G. Lonni
Department of Pharmaceutical Sciences, Health Sciences Center, Universidade Estadual de Londrina, Londrina, Paraná, Brazil

M. M. Miranda-Sapla
Department of Pathological Sciences, Biological Sciences Center, Universidade Estadual de Londrina, Londrina, Paraná, Brazil

F. Tomiotto-Pellissier
Carlos Chagas Institute (ICC), Fiocruz, Curitiba, Paraná, Brazil

© Springer Nature Switzerland AG 2020
M. Rai (ed.), *Nanotechnology in Skin, Soft Tissue, and Bone Infections*,
https://doi.org/10.1007/978-3-030-35147-2_4

4.1 Introduction

Metallic and metal oxide nanoparticles are part of a group of nanoparticles with different activities and characteristics that depend on their constituents. Metallic nanoparticles have been largely applied in industrial fields, engineering, and medicine, and are considered as a more efficient biotechnology tool (Mody et al. 2010).

According to the National Institute of Health, nanoparticles are referred to as "Nanomedicine" in the medical field, and these nanoparticles are intensively applied for diagnosis and treatment of infections using different strategies and types (Moghimi et al. 2005). Today, silver nanoparticles or nanosilver are incorporated into different material with biological properties, mainly as antimicrobial (Pulit-Prociak and Banach 2016).

Nanoparticles and nanoclusters have specific geometries and atoms number to reach an optimum stable configuration. These structures and their atom arrangement in protons or neutrons are described as "magic number," a unique property of metallic nanoparticles (Harish et al. 2018).

Spatial confinement of electrons depends on stabilization of nanoparticles. There are two types of stabilization: electrostatic (Vander Walls attraction and repulsion) and steric (polymeric stabilization) (Harish et al. 2018).

The synthesis of metallic nanoparticles is a very important step for efficient biological activities. There are two approaches to synthesize nanoparticles: "bottom-up" and "top-down" (Mandava 2017). Moreover, different methods can be used for synthesis of these nanoparticles (e.g., chemical, physical, and biological routes). The chemical process is usually expensive and non-eco-friendly, and physical methods tend to use equipment that expend a great amount of energy, besides the difficulty to produce nanoparticles on a large scale.

Silver nanoparticles are commonly synthesized chemically using a silver salt (e.g., silver nitrate) with a reducing agent as sodium borohydride. Various chemicals such as poly(vinylpyrrolidone), polyvinyl alcohol, bovine serum albumin, and citrate are used as stabilizers of nanoparticles (Mody et al. 2010).

The biological process or "green synthesis" has been much reported in the last years with great influence for biological effectiveness (Mandava 2017). Some features including pH and temperature are very important for the formation of these nanoparticles. The characterization of nanoparticles (size, shape, and zeta potential) is an important step after synthesis. There is always a necessity for standardization of this process (Lengke and Southam 2006; Makarov et al. 2014).

Silver nanoparticles are particles with size between 1 and 100 nm being used for different purposes due to their beneficial properties. According to the size, NPs can be selected for different function. NPs smaller than 4 nm can usually penetrate and permeate intact skin and reach deeper organs; however, NPs greater than 45 nm cannot penetrate or permeate the skin (Larese Filon et al. 2015) (Fig. 4.1).

Silver nanoparticles can be used as alternative to silver sulfadiazine for therapy of wounds (Mody et al. 2010). Biogenic silver nanoparticles showed a great antimicrobial activity against important pathogens including multidrug resistant bacteria

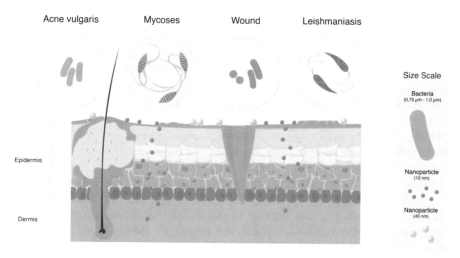

Fig. 4.1 Schematic drawing suggesting the action of NPs (greater than 45 nm) against cutaneous infections such as acne vulgaris, mycoses, cutaneous leishmaniasis, and wounds, without penetration and skin permeation, such as NP of 10 nm

also known as "superbugs" as well as antibiofilm effect (Cardozo et al. 2013; Biasi-Garbin et al. 2015; Longhi et al. 2016; Scandorieiro et al. 2016; Fanti et al. 2018; Bocate et al. 2019).

Silver metal has several applications in different fields (e.g., engineering, electronics, informatics, nanomaterials, cosmetics, and medicine). Due to the potent antimicrobial activity, nanosilver has been incorporated in materials such as food packaging (Nakazato et al. 2016) as well as pharmaceutical formulations (Mathur et al. 2018).

The characterization of silver nanoparticles is essential to compare efficiency of antimicrobial activity with existing data in the literature (Durán et al. 2016a) as well as to correlate with potential mechanisms of action (Durán et al. 2016b; Slavin et al. 2017). Some questions have been discussed with several studies about these mechanisms of antibacterial activity, such as silver ions or silver nanoparticles on the core of the antimicrobial activity, as well as sensitivity of different bacteria types (e.g., Gram-negative and Gram-positive bacteria) exposed to nanosilver action (Durán et al. 2016b; Slavin et al. 2017).

Antimicrobial resistance is a public health concern and some cautions about the NPs usage should be pointed to minimize adverse effects. Graves et al. (2015) reported a rapid evolution of nanoparticles resistance in *E. coli* strains. However, such cases are rare, therefore, silver nanoparticles can be utilized topically, in wound therapy.

Gold nanoparticles were synthetized by Michael Faraday in 1857 in the basement laboratory of Royal Institute (London, UK). Although considering NPs as a hot topic subject, the use of colloidal gold dates back to the Romanic Era, with application to stain glass for decorative purposes.

The synthesis of gold nanoparticles is performed mainly by chemical reduction. In 1994, AuNP synthesis was described by Burst-Schifrin and collaborators based on addition of organic thiol (S) with tetraoctylammonium bromide gold salt.

Gold nanoparticles present their main advantages as relatively simple synthesis with control of the size of the nanoparticles, besides the easy characterization due to the presence of their surface plasmon properties (Jain et al. 2007). An important feature about these nanoparticles is their biocompatibility, suggesting a safe use of gold nanoparticles in biomedical sciences (Karakoçak et al. 2016). Due to these features of gold nanoparticles, they are widely used in cancer treatment. Some therapeutic applications of these metallic nanoparticles are anti-leukemia, anti-rheumatoid arthritis, photothermal therapy, and radiotherapy (Elahi et al. 2018).

The shape of nanoparticles is very important for biological efficiency. The synthesis of gold nanoparticles enables to result different shapes of nanoparticles (nanorods, triangular, spherical, cubes and polygonal) (Mody et al. 2010). This characteristic property (higher surface area/volume ratio) is suitable to conjugate with functional groups (e.g., thiol) of antibodies, oligonucleotides, or antimicrobials (Mody et al. 2010).

Iron oxide nanoparticles composed of magnetite (Fe_3O_4) or maghemite (γ-Fe_2O_3) particles (size of 1 to 100 nm) have several applications, such as biosensors, drug-delivery strategy, and magnetic direction (Cordova et al. 2014).

Iron oxide nanoparticles can be synthesized by wet chemical, dry process and microbiological way (Hasany et al. 2012). Magnetite is commonly prepared with a base (OH^-) and aqueous solution of Fe^{+2} and Fe^{+3} chloride (Maity and Agrawal 2007).

The characterization of magnetic nanoparticles is an important aspect for their application. Fourier transform infrared spectroscopy, atomic force microscopy, X-ray photoelectron spectroscopy, thermal gravimetric and vibrating sample magnetometry are used to characterize magnetic nanoparticles (Xu et al. 2014).

In fact, nanometals have a great potential in medicine due to their different properties. One of these applications is on cutaneous infections, such as acne vulgaris, mycoses, cutaneous leishmaniasis, and wound, which will be discussed in this chapter (Fig. 4.1).

4.2   Acne Vulgaris: Conventional Treatment and Nanotherapy

Acne vulgaris is an inflammatory disease of the human sebaceous follicle, being the most common skin disease. It affects about 85% of adolescents in westernized populations (Melnik 2018).

Major factors involved in acne pathogenesis: (1) increased sebum production, (2) hypercolonization and biofilm formation of *Propionibacterium acnes* (*P. acnes*), (3) increased keratinocyte proliferation with comedo formation, (4) follicular and perifollicular inflammation. Sebum is the secretory product of holocrine secretion of sebaceous glands (Melnik 2018).

Treatment should be directed to the pathogenic factors involved in acne, commonly using comedolytic agents and antimicrobials (systemic and topical treatments). The severity of the acne helps in determining the most appropriate treatments (Dessinioti and Katsambas 2017; Melnik 2018).

In recent years, an increase in organisms that are resistant to conventionally used antibiotics and antifungal for skin has been observed. Therefore, there is a need to search for active antimicrobials with novel mechanisms of action.

Nanoparticles technology holds the state of the art of new products of advanced therapy for the skin. Nanoparticles bear the promise of revolutionizing the development of medical sciences and cosmetics by improving biological activity and regenerative properties. Furthermore, comprehension of the properties of nanoparticles and the nature they impart to the formulations that they are incorporated are necessary for to be safe and efficacious.

Silver nanoparticles (AgNPs) are nano-sized materials that bear unique and multi-functional properties including their thermoplasmonic capabilities, and superior surface Raman properties and antimicrobial activity. Many synthetic methods and review related to AgNP were already published ensuring its effectiveness (Durán et al. 2005, 2010; Marcato and Durán 2008; Rai et al. 2009, 2014; Wei et al. 2015).

Furthermore, triclosan (2,4,40-tricloro-20-hydroxydiphenyl ether) is a antimicrobial compound widely found in a variety of personal hygiene products such as soaps, body washes, deodorants, skin creams, toothpastes, cosmetics, and plastic packages to inhibit microbial growth. DeLorenzo et al. (2008) suggested that despite of triclosan poses low acute toxicity risk, the potential for chronic effects should be deeply investigated. At the end of 2018, 24 ingredients commonly used in over-the-counter (OTC) topical antiseptics were banned by the U.S. Food and Drug Administration (FDA). These active ingredients are now no longer recognized as safe and effective (Cantwell et al. 2010; Ul 2019).

In this way, AgNPs have been an interesting antimicrobial option because they have a broad spectrum of antibacterial action (Rai et al. 2014). Research in the pharmaceutical and cosmetic industry has demonstrated that for diseases and cosmetics, natural products represent an important source to development of new chemical compounds, due to their privileged structures.

Considering the increase of bacterial resistance to antibiotics, including topical antibiotics, the treatment with AgNP is an efficient alternative. Silver nanoparticles have demonstrated anti-inflammation and antibacterial effect against *P. acnes*. In a clinical study, AgNP gel was used for the treatment of acne vulgaris and demonstrated to be effective with a good safety profile. The study showed that there were no clinically significant differences between AgNP and clindamycin gel (1.0%) for the severe acne treatment when used in combination with 2.5% benzoyl peroxide (Jurairattanaporn et al. 2017).

Sathishkumar et al. (2016) proved that green synthesis of AgNP using *Coriandrum sativum* has great potential in biomedical applications such as anti-acne and anti-dandruff treatment.

Nanogel with AgNP synthesized from *Lawsonia inermis* showed activity against fungi and bacteria, including multidrug resistant microorganisms (Gupta et al. 2014).

Kokura et al. (2010) evaluated AgNPs as preservatives in cosmetics. They showed that AgNPs did not sediment after storage for more than 1 year, proving to be stable. The authors showed that AgNP is not able to penetrate human skin, implying that they function only as preservatives. However, when human skin erupts (e.g., allergy), it may be possible for a small amount of AgNPs to penetrate the skin (0.002–0.020 ppm), but these AgNP levels are not cytotoxic to keratinocytes. Thus, AgNPs are a good choice as a cosmetics preservative as they are safe, stable, and effective against a wide spectrum of microorganisms. Thus, a whole new horizon of possibilities remains to be explored in uses and applications for the healthy skin, which will hopefully lead to the development and implementation of new products containing AgNP.

Another promising candidate for the treatment of follicular skin diseases such as acne vulgaris is golden nanorod (GNR), once they have antibacterial activity against *Staphylococcus aureus* and *P. acnes* (Mahmoud et al. 2017).

4.3   Mycoses: Definition, Etiology, Conventional Treatment, Nanotherapy

More than 1.5 million people die from fungal diseases and over a billion people are affected every year. Most of the mycoses occur in developing countries but have global distribution. Predisposing conditions facilitate the development of fatal mycoses. These conditions include asthma, AIDS, cancer, organ transplantation, and immunosuppressive therapies. According to an estimate, a billion people suffer from skin, nail, and hair fungal infections, and nearly ten million have mucosal candidiasis and other 150 million people contain serious fungal diseases (Bongomin et al. 2017).

Mycoses may be classified according to the site and routes of infection. Thus, it can be classified as superficial, cutaneous, subcutaneous, and deep (opportunist fungi) mycoses.

Superficial mycoses are localized and limited to the stratum corneum. *Malassezia* species are yeasts that inhabit human and warm-blooded animal skin, causing a disease popularly known as dandruff. This basidiomycetous yeast comprises seventeen species which are lipophilic, occurring on scalps and other skin areas rich in lipid components. *Malassezia furfur* (*Pityrosporum ovale*) is a major cause of human skin disease (Theelen et al. 2018).

Cutaneous infections are caused by keratinophilic fungi involving tegmental system and their attachments (hair, nails), causing inflammation in response to products produced by dermatophyte fungi, which includes *Epidermophyton floccosum*; species from the genus *Microsporum*; and different species of *Trichophyton* (*T. rubrum* and *T. mentagrophytes*, in most cases). Infected individuals present itchy and sore skin rashes of the affected area. These fungi may spread to the scalp or nails causing hair loss and thickened or deformed fingernails (Kim et al. 2008; Gräser et al. 2018).

Onychomycosis affects up to 15% of the world population. The patient may be treated by oral or topical form. Oral treatment has the inconvenience of multiple side effects and drug interactions. A combination of methylene blue dye and gold nanoparticles (AuNPs) has shown to be an efficient delivery system for antifungal photodynamic therapy. In vitro inhibitory effect on dermatophyte spore germination was observed using gold nanoparticles (Tawfik et al. 2016; Rónavári et al. 2018). An attempt to access nanoparticles as carrier agents was done with lipid nanoparticles (SLNs) with terbinafine, a synthetic allylamine, broadly used as treatment for skin and nail mycoses. SLNs have occlusive properties, forming a film over the skin and avoiding loss of water, thus favoring penetration of terbinafine (Chen et al. 2012).

Subcutaneous mycoses are characterized by penetration of a heterogeneous group of fungi into dermis and deeply on subcutaneous tissue. There are several etiological agents present in soil, decaying matter, or animal excreta. The infection results from injuries following traumatic implantation, like those from wood splints penetration. Infections especially occur in low socioeconomic groups, on people living in rural areas (Queiroz-Telles et al. 2011).

Chromoblastomycosis, mycetoma, and sporotrichosis are examples of these infections. Chromoblastomycosis is caused by the genus *Fonsecaea, Phialophora,* and *Cladophialophora*. Mycetoma may be caused by *Madurella mycetomatis and Acremonium falciforme*. Sporotrichosis is the commonest subcutaneous infection, caused by the cosmopolitan agent *Sporothrix schenckii*, which penetrates in deep tissue, causing multiple lesions along lymphatic vessels (Lima Barros et al. 2011; Brito and Bittencourt 2018; Wang et al. 2019).

Untreated subcutaneous fungal infections may affect bones and joints, presenting difficult therapeutic challenges. Treatment involves antifungal agent administration and/or surgical excision. Development of new antifungal agents and combination therapies can result in improvement in the prognostic of subcutaneous mycoses (Koga et al. 2003). Cure rates, even with long thermotherapy, are low. Existing antifungal agents have significant toxicity and are poorly tolerated over an extended course of therapy; extensive surgical debridement is often required (Horsburgh et al. 1983). Amphotericin B, a classic antifungal drug for intravenous route or topical treatment, was combined with biogenic silver nanoparticles and tested against *Candida* species. As a result, antifungal activity was enhanced (Ahmad et al. 2016b). Amphotericin B is a nephrotoxic drug when given for a long time. Delivery system improves drug availability and reduces the risk of side effects. Nanosized magnetite used as a carrier overcomes amphotericin B associated risks.

Yeasts from genus *Candida* are common inhabitants of animal mucosa and cause candidiasis in the oral, gastrointestinal, and genital tracts. Silver nanoparticles were combined with fluconazole and itraconazole which showed efficacy against major fungal pathogens like *C. albicans* (Singh et al. 2013). Vaginal candidiasis is the commonest form of Candida infection. Intravaginal application of antifungal agents is the usual treatment regimen, as a cream or ointment. The use of nanostructures based on chitosan (a biodegradable polymer) has been explored by combination with miconazole, which is a drug of choice for vulvovaginal candidiasis (Amaral et al. 2019).

Pharmaceutical industry develops therapeutic agents with high efficacy, selective action, and which can be delivered at specific areas of human body. Nanomedicine tools, particularly nanoparticles, may be used, alone or in combination, acting directly or as carriers, to combat harmful microorganisms with high efficacy (Kingsley et al. 2006; Pulit-Prociak and Banach 2016; Berthet et al. 2017).

The combination of antibiotic and nanoparticles is a way to construct strategies for control of resistant microorganisms, at the same time avoiding putative toxicity of both agents. Combinations of antibiotics with nanoparticles resulted in a greater microbicidal effect than either of these antibacterial agents used alone (Herman and Herman 2014; Monowar et al. 2018).

Silver, since ancient times, has been known as effective antimicrobial agent. Silver nanoparticles (AgNPs) are known to have inhibitory and fungicidal effects (Auyeung et al. 2017). Nowadays, metallic nanoparticles are mostly prepared with silver, but other metals such as Pt, Au, and Zn are also used. Importantly, development of resistance in nanoparticles is unlikely, due to the multiple mechanisms of actions.

Depending on their size, nanomaterials may reach cells through the stratum corneum (particles smaller than 4 nm) and hair follicles (particles of 4–20 nm), or just settle on the skin surface (particles greater than 21 nm). Topical nanomedicines may be optimized, depending on their desired application on superficial mycoses (Pityriasis versicolor), dermatophytosis or subcutaneous mycoses (Joshi et al. 2013; Ebrahimnejad and Motaghi 2018).

Nanotechnology may impact pharmaceutical industry, offering many strategies to combat fungal infections. Nanoparticles may have direct antimicrobial function or be used as carriers. In both ways, nanoproducts are promising agents in pharmaceuticals, medical devices, and even in clothes. Also, nanomedicines used in combination with classical antifungal drugs have the advantage to reduce its side effects and toxicity.

4.4 Leishmaniasis: Definition, Etiology, Conventional Treatment, Nanotherapy

Leishmaniasis is a term applied to a group of vector-borne diseases caused by *Leishmania* spp. This protozoan has 18 species that are pathogenic to humans (Steverding 2017). The disease is transmitted to human or animal reservoir by the bite of female infected phlebotomine, and is endemic in 102 countries, areas, or territories worldwide with more than one billion people living at risk of infection (World Health Organization (WHO) 2018).

Distinct species of *Leishmania* cause different clinical manifestations, ranging in severity from self-curing. The clinical forms comprise the visceral (the most severe) and tegumentary forms (the most common) (WHO 2016; Steverding 2017).

Since the 1940s, the conventional treatment of leishmaniasis is based on the use of pentavalents such as N-methyl glucamine (Glucantime®) antimony and sodium stibogluconate (Pentostam®) as first-line drugs. Additional drugs that can be used are pentamidine, miltefosine, paromomycin, amphotericin B and its lipid formulations (Ponte-Sucre et al. 2017). The most of these drugs are highly toxic and cause serious systemic side effects, besides the expensive cost, invasive route of administration, and long treatment duration (Croft and Olliaro 2011).

In this sense, nanomaterials, especially the silver (AgNPs) and gold nanoparticles (AuNPs), are currently considered for several works showing the application of these on parasitic infections (Gutiérrez et al. 2016; Ovais et al. 2017; Benelli 2018). In particular, the use of green synthesis (biogenic) methods allowed several advantages over classic chemical and physical nano synthesis routes, being eco-friendly and not requiring the use of high energy inputs or hazardous substances (Lee et al. 2014).

Several mechanisms have been proposed for the antimicrobial property of metal nanoparticles. The Ag and Au nanoparticles as leishmanicidal agents act as a large reservoir of silver and gold ions, which provide a non-enzymatic source of reactive oxygen species (ROS), interacting with microbial cell surface, penetrating into the cytoplasm and binding with the target sites destroying the invaded parasite (Durán et al. 2016a). Previous studies also indicate that Au and AgNPs can act in the parasite's redox metabolism, affecting the levels of trypanothione reductase, essential enzyme for *Leishmania* survival (Baiocco et al. 2011).

About the current decade, different reports were published with in vitro studies showing the effect of biogenic AgNP on different dermotropic *Leishmania* species. A research group tested AgNP produced using *Sargentodoxa cuneata* and *Isatis tinctoria* plants against promastigote forms of *L. tropica*. They found that the AgNPs formed from both plants have a promising antileishmanial activity, with an IC_{50} of 4.37 and 4.2 µg/mL, respectively. The authors believe that the effect is not only by the Ag but also by the plant macromolecules carried on the nanoparticle surfaces (Ahmad et al. 2015, 2016a). They also found that the leishmanicidal activity of AgNPs formed from *I. tinctoria* was considerably enhanced by conjugation with amphotericin B, providing a new, more economic and safe use of amphotericin B (Ahmad et al. 2016a).

In a different study, authors used AgNPs produced using *Anethum graveolens,* which showed that the nanoparticles alone (50 µM) have not shown antileishmanial effect on *L. donovani* promastigotes, but its combination with miltefosine (12.5 and 25 µM) magnified the leishmanicidal effect of miltefosine (Kalangi et al. 2016).

Another plant, *Olax nana* Wall. ex Benth, was used to produce AgNPs. These nanoparticles were effective against *L. tropica* amastigotes and promastigotes (IC_{50} of 12.56 and 17.44 µg/mL, respectively). AgNPs formed from extract of this plant were also biocompatible with red blood cells and macrophages (high percentage of viability after treatment) (Ovais et al. 2018). Similar results were found when AgNPs produced from extract of *Sechium edule* were used against *L. donovani* promastigotes (IC$_{50}$ value of 51.88 µg/mL), having biocompatibility with normal mammalian monocyte cell line (U937) (Baranwal et al. 2018).

In an in vivo study, AgNPs produced using *Moringa oleifera* leaf extract were tested against cutaneous leishmaniasis in *L. major* murine model. The higher and faster clinical efficacy in AgNPs-treated mice was recorded than standard pentavalent antimonial treatment (El-Khadragy et al. 2018).

Different species of fungi have also been reported as useful in the biotransformation of silver nanoparticles. Fanti et al. (2018) showed that *Fusarium oxysporum*-produced AgNPs acted on *L. amazonensis* promastigotes by apoptosis-like events due an increased production of reactive oxygen species, loss of mitochondrial integrity, phosphatidylserine exposure, and promastigotes membrane damage. These AgNPs were still able to act in intracellular amastigotes, suggesting that the compound has a direct effect on intracellular amastigotes. The fungus *Aspergillus flavus* was also used to produce nanocomposites containing AgNPs and glucantime. The nanocomposites showed a potent inhibitory effect on the cellular viability of *L. amazonensis* promastigote and amastigote forms and the absence of cytotoxicity in macrophages (Gélvez et al. 2018).

In this sense, we can infer that AgNPs produced using different biological sources may be useful in the treatment of cutaneous leishmaniasis, promoting both direct effect on the parasite and effect on lesion reduction. Such nanoparticles can still be combined with traditional drugs, enhancing their leishmanicidal action while reducing cytotoxicity on host cells.

On the other hand, Lopes et al. (2018) synthesized AgNPs by using two chemical methods in which they found that both citric acid and tannic acid are good reducing agents in the production of nanoparticles. However, AgNPs produced using tannic acid were most effective against *L. amazonensis* promastigotes and attenuates nanosilver toxicity comparatively to its precursor (Ag$^+$). In another work addressed the effect of chemically synthesized AgNPs, decanethiol functionalized against *L. mexicana* and *L. major*. The authors found a remarkable leishmanicidal effect in both strains of parasites without toxicity to J774A.1 macrophage (Isaac-Márquez et al. 2018).

Dolat et al. (2015) reported that the use of electroporation combined with chemically synthesized AgNPs can induce greater accumulation of particles in the promastigote forms and infected cells, and thus promoted a higher effect of the AgNPs in the *L. major* elimination. However, limitations of the use of electroporation in in vivo systems should be considered.

Some other groups also demonstrated the efficacy of AgNPs combined with ultra-violet (UV) and infra-red (IR) light against parasites causing cutaneous leishmaniasis. One of the pioneers in the AgNPs study with *Leishmania* showed that the combination of UV and IR light increased antileishmanial properties of commercial AgNPs on *L. major* (Jebali and Kazemi 2013). The effect of chemically synthesized AgNPs under UV light was also tested and was verified that the nanoparticles were effective against promastigotes and amastigotes of *L. tropica*, and those effects were more significant in the presence of UV light (Allahverdiyev et al. 2011).

Another in vivo study also showed enhanced efficacy of chemically produced AgNPs in presence of UV light. In this work, *L. major*-infected mice were treated with AgNPs or AgNPs plus UV light. The results showed that AgNPs alone can control the parasitic burden, leishmaniotic lesions, and visceral progression rate, but the effect was pronounced by the UV light application (Mayelifar et al. 2015).

The comparative antileishmanial activities between chemically and biological synthesized AgNPs (from *Teucrium stocksianum* Boiss) showed that the biological AgNPs were more effective than the chemically synthesized AgNPs, with IC_{50} of 30.71 and 51.23 µg/mL, respectively (Ullah et al. 2018). The pronounced effect can be explained by the fact that biological nanoparticles carry molecules of the organism used in the synthesis (Ahmad et al. 2015, 2016a).

Regarding the gold nanoparticles, some studies also reported the in vitro antileishmanial effect of these metallic nanoparticles alone or associated with other compounds. The AuNPs action showed a satisfactory effect in most of the studies, although in general, when it was possible to compare AuNPs to AgNPs, the AuNP-effect seems to be lower. This was reported by Ahmad et al. (2015) and Ovais et al. (2018) who evaluated AuNPs produced by *Sargentodoxa cuneata* and *Olax nana*, respectively, against *Leishmania tropica* forms. The AuNPs from *Sargentodoxa cuneata* inhibited 30% less growth of promastigote forms when compared to AgNPs after 24 h of treatment, being determined the AuNPs IC50 value of 5.29 µg/mL. The AuNPs from *Olax nana*, although the effect on promastigote forms was similar to AgNPs, the IC50 determined for the amastigote forms was 2× higher for the AuNPs when compared to the AgNPs from the same plant source (Ovais et al. 2018).

Ahmad et al. (2017) also demonstrated that AuNPs from another plant source, *Rhazya stricta* (medicinal herb), showed activity on macrophages (THP-1) cells infected with amastigotes of *L. tropica*. AuNPs inhibited the growth of intra-THP-1 amastigotes at 100 µg/mL concentration (IC50 = 43 µg/mL) after 48-h incubation.

Ghosh et al. (2015) reported the synthesis of Au^{core} Ag^{shell} NPs (Au core: 9 nm, total diameter: 15 nm) from *Dioscorea bulbifera* L., a traditional medicinal plant from Asia, against *L. donovani* promastigotes. The scanning electron microscopy showed that 32 µg/mL-Au^{core} Ag^{shell} NP treatment altered cell body morphology resulting in spherical change. Barboza-Filho et al. (2012) showed the leishmanicidal effect of AuNPs incorporated with natural rubber membranes on promastigotes of *Leishmania braziliensis*, suggesting new studies to evaluate the application of such membranes as flexible band-aids for skin lesion models.

However, Lopes et al. (2018) who tested two chemical methods based on citric acid and tannic acid for the production of AgNPs and AuNPs found no leishmanicidal effect against *Leishmania amazonensis* promastigote forms under studied conditions.

Some studies show that gold nanoparticles when associated with other components have their effect enhanced. Jabir et al. (2018) showed in their work that the synthesis of glutathione modified gold nanoparticles associated or not with linalool, an essential oil extensively used in the pharmaceutical industry (Kamatou and

Viljoen 2008), reported antileishmanial effect on axenic amastigotes of *Leishmania tropica*. Glutathione-AuNPs (10 μg/mL) inhibited 38.5% of the amastigotes growth after 48 h of treatment; however, this effect was potentiated by the association with linalool (LIN-glutathione-AuNP), reaching 72.4% of parasite cytotoxicity.

The association of AuNPs with ultra-violet (UV) and infra-red (IR) light (Jebali and Kazemi 2013) and microwave radiation (Sazgarnia et al. 2013) against *L. major* parasites and macrophages was also studied. AuNPs demonstrated effect against promastigotes of *L. major*; however, when associated to UV and IR there was an increase on the cytotoxicity of both promastigotes and macrophages, showing that these associations were not good candidates for treatment of leishmaniasis (Jebali and Kazemi 2013). On the other hand, the effectiveness of AuNP coupled with microwave radiation on promastigotes and amastigotes of *L. major* decreased significantly as the microwave irradiation time increase (Sazgarnia et al. 2013).

In conclusion, silver and gold nanoparticles of chemical or biological origin, combined or not with other compounds, have proved to be effective against parasites that cause cutaneous leishmaniasis. However, few studies showed in vivo activity of metallic nanoparticles on *Leishmania* model. New studies exploring the action mechanisms and the involvement of different pathways will help in the understanding of how these nanomedicines will be able to act on leishmaniasis. Anyway, it is worth emphasizing the importance of nanotechnology in the development of new drugs, with more directed action to the parasite and, consequently, less toxic to the host.

4.5 Wounds: Definition, Etiology, Conventional Treatment, Nanotherapy

Wounds are an interruption in the continuity of a corporeal tissue (epithelial tissue, mucosa, or organ), compromising the basic functions of the tissue (Lazarus et al. 1994). Wounds can be caused by surgical, traumatic, and ulcerative processes.

As for the presence of microorganisms, the wounds are classified as clean, contaminated clean, contaminated, or infected. Clean wounds are those that present aseptic conditions and therefore, there is no presence of microorganisms. When the time between trauma and care is less than 6 h and the wound does not present significant microbial contamination, the wound is classified as contaminated clean; contaminated wounds are injuries that occurred more than 6 h between trauma and care, with no sign of infection; and finally, infected wounds are those with the presence of microorganisms at the trauma site, with evidence of inflammatory reaction and tissue damage, and these cases are more severe (Tazima et al. 2008).

The bacteria present in the wound compete for oxygen and nutrients with normal cells. Moreover, bacteria and bacterial products, such as endotoxins and proteolytic enzymes, can cause harm in all stages of wound healing (Warriner and Burrell 2005), hence prolonging the patient's hospitalization time and increasing hospitalization costs (Pollack et al. 2015; Warriner and Burrell 2005). Therefore, bacterial infection is one of the major obstacles to proper wound healing and keeping the wound free of bacteria is fundamental for proper tissue repair to occur (Nam et al. 2015).

Currently, several products are used to combat and prevent wound infections, and among them we can mention products containing iodine (iodine and iodopovidone cadexomer) and other products containing silver (silver sulfadiazine and ionic silver impregnated dressings) (Vowden and Vowden 2017). However, with the advent of nanotechnology, new alternatives for the treatment of skin infections are being developed as is the case of silver nanoparticles and gold nanoparticles.

Silver nanoparticles may exhibit different toxicological and antimicrobial properties, depending on the method of synthesis and particle sizes. Several studies have demonstrated the antimicrobial activity of silver nanoparticles, including activity against multidrug resistant bacteria (Cardozo et al. 2013; Ansari et al. 2014; Palanisamy et al. 2014; Singh et al. 2014; Scandorieiro et al. 2016).

The mechanism by which silver nanoparticles exert their antibacterial activity has not yet been fully elucidated. Studies indicate that silver nanoparticles increase cell membrane permeability, inactivate enzymes, interfere with intracellular ATP levels, cause DNA damage and induce the formation of reactive oxygen species (Feng et al. 2000; Dibrov et al. 2002; Lok et al. 2006; Kim et al. 2011).

In addition to presenting antimicrobial activity and acting as a barrier to protect against infection wounds, several studies have shown that silver nanoparticles can be incorporated into different matrices and assist in the healing of wounds.

Boonkaew et al. (2014) introduced a dressing containing silver nanoparticles for treatment of infected burns. In the cytotoxicity assessment, none of the silver nanoparticle-containing hydrogels were toxic to rat fibroblast cell lines tested. In addition, the nanoparticle-containing hydrogels showed antibacterial activity against *S. aureus* (ATCC 25923) and MRSA. Therefore, the results support its use as a potential curative for combating wound infections.

The study by Pourali and Yahyae (2016) has shown that silver nanoparticles produced using the bacterial culture supernatant of *Bacillus cereus* and *Escherichia fergusonii* had low cytotoxic effects on NIH-3T3 D4 fibroblast lineage cells. Results showed that silver nanoparticles had excellent wound healing properties in the animal model, accelerating collagen formation, epithelization, and fibroplasia, and slowed angiogenesis and duration of epithelial filling.

Another study (Kim et al. 2017) reported the production of cotton coated with silver nanoparticles, which exhibited excellent antibacterial activity against *Escherichia coli* and *Staphylococcus aureus*. The cotton samples prepared in this study are expected to be used in the future to prevent and treat wound bed infections.

In the study of Mekkawy et al. (2017), silver nanoparticles were synthesized from the biomass of *Fusarium verticillioides* and were incorporated into hydrogels. Silver nanoparticles were effective against Gram-positive (MRSA and MSSA) and Gram-negative (*E. coli*) bacteria. In this study, the healing time of the silver nanoparticles containing hydrogel and 1% silver sulfadiazine (commercial ointment) was compared and the first group showed a faster wound closure compared to the second group.

Salomoni et al. (2017) evaluated the antimicrobial activity of 10 nm silver nanoparticles against multidrug resistant and non-resistant strains of *Pseudomonas aeruginosa*, showing good activity against these strains in a concentration safe to cell lines tested. The application of nanoparticles treating wounds infected by *Pseudomonas aeruginosa* is assessed in a in vivo study of Ahmadi and Adibhesami (2017), in which they created 500 mm^2 wounds on the back of mice, infected them with *Pseudomonas aeruginosa,* and treated them with 20 nm silver nanoparticles alone and along with tetracycline, evaluating bacterial population and wound closure over 12 days. Although nanoparticles and tetracycline alone showed better results than the control group, the treatment using silver nanoparticles along with tetracycline was more efficient in lowering bacterial population and wound macroscopic contraction.

As seen previously, many studies have been made using silver nanoparticles for the prevention and treatment of wound infections, precisely because these particles exhibit excellent antimicrobial activity and assist in the wound healing process.

Among the different types of metallic nanoparticles, we can highlight the gold nanoparticles, which have attracted interest from researchers due to their excellent biocompatibility with human cells, simple routes of synthesis, easy bioconjugation with several molecules (DNA, RNA, antibodies, peptides, etc.), chemical stability, and antimicrobial properties (Shah et al. 2014; Elahi et al. 2018). However, gold nanoparticles are widely used as bioactive carriers or carriers of antibiotics, thus increasing the antibacterial effect of these particles (Zhang et al. 2015).

Zhou et al. (2012) demonstrated that gold and silver nanoparticles exhibit excellent antibacterial potential for Gram-negative *E. coli* bacteria and *Bacillus* Calmette–Guérin Gram-positive bacteria. In another study (Shamaila et al. 2016), chemically synthesized gold nanoparticles with a size of 6–40 nm demonstrated high antibacterial activity against four human pathogenic bacteria, *Bacillus subtilis*, *Staphylococcus aureus*, *Klebsiella pneumoniae*, and *Escherichia coli*.

In addition to presenting isolated antimicrobial activity and when associated with other antimicrobials, gold nanoparticles can act as a barrier to protect against infection wounds, studies have shown that gold nanoparticles can also be incorporated into different matrices and assist in wound healing.

In the study of Akturk et al. (2016), gold nanoparticles were incorporated into collagen scaffolds to be applied in wound healing. The group treated with gold nanoparticle presented suppressed the inflammation and significantly promoted the formation of granulation tissue and formation of new blood vessels when compared to the control group. In addition, wound closure of the group of animals treated with gold nanoparticle was better than untreated controls.

In this section of the chapter, we have discussed antimicrobial activity of silver and gold nanoparticles, and the exact mechanisms of action of these particles on microorganisms are not yet fully understood, so further studies are needed. In addition to the antimicrobial property, the application of these particles in the wound healing process was also discussed. Because combining the antimicrobial property plus the fact of accelerating the process of wound recovery, these nanoparticles would be of great potential for the combat and treatment of wound infections.

4.6   Toxicity of Metallic and Metal Oxide Nanoparticles

The skin is the largest organ of the human body and has, as main functions, to act as a barrier, protecting the human body from external injuries. However, some compounds or occurrences, such as skin continuity solution or tissue injury, may facilitate the transposition of this barrier, facilitating the penetration and permeation of these compounds, causing local effects such as irritation or even translocation to blood vessels reaching the systemic circulation. The applications of nanometals in cutaneous infections, mainly metallic and metal oxide nanoparticles, are very useful due to dermal exposure, which can become a entry sites of the human body. Therefore, the evaluation of the cytotoxicity and genotoxicity of these compounds, as well as the evaluation of the passage of these compounds through the skin, is extremely important (Larese Filon et al. 2015).

Characteristics such as size, shape, charge and surface properties of nanoparticles (NPs) seem influence, and eventually, can affect skin penetration and permeation. However, it is important to point out that physiological media, temperature, vehicle, and other extrinsic factors may, in some cases, shift NPs characteristics causing aggregation and agglomeration and consequently changing the particle sizes and their performance (Larese Filon et al. 2015).

Thus, NP size in physiological media is one of the main characteristics that affect NP penetration and permeation efficiency (Fig. 4.1). Larese Filon et al. (2015) concluded that NPs smaller than 4 nm can usually penetrate and permeate intact skin; NPs of 4–20 nm can permeate intact and damaged skin; NPs of 21 to 45 nm can penetrate and permeate only damaged skin; NPs greater than 45 nm cannot penetrate or permeate the skin.

According to Larese Filon et al. (2015), another aspect to be considered is the nature of the NP. Metallic and non-metallic NPs behave differently. NPs of TiO_2 and ZnO cannot pass through the skin causing pathological effects. Already metal-based NPs can easily release ions, resulting in a high permeation of the metal through the skin. AgNPs can penetrate and permeate the skin when used in dressings or tissues and a large surface area of the skin is covered, causing a high absorption of silver by the skin, which can exceptionally cause effects on internal organs. The AuNPs can penetrate the skin. However, being a noble metal, in general, it presents low toxicity to human health.

The size of NP influences not only the dermal pathway but also other pathways. Cho et al. (2018) evaluated variations in toxicity of silver nanoparticles according to different sizes (10, 60, or 100 nm diameter) administered intraperitoneally (AgNPs) in mice (0.2 mg/mouse). Mice administered with 10 nm AgNPs showed histopathological changes of congestion, vacuolation, focal necrosis in the liver; congestion in the spleen; and apoptosis in the thymus cortex and died after 24 h. These histopathological changes were not detected after 60 or 100 nm AgNPs administration and in these groups no mice died after 24 h.

There are some studies demonstrating the toxicity of AgNPs administered intravascularly (Wen et al. 2017). These studies confirmed that the AgNPs can be regarded as weak skin sensitizer when these are administered by the dermal route (Kim et al. 2015). Therefore, many factors should be considered, such as NP size, routes of administration, and NP nature (dos Santos et al. 2014). Thus, there is a need for further studies to prove the safety for use of this route of administration.

4.7 Conclusion and Future Perspectives

It can be concluded that nanoparticles are an excellent option in the treatment of cutaneous infections such as acne vulgaris, mycoses, cutaneous leishmaniasis, and other types of skin wounds, but more studies are needed to evaluate the effectiveness of the antimicrobial action in vivo. Another positive factor for the study of silver nanoparticles in cutaneous infections is the possibility of using nanoparticles larger than 45 nm, since they supposedly have an antimicrobial action, offering a low penetration and permeation risk on the skin, compared to NP less than 10 nm, reinforcing the possibility of use against cutaneous infections discussed in this chapter.

Nanotechnology has a promising potential to improve many sectors of society, with the possibility of bringing a substantial positive impact mainly in health/medical category. Nanomaterials can be incorporated not only to treat but also to prevent infections. They can also offer an alternative to ineffective treatments due to multidrug resistant microbial strains, as researchers are proving the activity of nanometals against MDR strains. Application of nanometals in treatment of cutaneous infections demands great knowledge of the action mechanism of these nanomaterials and how they can interact with molecules, substances, cells, metabolism, and the patient's organism. To achieve this comprehension, more in vivo studies are required, so science can effectively guarantee efficacy and safety in clinical treatments of cutaneous infections using nanometals.

References

Ahmad A, Syed F, Shah A, Khan Z, Tahir K, Khan AU, Yuan Q (2015) Silver and gold nanoparticles from *Sargentodoxa cuneata*: synthesis, characterization and antileishmanial activity. RSC Adv 5:73793–73806

Ahmad A, Wei Y, Syed F, Khan S, Khan GM, Tahir K, Khan AU, Raza M, Khan FU, Yuan Q (2016a) *Isatis tinctoria* mediated synthesis of amphotericin B-bound silver nanoparticles with enhanced photoinduced antileishmanial activity: a novel green approach. J Photochem Photobiol B Biol 161:17–24

Ahmad A, Wei Y, Syed F, Tahir K, Taj R, Khan AU, Hameed MU, Yuan Q (2016b) Amphotericin B-conjugated biogenic silver nanoparticles as an innovative strategy for fungal infections. Microb Pathog 99:271–281

Ahmad A, Wei Y, Ullah S, Shah SI, Nasir F, Shah A, Iqbal Z, Tahir K, Khan UA, Yuan Q (2017) Synthesis of phytochemicals-stabilized gold nanoparticles and their biological activities against bacteria and Leishmania. Microb Pathog 110:304–312

Ahmadi M, Adibhesami M (2017) The effect of silver nanoparticles on wounds contaminated with *Pseudomonas aeruginosa* in mice: an experimental study. Iran J Pharmaceut Res 16(2):661–669

Akturk O, Kismet K, Yasti AC, Kuru S, Duymus ME, Kaya F, Caydere M, Hucumenoglu S, Keskin D (2016) Collagen/gold nanoparticle nanocomposites: a potential skin wound healing biomaterial. J Biomater Appl 31(2):283–301

Allahverdiyev A, Abamor ES, Bagirova M, Ustundag CB, Kaya C, Kaya F, Rafailovich M (2011) Antileishmanial effect of silver nanoparticles and their enhanced antiparasitic activity under ultraviolet light. Int J Nanomedicine 6:2705–2714

Amaral AC, Saavedra PH, Souza ACO, de Melo MT, Tedesco AC, Morais PC, Soares Felipe MS, Bocca AL (2019) Miconazole loaded chitosan-based nanoparticles for local treatment of vulvovaginal candidiasis fungal infections. Colloids Surf B Biointerfaces 174:409–415

Ansari MA, Khan HM, Khan AA, Cameotra SS, Saquib Q, Musarrat J (2014) Gum arabic capped-silver nanoparticles inhibit biofilm formation by multi-drug 16 resistant strains of *Pseudomonas aeruginosa*. J Basic Microbiol 54(7):688–699

Auyeung A, Casillas-Santana MÁ, Martínez-Castañón GA, Slavin YN, Zhao W, Asnis J, Hafeli UO, Bach H (2017) Effective control of molds using a combination of nanoparticles. PLoS One 12(1):e0169940

Baiocco P, Ilari A, Ceci P, Orsini S, Gramiccia M, Di Muccio T, Colotti G (2011) Inhibitory effect of silver nanoparticles on trypanothione reductase activity and *Leishmania infantum* proliferation. ACS Med Chem Lett 2:230–233

Baranwal A, Chiranjivi AK, Kumar A, Dubey VK, Chandra P (2018) Design of commercially comparable nanotherapeutic agent against human disease-causing parasite, Leishmania. Sci Rep 8:8814

Barboza-Filho CG, Cabrera FC, dos Santos RJ, de Saja Saez JA, Job AE (2012) The influence of natural rubber/Au nanoparticle membranes on the physiology of *Leishmania brasiliensis*. Exp Parasitol 130:152–158

Benelli G (2018) Gold nanoparticles—against parasites and insect vectors. Acta Trop 178:73–80

Berthet M, Gauthier Y, Lacroix C, Verrier B, Monge C (2017) Nanoparticle-based dressing: the future of wound treatment? Trends Biotechnol 35(8):770–784

Biasi-Garbin RP, Otaguiri ES, Morey AT, Silva MF, Morguete AEB, Contreras CCL, Kian D, Perugini MRE, Nakazato G, Durán N, Nakamura CV, Yamauchi LM, Yamada-Ogatta SF (2015) Effect of eugenol against *Streptococcus agalactiae* and synergistic interaction with biologically produced silver nanoparticles. Evid Based Complement Alternat Med 2015:861497

Bocate KP, Reis GF, de Souza PC, Oliveira AG, Durán N, Nakazato G, Furlaneto MC, Almeida RSC, Panagio LA (2019) Antifungal activity of silver nanoparticles and simvastatin against toxigenic species of *Aspergillus*. Int J Food Microbiol 291:79–86

Bongomin F, Gago S, Oladele R, Denning D (2017) Global and multi-national prevalence of fungal diseases estimate precision. J Fungi 3(4):57

Boonkaew B, Suwanpreuksa P, Cuttle L, Barber PM, Supaphol P (2014) Hydrogels containing silver nanoparticles for burn wounds show antimicrobial activity without cytotoxicity. J Appl Polym Sci 131(9):1

Brito ACD, Bittencourt MDJS (2018) Chromoblastomycosis: an etiological, epidemiological, clinical, diagnostic, and treatment update. An Bras Dermatol 93(4):495–506

Cantwell MG, Wilson BA, Zhu J, Wallace GT, King JW, Olsen CR, Burgess RM, Smith JP (2010) Temporal trends of triclosan contamination in dated sediment cores from four urbanized estuaries: evidence of preservation and accumulation. Chemosphere 78:347–352

Cardozo VF, Oliveira AG, Nishio EK, Perugini MRE, Andrade CGTJ, Silveira WD, Durán N, Andrade G, Kobayashi RKT, Nakazato G (2013) Antibacterial activity of extracellular compounds produced by a Pseudomonas strain against methicillin-resistant *Staphylococcus aureus* (MRSA) strains. Ann Clin Microbiol Antimicrob 12:12

Chen YC, Liu DZ, Liu JJ, Chang TW, Ho HO, Sheu MT (2012) Development of terbinafine solid lipid nanoparticles as a topical delivery system. Int J Nanomedicine 7:4409

Cho Y-M, Mizuta Y, Akagi J, Toyoda T, Sone M, Ogawa K (2018) Size-dependent acute toxicity of silver nanoparticles in mice. J Toxicol Pathol 31:73–80

Cordova G, Attwood S, Gaikwad R, Gu F, Leonenko Z (2014) Magnetic force microscopy characterization of superparamagnetic iron oxide nanoparticles (SPIONs). Nano Biomed Eng 6(1):31–39

Croft SL, Olliaro P (2011) Leishmaniasis chemotherapy-challenges and opportunities. Clin Microbiol Infect 17:1478–1483

DeLorenzo ME, Keller JM, Arthur CD, Finnegan MC, Harper HE, Winder VL, Zdankiewicz DL (2008) Toxicity of the antimicrobial compound triclosan and formation of the metabolite methyl-triclosan in estuarine systems. Environ Toxicol 23:224–232

Dessinioti C, Katsambas A (2017) *Propionibacterium acnes* and antimicrobial resistance in acne. Clin Dermatol 35(2):163–167

Dibrov P, Dzioba J, Gosink KK, Häse CC (2002) Chemiosmotic mechanism of antimicrobial activity of Ag+ in *Vibrio cholerae*. Antimicrob Agents Chemother 46:8–11

Dolat E, Rajabi O, Salarabadi SS, Yadegari-Dehkordi S, Sazgarnia A (2015) Silver nanoparticles and electroporation: their combinational effect on *Leishmania major*. Bioelectromagnetics 36:586–596

dos Santos CA, Seckler MM, Ingle AP, Gupt I, Galdiero S, Galdiero M, Gade A, Rai M (2014) Silver nanoparticles: therapeutical uses, toxicity, and safety issues. J Pharm Sci 103(7):1931–1944

Durán N, Marcato PD, Alves OL, Souza GIH, Esposito E (2005) Mechanistic aspects of biosynthesis of silver nanoparticles by several *Fusarium oxysporum* strains. J Nanobiotechnol 3(8):1–7

Durán N, Marcato PD, de Conti R, Alves OL, Costa FTM, Brocchi M (2010) Potential use of silver nanoparticles on pathogenic bacteria, their toxicity and possible mechanisms of action. J Braz Chem Soc 21:949–959

Durán N, Nakazato G, Seabra AB (2016a) Antimicrobial activity of biogenic silver nanoparticles, and silver chloride nanoparticles: an overview and comments. Appl Microbiol Biotechnol 100(15):6555–6570

Durán N, Durán M, de Jesus MB, Seabra AB, Fávaro WJ, Nakazato G (2016b) Silver nanoparticles: a new view on mechanistic aspects on antimicrobial activity. Nanomedicine 12:789–799

Ebrahimnejad H, Motaghi S (2018) Influence of nanomaterials on human health. In: Kumar V, Dasgupta N, Ranjan S (eds) Nanotoxicology: toxicity evaluation, risk assessment and management. CRC, Boca Raton, FL, p 228

Elahi N, Mehdi K, Baghersad MH (2018) Recent biomedical applications of gold nanoparticles: a review. Talanta 184:537–556

El-Khadragy M, Alolayan E, Metwally D, El-Din M, Alobud S, Alsultan N, Alsaif S, Awad M, Abdel Moneim A (2018) Clinical efficacy associated with enhanced antioxidant enzyme activities of silver nanoparticles biosynthesized using moringa oleifera leaf extract, against cutaneous leishmaniasis in a murine model of *Leishmania major*. Int J Environ Res Public Health 15(5):1037

Fanti JR, Pelissier F, Cataneo AHD, Andrade CGTJ, Panis C, Rodrigues JHS, Wowk KP, Kuczera D, Nazareth I, Nakamura CV, Nakazato G, Durán N, Pavanelli WR, Costa IC (2018) Biogenic silver nanoparticles inducing *Leishmania amazonensis* promastigote and amastigote death *in vitro*. Acta Trop 178:46–54

Feng Q, Wu J, Chen G (2000) A mechanistic study of the antibacterial effect of silver ions on *Escherichia coli* and *Staphylococcus aureus*. J Biomed Mater Res 52(4):662–668

Gélvez APC, Farias LHS, Pereira VS, da Silva ICM, Costa AC, Dias CGBT, Costa RMR, da Silva SHM, Rodrigues APD (2018) Biosynthesis, characterization and leishmanicidal activity of a biocomposite containing AgNPs-PVP-glucantime. Nanomedicine 13:373–390

Ghosh S, Jagtap S, More P, Shete UJ, Maheshwari NO, Rao SJ, Kitture R, Kale S, Bellare J, Patil S, Pal JK, Chopade BA (2015) *Dioscorea bulbifera* mediated synthesis of novel Au $_{core}$ Ag $_{shell}$ nanoparticles with potent antibiofilm and antileishmanial activity. J Nanomater 2015:1–12

Gräser Y, Monod M, Bouchara JP, Dukik K, Nenoff P, Kargl A, Kupsch C, Zhan P, Packeu A, Chaturvedi V, de Hoog S (2018) New insights in dermathophyte research. Med Mycol 56(suppl_1):2–9

Graves JL, Tajkarimi M, Cunningham Q, Campbell A, Nonga H, Harrison SH, Barrick JE (2015) Rapid evolution of silver nanoparticle resistance in *Escherichia coli*. Front Genet 6:42

Gupta A, Bonde SR, Gaikwad S, Ingle A, Gade AK, Rai M (2014) *Lawsonia inermis*-mediated synthesis of silver nanoparticles: activity against human pathogenic fungi and bacteria with special reference to formulation of an antimicrobial nanogel. IET Nanobiotechnol 8(3):172–178

Gutiérrez V, Seabra AB, Reguera RM, Khandare J, Calderón M (2016) New approaches from nanomedicine for treating Leishmaniasis. Chem Soc Rev 1:1–28

Harish KK, Nagasamy V, Himangshu B, Anuttam K (2018) Metallic nanoparticle: a review. Biomed J Sci Tech Res 4(2):3765–3775

Hasany SF, Ahmed I, Rajan J, Rehman A (2012) Systematic review of the preparation techniques of iron oxide magnetic nanoparticles. Nanosci Nanotechnol 2(6):148–158

Herman A, Herman AP (2014) Nanoparticles as antimicrobial agents: their toxicity and mechanisms of action. J Nanosci Nanotechnol 14(1):946–957

Horsburgh CR Jr, Cannady PB Jr, Kirkpatrick CH (1983) Treatment of fungal infections in the bones and joints with ketoconazole. J Infect Dis 147(6):1064–1069

Isaac-Márquez AP, Talamás-Rohana P, Galindo-Sevilla N, Gaitan-Puch SE, Díaz-Díaz NA, Hernández-Ballina GA, Lezama-Dávila CM (2018) Decanethiol functionalized silver nanoparticles are new powerful leishmanicidals *in vitro*. World J Microbiol Biotechnol 34(3):38

Jabir MS, Taha AA, Sahib UI (2018) Linalool loaded on glutathione-modified gold nanoparticles: a drug delivery system for a successful antimicrobial therapy. Artif Cells Nanomed Biotechnol 46(sup2):345–355

Jain PK, El-Sayed IH, El-Sayed MA (2007) Au nanoparticles target cancer. Nano Today 2(1):18–29

Jebali A, Kazemi B (2013) Nano-based antileishmanial agents: a toxicological study on nanoparticles for future treatment of cutaneous leishmaniasis. Toxicol In Vitro 27:1896–1904

Joshi PA, Bonde SR, Gaikwad SC, Gade AK, Abd-Elsalam K, Rai MK (2013) Comparative studies on synthesis of silver nanoparticles by *Fusarium oxysporum* and *Macrophomina phaseolina* and it's efficacy against bacteria and *Malassezia furfur*. J Bionanosci 7(4):378–385

Jurairattanaporn N, Chalermchai T, Ophaswongse S, Udompataikul M (2017) Comparative trial of silver nanoparticle gel and 1% clindamycin gel when use in combination with 2.5% benzoyl peroxide in patients with moderate acne vulgaris. J Med Assoc Thai 100(1):78–85

Kalangi SK, Dayakar A, Gangappa D, Sathyavathi R, Maurya RS, Narayana Rao D (2016) Biocompatible silver nanoparticles reduced from *Anethum graveolens* leaf extract augments the antileishmanial efficacy of miltefosine. Exp Parasitol 170:184–192

Kamatou GPP, Viljoen AM (2008) Linalool—a review of a biologically active compound of commercial importance. Nat Prod Commun 3(7):1183–1192

Karakoçak BB, Raliya R, Davis JT, Chavalmane S, Wang WN, Ravi N, Biswas P (2016) Biocompatibility of gold nanoparticles in retinal pigment epithelial cell line. Toxicol In Vitro 37:61–69

Kim KJ, Sung WS, Moon SK, Choi JS, Kim JG, Lee DG (2008) Antifungal effect of silver nanoparticles on dermatophytes. J Microbiol Biotechnol 18(8):1482–1484

Kim SH, Lee HS, Ryu DS, Choi SJ, Lee DS (2011) Antibacterial activity of silver-nanoparticles against *Staphylococcus aureus* and *Escherichia coli*. J Microbiol Biotechnol 39(1):77–85

Kim E, Lee JH, Kim JK, Lee GH, Ahn K, Park JD, Yu IJ (2015) Case study on risk evaluation of silver nanoparticle exposure from antibacterial sprays containing silver nanoparticles.
J Nanomater 346586:1–8

Kim TS, Cha JR, Gong MS (2017) Investigation of the antimicrobial and wound healing properties of silver nanoparticle-loaded cotton prepared using silver carbamate. Textile Res
J 88(7):766–776

Kingsley JD, Dou H, Morehead J, Rabinow B, Gendelman HE, Destache CJ (2006) Nanotechnology:
a focus on nanoparticles as a drug delivery system. J Neuroimmune Pharmacol 1(3):340–350

Koga T, Matsuda T, Matsumoto T, Furue M (2003) Therapeutic approaches to subcutaneous mycoses. Am J Clin Dermatol 4(8):537–543

Kokura S, Handa O, Takagi T, Ishikawa T, Naito Y, Yoshikawa T (2010) Silver nanoparticles as a
safe preservative for use in cosmetics. Nanomed Nanotechnol Biol Med 6:570–574

Larese Filon F, Mauro M, Adami G, Bovenzi M, Crosera M (2015) Nanoparticles skin absorption:
new aspects for a safety profile evaluation. Regul Toxicol Pharmacol 72(2):310–322

Lazarus GS, Cooper DM, Knighton DR, Margolis DJ, Percoraro RE, Rodeheaver G, Robson MC
(1994) Definitions and guidelines for assessment of wounds and evaluation of healing. Arch
Dermatol 130(4):489–493

Lee J, Park EY, Lee J (2014) Non-toxic nanoparticles from phytochemicals: preparation and biomedical application. Bioprocess Biosyst Eng 37:983–989

Lengke M, Southam G (2006) Bioaccumulation of gold by sulphate-reducing bacteria cultured in
the presence of gold (I)-thiosulfate complex. Geochim Cosmochim Acta 70(14):3646–3661

Lima Barros MB, Almeida Paes R, Schubach AO (2011) *Sporothrix schenckii* and Sporotrichosis.
Clin Microbiol Rev 24(4):633–654

Lok CN, Ho CM, Chen R, He QY, Yu WY, Sun H, Tam PK, Chiu JF, Che CM (2006) Proteomic
analysis of the mode of antibacterial action of silver nanoparticles. J Proteome Res 5(4):916–924

Longhi C, Santos JP, Morey AT, Marcato PD, Durán N, Pinge-Filho P, Nakazato G, Yamada-Ogatta
SF, Yamauchi LM (2016) Combination of fluconazole with silver nanoparticles produced by
Fusarium oxysporum improves antifungal effect against planktonic cells and biofilm of drug-
resistant *Candida albicans*. Med Mycol 54:428–432

Lopes LCS, Brito LM, Bezerra TT, Gomes KN, Carvalho FADA, Chaves MH, Cantanhêde W
(2018) Silver and gold nanoparticles from tannic acid: synthesis, characterization and evaluation of antileishmanial and cytotoxic activities. An Acad Bras Cienc 90:2679–2689

Mahmoud NN, Alkilany AM, Khalil EA, Gal-Bakri A (2017) Antibacterial activity of gold
nanorods against *Staphylococcus aureus* and *Propionibacterium acnes*: misinterpretations and
artifacts. Int J Nanomedicine 12:7311–7322

Maity D, Agrawal D (2007) Synthesis of iron oxide nanoparticles under oxidizing environment
and their stabilization in aqueous and non-aqueous media. J Magn Magn Mater 308(1):46–55

Makarov VV, Love AJ, Sinitsyna OV, Makarova SS, Yaminsky IV, Taliansky ME et al. (2014)
"Green" nanotechnologies: synthesis of metal nanoparticles using plants. Acta Naturae 6:35–44

Mandava K (2017) Biological and non-biological synthesis of metallic nanoparticles: scope for
current pharmaceutical research. Indian J Pharm Sci 79(4):501–512

Marcato P, Durán N (2008) New aspects of nanopharmaceutical delivery systems. J Nanosci
Nanotechnol 8:2216–2229

Mathur P, Jha S, Ramteke S, Jain NK (2018) Pharmaceutical aspects of silver nanoparticles. Artif
Cells Nanomed Biotechnol 46:115–126

Mayelifar K, Taheri AR, Rajabi O, Sazgarnia A (2015) Ultraviolet B efficacy in improving antileishmanial effects of silver nanoparticles. Iran J Basic Med Sci 18(7):677–683

Mekkawy AI, El-Mokhtar MA, Nafady NA, Yousef N, Hamad MA, El-Shanawany SM, Ibrahim
EH, Elsabahy M (2017) In vitro and in vivo evaluation of biologically synthesized silver
nanoparticles for topical applications: effect of surface coating and loading into hydrogels. Int
J Nanomedicine 12:759–777

Melnik BC (2018) Acne vulgaris: the metabolic syndrome of the pilosebaceous follicle. Clin
Dermatol 36(1):29–40

Mody VV, Siwale R, Singh A, Mody HR (2010) Introduction to metallic nanoparticles. J Pharm Bioallied Sci 2(4):282–289

Moghimi SM, Hunter AC, Murray JC (2005) Nanomedicine: current status and future prospects. FASEB J 19(3):311–330

Monowar T, Rahman M, Bhore S, Raju G, Sathasivam K (2018) Silver nanoparticles synthesized by using the endophytic bacterium *Pantoea ananatis* are promising antimicrobial agents against multidrug resistant bacteria. Molecules 23(12):3220

Nakazato G, Kobayashi RKT, Seabra AB, Durán N (2016) Use of nanoparticles as a potential antimicrobial for food packaging (ISBN 9780128043035). Food preservation, vol 2, 1st edn. Elsevier, Amsterdam, pp 413–447

Nam G, Rangasamy S, Purushothaman B, Song JM (2015) The application of bactericidal silver nanoparticles in wound treatment. Nanomater Nanotechnol 5(23):1–14

Ovais M, Nadhman A, Khalil AT, Raza A, Khuda F, Sohail MF, Islam NU, Sarwar HS, Shahnaz G, Ahmad I, Saravanan M, Shinwari ZK (2017) Biosynthesized colloidal silver and gold nanoparticles as emerging leishmanicidal agents: an insight. Nanomedicine 12(24):2807–2819

Ovais M, Khalil AT, Raza A, Islam NU, Ayaz M, Saravanan M, Ali M, Ahmad I, Shahid M, Shinwari ZK (2018) Multifunctional theranostic applications of biocompatible green-synthesized colloidal nanoparticles. Appl Microbiol Biotechnol 102:4393–4408

Palanisamy NK, Ferina N, Amirulhusni AN, Mohd-Zain Z, Hussaini J, Ping LJ, Durairaj R (2014) Antibiofilm properties of chemically synthesized silver nanoparticles found against *Pseudomonas aeruginosa*. J Nanobiotechnol 12(2):1–7

Pollack CV Jr, Amin A, Ford WT Jr, Finley R, Kaye KS, Nguyen HH, Rybak MJ, Talan D (2015) Acute bacterial skin and skin structure infections (ABSSSI): practice guidelines for management and care transitions in the emergency department and hospital. J Emerg Med 48(4):508–519

Ponte-Sucre A, Gamarro F, Dujardin JC, Barrett MP, López-Vélez R, García-Hernández R, Pountain AW, Mwenechanya R, Papadopoulou B (2017) Drug resistance and treatment failure in leishmaniasis: a 21st century challenge. PLoS Negl Trop Dis 11(12):e0006052

Pourali P, Yahyae B (2016) Biological production of silver nanoparticles by soil isolated bacteria and preliminary study of their cytotoxicity and cutaneous wound healing efficiency in rat. J Trace Elem Med Biol 34:22–31

Pulit-Prociak J, Banach M (2016) Silver nanoparticles—a material of the future…? Open Chem 14:76–91

Queiroz-Telles F, Nucci M, Colombo AL, Tobón A, Restrepo A (2011) Mycoses of implantation in Latin America: an overview of epidemiology, clinical manifestations, diagnosis and treatment. Med Mycol 49(3):225–236

Rai M, Yadav A, Gade A (2009) Silver nanoparticles as a new generation of antimicrobials. Biotechnol Adv 27(1):76–83

Rai M, Kon K, Ingle A, Duran N, Galdiero S, Galdiero M (2014) Broad-spectrum bioactivities of silver nanoparticles: the emerging trends and future prospects. Appl Microbiol Biotechnol 98(5):1951–1961

Rónavári A, Igaz N, Gopisetty MK, Szerencsés B, Kovács D, Papp C, Vágvölgyi C, Boros IM, Kónya Z, Kiricsi M, Pseiffer I (2018) Biosynthesized silver and gold nanoparticles are potent antimycotics against opportunistic pathogenic yeasts and dermatophytes. Int J Nanomedicine 13:695–703

Salomoni R, Léo P, Montemor A, Rinaldi B, Rodrigues M (2017) Antibacterial effect of silver nanoparticles in *Pseudomonas aeruginosa*. Nanotechnol Sci Appl 10:115–121

Sathishkumar P, Preethi J, Vijayan R, Yusoff ARMY, Ameend F, Suresh S, Balagurunathan R, Palvannan T (2016) Anti-acne, anti-dandruff and anti-breast cancer efficacy of green synthetised silver nanoparticles using *Coriandrum sativum* leaf extract. J Photochem Photobiol B Biol 163:69–76

Sazgarnia A, Taheri AR, Soudmand S, Parizi AJ, Rajabi O, Darbandi MS (2013) Antiparasitic effects of gold nanoparticles with microwave radiation on promastigotes and amastigotes of *Leishmania major*. Int J Hyperthemia 29:79–86

Scandorieiro S, Camargo LC, Contreras CA, Yamada-Ogatta SF, Nakamura CV, de Oliveira AG, Andrade CG, Duran N, Nakazato G, Kobayashi RKT (2016) Synergistic and additive effect of oregano essential oil and biological silver nanoparticles against multidrug resistant bacterial strains. Front Microbiol 7:760

Shah M, Badwaik V, Kherde Y, Waghwani HK, Modi T, Aguilar ZP, Rodgers H, Hamilton W, Marutharaj T, Webb C, Lawrenz MB, Dakshinamurthy R (2014) Gold nanoparticles: various methods of synthesis and antibacterial applications. Front Biosci 19:1320–1344

Shamaila S, Zafar N, Riaz S, Sharif R, Nazir J, Naseem S (2016) Gold nanoparticles: an efficient antimicrobial agent against enteric bacterial human pathogen. Nanomaterials 6(4):71

Singh M, Kuma M, Kalaivani R, Manikandan S, Kumaraguru AK (2013) Metallic silver nanoparticle: a therapeutic agent in combination with antifungal drug against human fungal pathogen. Bioprocess Biosyst Eng 36(4):407–415

Singh K, Panghal M, Kadyan S, Chaudhary U, Yadav J (2014) Green silver nanoparticles of *Phyllanthus amarus*: as an antibacterial agent against multi drug resistant clinical isolates of *Pseudomonas aeruginosa*. J Nanobiotechnol 12:40

Slavin YN, Asnis J, Häfeli UO, Bach H (2017) Metal nanoparticles: understanding the mechanisms behind antibacterial activity. J Nanobiotechnol 15(1):65

Steverding D (2017) The history of leishmaniasis. Parasit Vectors 10:82

Tawfik AA, Noaman I, El-Elsayyad H, El-Mashad N, Soliman M (2016) A study of the treatment of cutaneous fungal infection in animal model using photoactivated composite of methylene blue and gold nanoparticle. Photodiagnosis Photodyn Ther 15:59–69

Tazima MFGS, Vicente YAMVA, Moriya T (2008) Biologia da ferida e cicatrização. Med Ribeirão Preto 41(3):259–264

Theelen B, Cafarchia C, Gaitanis G, Bassukas ID, Boekhout T, Dawson TL Jr (2018) Malassezia ecology, pathophysiology, and treatment. Med Mycol 56(suppl 1):10–25

Ul (2019) U.S. FDA bans use of Triclosan in health care antiseptics. https://psi.ul.com/en/resources/article/u.s.-fda-bans-use-of-triclosan-in-health-care-antiseptics/. Accessed 9 Jan 2019

Ullah I, Cosar G, Abamor ES, Bagirova M, Shinwari ZK, Allahverdiyev AM (2018) Comparative study on the antileishmanial activities of chemically and biologically synthesized silver nanoparticles (AgNPs). 3 Biotech 8:98

Vowden K, Vowden P (2017) Wound dressings: principles and practice. Surgery 35(9):489–494

Wang R, Yao X, Li R (2019) Mycetoma in China: a case report and review of the literature. Mycopathologia 184:327–334

Warriner R, Burrell R (2005) Infection and the chronic wound: a focus on silver. Adv Skin Wound Care 18:2–12

Wei L, Lu J, Xu H, Patel A, Chen Z, Chen G (2015) Silver nanoparticles: synthesis, properties, and therapeutic applications. Drug Discov Today 20(5):595–601

Wen H, Dan M, Yang Y, Lyu J, Shao A, Cheng X, Chen L, Xu L (2017) Acute toxicity and genotoxicity of silver nanoparticle in rats. PLoS One 12(9):e0185554

WHO (2016) Leishmaniasis in high-burden countries: an epidemiological update based on data reported in 2014. Wkly Epidemiol Rec 91:285–296

World Health Organization (WHO) (2018) Leishmaniasis [WWW Document]

Xu J, Sun J, Wang Y, Sheng J, Wang F, Sun M (2014) Application of iron magnetic nanoparticles in protein immobilization. Molecules 19(4):11465–11486

Zhang Y, Shareena Dasari TP, Deng H, Yu H (2015) Antimicrobial activity of gold nanoparticles and ionic gold. J Environ Sci Health C 33(3):286–327

Zhou Y, Kong Y, Kundu S, Cirillo JD, Liang H (2012) Antibacterial activities of gold and silver nanoparticles against *Escherichia coli* and bacillus Calmette-Guérin. J Nanobiotechnol 10(1):19

Chapter 5
Antifungal Nanotherapy: A Novel Approach to Combat Superficial Fungal Infections

Farnoush Asghari-Paskiabi, Zahra Jahanshiri,
Masoomeh Shams-Ghahfarokhi, and Mehdi Razzaghi-Abyaneh

Abstract Superficial fungal infections (SFIs) affect up to 25% of population all over the world. Although dermatophytosis is the main SFIs with worldwide distribution, tinea versicolor caused by *Malassezia* species and *Candida*-related infections are also common. SFIs have diverse etiologic agents, which differ in pathogenesis and geographic distribution with increasing rate of resistant species to current antifungal therapy. Nowadays, the conventional antifungal therapy of SFIs using current antifungals of azoles, allylamines, and griseofulvin have some drawbacks like liver toxicity, skin problem, severe headaches and sometimes recurrences and drug–drug interactions especially in patients who are under drug treatment for other diseases. The problem is more complicated in immunocompromised patients who undergone systemic immunosuppressive therapies. On the other hand, low penetration of antifungal drugs in hard tissues of nail in onychomycoses caused by the dermatophytes and *Candida* species in local therapies and drug resistance in emerging causative species are considered as other important limitations of current antifungal therapy against SFIs. Novel formulations of antifungals or new devices that increase the chance of the delivery of the drug into the site of the infection seem necessary in order to enhance the drug efficiency. Recently, nanotechnology has contributed into this area and proposes great opportunities for more effective treatments of SFIs. In this chapter, we highlight current status of antifungal nanotherapy using advanced nanoformulations to combat SFIs and discuss in details their application in future medicine.

Keywords Nanotechnology · Fungal infections · Antifungal activity · Nanocarriers · Nanoparticles · Dermatophytosis · Candidiasis

F. Asghari-Paskiabi · Z. Jahanshiri · M. Razzaghi-Abyaneh (✉)
Department of Mycology, Pasteur Institute of Iran, Tehran, Iran
e-mail: mrab442@pasteur.ac.ir

M. Shams-Ghahfarokhi
Department of Mycology, Faculty of Medical Sciences, Tarbiat Modares University, Tehran, Iran

© Springer Nature Switzerland AG 2020
M. Rai (ed.), *Nanotechnology in Skin, Soft Tissue, and Bone Infections*,
https://doi.org/10.1007/978-3-030-35147-2_5

Nomenclature

CLSI   Clinical and Laboratory Standards Institute
CLSM   Confocal Laser Scanning Microscopy
FBS   Fetal Bovine Serum
IC_{80} 80% Inhibitory Concentration
MGYP   Malt extract, Glucose, Yeast extract and Peptone
NPs   Nanoparticles
PAN   Polyacrylonitrile
PCL   Polycaprolactone
PEG   Poly Ethylene Glycol
PEO   Poly(Ethylene Oxide)
PG   Propylene Glycol
ROS   Reactive Oxygen Species
SEM   Scanning Electron Microscope
XRD   X-ray diffraction
YPD   Yeast extract/Peptone/Dextrose

5.1   Introduction

There are many fungi that cause superficial fungal infections in various parts of human body which mainly belong to dermatophytes and species of *Candida* and *Malassezia* genera (Havlickova et al. 2008; Seebacher et al. 2008; Kaushik et al. 2015; Salehi et al. 2018). In superficial fungal infections, the pathogenic fungus is confined to the stratum corneum, skin, or mucosa (Schwartz 2004; Zamani et al. 2016). Dermatophytes invade keratinized epithelium, nail apparatus, and hair follicles (Fig. 5.1). They are distributed to three principal genera of them, namely *Trichophyton*, *Microsporum*, and *Epidermophyton*.

Candida and *Malassezia* species as causative agents of superficial mycoses and normal flora of skin and mucosa grow in a warm moist space all over the world (Kaushik et al. 2015; Sadeghi et al. 2018). *Candida albicans* is mainly responsible for superficial infections in the vagina, gastrointestinal tract, and mouth. Common surface commensal of grease skin is *Malassezia* spp., which are related to folliculitis, seborrhoeic dermatitis, and pityriasis versicolor (Hay 2017).

Superficial fungal infections have risen drastically from late 1960s after development of antibiotic therapies (Ameen 2010; Razzaghi-Abyaneh et al. 2015; Asghari-Paskiabi et al. 2016). Now they threaten the global health especially in association with emergence of immunodeficient diseases or situations such as cancer, AIDs, diabetes, organ transplants, old age, and cystic fibrosis (Vandeputte et al. 2012). Many local and systemic therapies have been applied for treatment of fungal infections. Ketoconazole, fluconazole, itraconazole, griseofulvin, and terbinafine are the main conventional drugs which are being prescribed for patients suffering from superficial fungal infections (Dias et al. 2013).

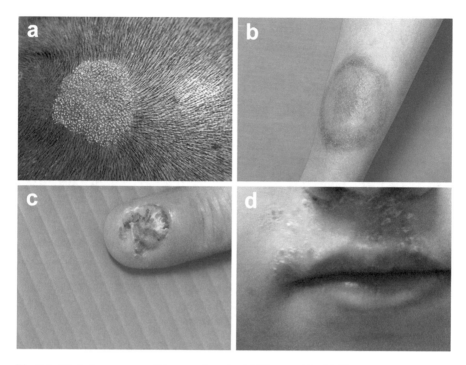

Fig. 5.1 Clinical appearance of dermatophytosis: (**a**) *Tinea capitis*, (**b**) *Tinea manuum*, (**c**) *Tinea unguium*, and (**d**) *Tinea barbae*

Despite many common existing antifungals, developing resistance in fungi as biofilm formation and efflux pump proteins insist the necessity of new treatment strategies. Combination of antifungals, new formulations for old antifungals using nanocarriers, chemical modification of traditional drugs, and improvement of pharmacokinetic of drugs have been carried out by the researchers in the recent past (Asghari-Paskiabi et al. 2016). Recently, nanotechnology has contributed into this area and proposes some opportunities for more effective treatments of superficial fungal infections (Fig. 5.2).

In fact, there is a bidirectional relationship between mycology and nanotechnology. On one hand, it has been demonstrated that many metal NPs have antifungal activity and on the other hand many fungi are able to produce metal NPs from their initial salts (Asghari-Paskiabi et al. 2016). Silver NPs displayed synergistic antifungal property with amphotericin B against *Candida tropicalis* and *C. albicans* (Ahmad et al. 2016). Magnetic NPs and polyenes were combined to obtain a bioactive nano formulation which demonstrated augmented effect against *Candida* sp. (Niemirowicz et al. 2016; Scorzoni et al. 2017). This chapter highlights different cases of nanotechnology applications in the treatment of superficial fungal infections and introduces new treatments in novel formulations for such infections in comparison with older conventional drugs.

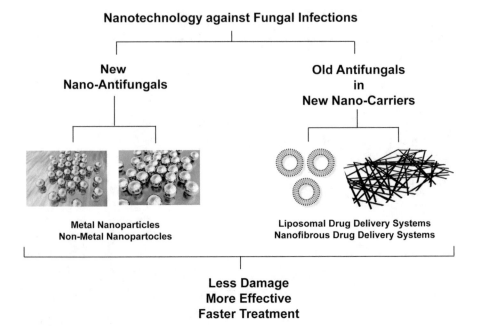

Fig. 5.2 Nanotechnology to combat fungal infections

5.2 Nanoparticles for Superficial Fungal Infections

5.2.1 Antifungal Metal Nanoparticles

5.2.1.1 Chemically Synthesized Nanoparticles

Kim et al. (2008) synthesized silver NPs by first dissolving solid silver in nitric acid at 90 °C and then adding sodium chloride to reduce Ag ions into Ag-NPs. The obtained Ag-NPs were in size of 3 nm in transmission electron microscope micrographs. Antifungal susceptibility pattern of 44 strains of species of *C. albicans*, *C. tropicalis*, *C. glabrata*, *C. parapsilosis*, *C. krusei*, and *Trichophyton mentagrophytes* was determined. The MICs were measured according to Clinical and Laboratory Standards Institute (CLSI) by a broth microdilution method. Amphotericin B and fluconazole were applied as positive control (Kim et al. 2008). Amphotericin B is widely used for systemic fungal infections (Hartsel and Bolard 1996) while fluconazole is used to dermatophytes and *Candida* species based superficial skin infections. The authors observed that Ag-NPs demonstrated antifungal activity against *Candida* species and *T. mentagrophytes* significantly in an IC_{80} range of 1–7 μg/mL. Antifungal activity of Ag-NPs was similar with amphotericin B whose IC_{80} values were in range of 1–5 μg/mL for all fungal strains. Ag-NPs showed more potent activity than fluconazole with IC_{80} values of 10–30 μg/mL.

Authors cultured the yeast cells of *C. albicans* in the liquid medium of yeast extract/peptone/dextrose (YPD) at 37 °C and supplemented the medium with 20% of fetal bovine serum (FBS) in order to induce mycelial formation. They determined dimorphic transition to mycelia in experiments containing Ag-NPs in concentration of 2 μg/mL (IC_{80}) by phase contrast light microscopy. They observed that the presence of Ag-NPs significantly inhibited formation and extension of the serum-induced mycelia. These findings suggested that Ag-NPs are able to treat or stop superficial fungal infections mediated by *T. mentagrophytes* and *Candida* species which were investigated in that research (Kim et al. 2008).

Lee et al. (2010) synthesized 3 nm spherical silver NPs through chemical method as described earlier. The MIC of the Ag-NPs was determined by broth microdilution method for *Candida* spp. and *T. mentagrophytes*. Antifungal activity of Ag-NPs was observed against *C. albicans*, *C. tropicalis*, *C. glabrata*, *C. parapsilosis*, *C. krusei*, and 30 species of *T. mentagrophytes* (the total species were 44) whose IC_{80} range was 1–25 μg/mL (Lee et al. 2010).

In a study to investigate the effect of NPs on the treatment of keratitis, silver NPs with a particle size of 20–30 nm were stabilized with a polymer and for comparison, natamycin was used. The antifungal activity of silver NPs was tested against 216 fungal species isolated from patients diagnosed with fungal keratitis from the Henan Eye Institute in Zhengzhou, China. Silver NPs compared with natamycin had a high antimicrobial activity against the filamentous fungi that had caused eye keratitis. Silver NPs showed 8, 32, and 4 times more activity against *Fusarium* spp. *Aspergillus* spp., and *Alternaria alternata*, respectively, in comparison with natamycin. The authors believed that Ag-NPs can be used to eradicate ocular filamentous fungal pathogens (Li et al. 2013).

Li et al. (2013) added silver nitrate ($AgNO_3$) into graphene oxide (GO) solution drop by drop, which resulted in reduction of silver nitrate to silver NPs. The NPs attached to the graphene oxide through oxygen functional groups and the defects of the surface. They used sonication to make carbon nanoscrolls (CNSs) and silver NPs hybrids. They observed that GO-Ag-NPs and CNSs-Ag-NPs demonstrated enhanced antifungal activity against *C. tropicalis* and *C. albicans*. CNSs-Ag-NPs hybrids can be candidates for treatment of fungal infections caused by clinical resistant strains in many surgeries of abdomen, *Candida* vaginitis, and burn wounds (Li et al. 2013).

Kumar et al. (2015) synthesized copper oxide NPs (CuO-NPs) chemically and evaluated their structure and antifungal properties. First the precursor, copper (II) sulfate pentahydrate, was dissolved in deionized water. Then Poly Ethylene Glycol (PEG) 6000 was added in a concentration of 0.02 M. Next, the reducing agents, sodium hydroxide and ascorbic acid, were added to the solution in the concentrations of 0.1 M and 0.02 M, respectively. Finally, sodium borohydride ($NaBH_4$) was added to the synthesis solution as a source of electrons. The obtained nanorods copper oxide particles were characterized by XRD and SEM. Antifungal activity of the NPs was determined by broth microdilution antifungal susceptibility method based on CLSI recommendation, which demonstrated an excellent anti-dermatophyte activity against *T. mentagrophytes* and *T. rubrum*. In electron microscopy examinations, deformity of morphology and lysis of mycelium of *T. rubrum* was observed. The high antifungal activity of these NPs was attributed to the existence of the carboxyl and amine groups on the cell surfaces which caused a great affinity towards the copper ions. The large surface area of CuO-NPs caused a proper contact with the pathogen. NPs with sizes more than 30 nm are not able to penetrate through skin and enter in bloodstream, while chemicals in molecular size are absorbed into the skin (Kumar et al. 2015).

Mousavi et al. (2015) investigated the antifungal activity of Ag-NPs against *Microsporum canis*, *T. mentagrophytes*, and *M. gypseum*. In their study, the anti-dermatophyte activity of Ag-NPs was not as much as griseofulvin. *M. Canis* was the most susceptible followed by *T. mentagrophytes* and *M. gypseum*.

Ouf et al. (2017) conjugated the Ag-NPs with monoclonal antibody and treated with Q-switched Nd: YAG. In comparison with fluconazole, all the dermatophytes species showed significant sensitivity to Ag-NPs. Combination of Ag-NPs with Q-switched Nd-YAG laser caused antifungal activity in lower concentration of Ag-NPs. They suggested that the laser by making pits in the cell wall of the fungi caused the NPs to penetrate easier into the cells. Also the thermal effect of laser radiation caused electron excitation in Ag-NPs which in reaction with oxygen on the active site of the NPs, produced superoxide radicals. These radicals induce reactive oxygen species (ROS) which do the antifungal activity. They also observed a decrease in keratinase activity of dermatophytes when a combination of Ag-NPs and Nd: YAG laser was applied. Among the tested dermatophytes, *Epidermophyton floccosum* and *T. rubrum* were the most sensitive and the most tolerant species, respectively (Ouf et al. 2017).

5.2.1.2 Biologically Synthesized Nanoparticles

The antifungal properties of silver nanoparticles that had been bio-produced were also studied. Silver NPs have been produced by *F. oxysporum* and were examined against *T. rubrum* and *T. mentagrophytes*. The spherical, 2 nm Ag-NPs were able to show antifungal activity against dermatophytes in range of 1 to 2 μg/mL and 1 to 5 μg/mL alone and in combination with amphotericin B, respectively (Marcato et al. 2012). Rathna et al. (2013) biosynthesized Ag-NPs by *Aspergillus terreus* isolated from the mangrove leaves of *Rhizophora annamalayana* and analyzed their antifungal activity against *T. mentagrophytes*, *E. floccosum*, and *T. rubrum* by well diffusion method. The NPs displayed the most antifungal activity against *E. floccosum* (Rathna et al. 2013). It is reported that Ag-NPs disrupted *C. albicans* membrane and increased its permeability. The NPs perturbed the lipid bilayers of the membrane, caused ions transfer and pore formation and decayed the membrane electrical potential (Kim et al. 2009). Joshi et al. (2013) compared the efficiency of Ag-NPs obtained from *F. oxysporum* and *Macrophomina phaseolina*. The Ag-NPs obtained from *M. phaseolina* showed more antifungal activity against *Malassezia furfur* (Joshi et al. 2013). In study of Wypij et al. (2017), the antifungal activity of Ag-NPs against *M. furfur* was higher than ketoconazole and amphotericin B.

Silver nanoparticles were obtained from nitrate reductase activity of *Fusarium oxysporum* on silver nitrate. The mean diameter of the nanoparticles was 50 nm and they successfully hindered the growth of *M. gypseum, T. mentagrophytes,* and *Paecilomyces variotii* with minimum inhibition zones between 17 and 25 mm. The inhibition zone was strongly larger than that of azoles and amphotericin B (Gholami-Shabani et al. 2014).

The antifungal properties of biosynthesized gold NPs have also been studied. The NPs were obtained from the activity of sulfite oxidoreductase enzyme of *F. oxysporum* on $HAuCl_4.3H_2O$. The mean diameter of these particles was 20 nm and the NPs successfully hinder the growth of several pathogenic fungi such as *M. gypseum, T. mentagrophytes, C. glabrata,* and *C. albicans* (Gholami-Shabani et al. 2016).

Edwin et al. (2017) from India biosynthesized Ag-NPs using the leaves of *Lawsonia inermis,* henna. Antifungal activity of the obtained NPs was evaluated through agar dilution method. They observed that in 6 ppm concentration, the Ag-NPs were able to inhibit only *C. albicans* where in 10 ppm and more all the fungal species were inhibited completely. The suitability of *Phaffia rhodozyma,* basidiomycetous red yeast, to biosynthesize Ag-NPs and Au-NPs was investigated. The formation of the NPs happened with an effective antioxidant, astaxanthin, existing in the microorganism. In evaluation of biological activity of the NPs, Ag-NPs were able to inhibit approximately all the pathogenic fungi which were examined in the research. These Ag-NPs were recognized highly potent for antifungal activity against the dermatophytes *Trichophyton* and *Microsporum*. No toxicity of these NPs was observed against HaCat keratinocytes. Au-NPs exhibited antifungal activity against *Cryptococcus neoformans,* but dermatophyte species were resistant against Au-NPs in concentrations of 10 or 30 µg/mL (Rónavári et al. 2018).

Pereira et al. (2014) synthesized Ag-NPs both biologically and chemically. They aimed to compare the efficacy of the Ag-NPs with other antifungal drugs. To produce chem-Ag-NPs they reduced $AgNO_3$ in an aqueous solution of polyvinyl pyrrolidone (PVP) and glucose. The solution was heated up to 70 °C and then Milli-Q deionized water was added in a rate of one drop per second. The NPs were obtained from centrifugation. Bio-Ag-NPs were achieved by culturing the fungal cells in malt extract, glucose, yeast extract, and peptone (MGYP) liquid medium and harvesting fungal biomass after 72 h. The biomass was washed and incubated with Milli-Q deionized water for another 72 h. Biosynthesis of bio-Ag-NPs was obtained by confronting $AgNO_3$ and the filtrate of abovementioned biomass suspension which took 96 h. They used *Penicillium chrysogenum* and *Aspergillus oryzae* for extracellular biosynthesis of Ag-NPs. Antifungal activity of bio-Ag-NPs and chem-Ag-NPs against clinical and reference strains of *T. rubrum* was evaluated. MIC range of chem-Ag-NPs was lower than bio-Ag-NPs produced by both fungi. Chem-Ag-NPs were smaller than the bio-Ag-NPs produced by both fungi, so their higher antifungal activity was attributed to their larger surface-to-volume ratio. Also the coating of the bio-Ag-NPs may cause this decrease of antifungal activity. Both chem-Ag-NPs and bio-Ag-NPs were tenfold more efficient than fluconazole against dermatophytes (Pereira et al. 2014). Antifungal activity of biosynthesized ZnO-NPs was examined against T. mentagrophytes and *M. canis* alone and in combination

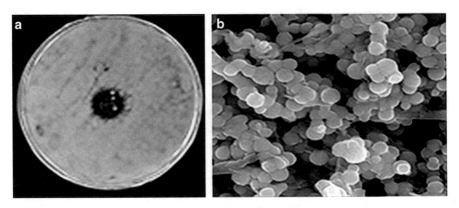

Fig. 5.3 (**a**) Inhibition zone of the growth of *M. canis* by a blank disk contained selenium sulfide NPs. (**b**) SEM micrograph of the selenium sulfide NPs shows spherical shapes with uniform size

with ketoconazole. The experiments showed that biosynthesized ZnO-NPs had antifungal activity against dermatophytes and were able to enhance the antifungal activity of ketoconazole. The size of NPs was approximately 100 nm in TEM micrographs (Tiwari et al. 2016). Recently, selenium sulfide NPs has been biosynthesized (Asghari-Paskiabi et al. 2018; Asghari-Paskiabi et al. 2019). As shown in Fig. 5.3, the spherical NPs originated from selenous acid and sodium sulfite and biosynthesized by *Saccharomyces cerevisiae* were able to inhibit pathogenic saprophytes, yeasts, and dermatophytes (Asghari-Paskiabi et al. 2019).

5.2.2 Non-metal Antifungal Nanoparticles

A nanoemulsion called NB-002 has also been employed to fight against superficial fungal infections. A cationic quaternary ammonium compound, cetylpyridinium chloride (CPC) in NB-002 causes both antifungal activity and stability of nanoemulsion droplets. Pannu et al. (2009) assessed antifungal activity of NB-002 against *C. albicans*, dermatophytes, and other filamentous fungi. They demonstrated that NB-002 has a wide and uniformly fungicidal activity. This antifungal activity was against causative agents of tinea cruris, tinea pedis, tinea capitis, tinea corporis, and onychomycosis. Antifungal effect of NB-002 against *T. rubrum*, *T. mentagrophytes*, and *E. floccosum* was compared to orally administered compound of terbinafine, griseofulvin, and itraconazole. The results showed a remarkable heterogeneity in the oral compounds' antifungal activity. They also demonstrated antifungal activity of NB-002 against other filamentous genera which were resistant to many drugs. These fungi had been isolated from immunocompromised patients. NB-002 showed impressive activity against *Paecilomyces*, *Scedosporium* spp., *Scopulariopsis* spp., and *Fusarium* spp. NB-002 had strong activity against azole-resistant *C. albicans* isolates, terbinafine-resistant *T. rubrum* isolates, and multidrug-resistant molds.

NB-002 was able to kill both microconidia and mycelia. Its fungicidal activity was fast even for dormant forms of fungal cells (Pannu et al. 2009).

5.3 Nanoparticles as Antifungal-Carriers for Superficial Fungal Infections

Many nanocarriers have been examined for topical delivery of antibiotics against dermatophytes. Nanocarriers are supposed to deliver the antifungal to the target's point, without causing damage to the liver through bloodstream or rapidly passing off the kidneys. By controlled release of the antifungal, the nanocarriers cause a prolonged drug-lesion confrontation and help heal the wounds.

5.3.1 Liposomal Drug Delivery Systems

One of the most widely used nanocarriers is the liposome. Liposomes can penetrate into the invasion site of dermatophytes. They can penetrate into stratum corneum, the part of the tissue that is being attacked by dermatophytes. Sudhakar et al. (2014) produced liposomes in which terbinafine hydrochloride was loaded. These liposomes were dispersed in gum karaya gel and tested ex vivo on the rabbit's skin. In comparison with gum karaya gel containing terbinafine hydrochloride, without liposome, the type that contained a drug-loaded liposome showed more durability of the drug on the rabbit's skin.

Elmoslemany et al. (2012) compared the efficacy of transdermal delivery between conventional liposomes and propylene glycol (PG) liposomes which were loaded with miconazole nitrate. The minimum inhibitory concentration (MIC) value for propylene glycol liposomes loaded with miconazole nitrate was 1.46 µg/mL while the MIC value of conventional liposomes was 2.93 µg/mL against *C. albicans*. Penetration and skin retention of miconazole nitrate in human skin for PG liposomes was higher in comparison with miconazole nitrate suspension and conventional liposomes.

Other types of phospholipid-based vesicle nanocarrier are ethosomes which due to their high ethanol content fluidizes the lipids of stratum corneum and causes the penetration of the vesicles into the skin (Blume et al. 1993). The sizes of ethosomes are controllable by changing the proportion of the ethanol and phospholipids. More amount of ethanol causes the reduction of the size of the nanocarriers (Campani et al. 2016). Fluconazole has been loaded into the ethosomes for treatment of superficial candidiasis during a month. In comparison with commercial fluconazole cream (25–30%) and liposomes (30–60%), the ethosomes showed a high reduction in skin candidiasis (50–70%) (Bhalaria et al. 2009). Verma and Pathak (2012) compared the penetration of ethosomes and liposomes when both were loaded with econazole nitrate. Ethosomes diffused into the albino rat skin twofold more than liposomes which make them an appropriate candidate for the treatment of deep fungal infection.

Transfersomes are kinds of liposomes which are modified by the addition of edge activators (Cevc and Blume 1992) such as Tween 20, Tween 60, Tween 80, dipotassium glycyrrhizinate, sodium cholate, sodium deoxycholate, Span 60, Span 65, and Span 80 (Benson 2006). Edge activators cause the weakening of lipid bilayers of the transfersomes which leads to their enhanced deformability (Benson 2009). In comparison with conventional liposomes, higher penetration of transfersomes into the skin was observed (Hussain et al. 2017). Also, miconazole nitrate loaded transfersomes showed very effective in vivo antifungal activity in comparison with free drug solution and conventional liposomes (Pandit et al. 2014).

Transethosomes are similar to ethosomes except that they have an edge activator or a penetration enhancer (Kumar et al. 2016). Voriconazole loaded transethosomes were evaluated for the drug skin deposition in mice. The results showed that compared to conventional liposomes, polyethylene glycol drug solution and ethosomes, there was an increase of voriconazole deposition in the epidermis and dermis (Song et al. 2012).

Niosomes which are made of alkyl chain non-ionic surfactants are kinds of bilayer vesicular system (Hamishehkar et al. 2013). Both lipophilic and hydrophilic drugs can be encapsulated into the niosomes (Thakkar 2016). A comparative assessment was carried out between liposomal gel loaded with griseofulvin and niosomal gel loaded with the same. Liposomal gel showed 50% cure rate, while the cure rate of niosomal gel was approximately 80% (Kassem et al. 2006). Spanlastics contain edge activator in their niosomal structure and are called "modified niosomes." Spanlastics have been loaded with terbinafine hydrochloride and have been examined for treatment of nail fungal infection (onychomycosis). In confocal laser scanning microscopy (CLSM) examinations, it was revealed that spanlastic formulation had permeated into ex vivo nail efficiently (Elsherif et al. 2017; Verma and Utreja 2018).

5.3.2 Nanofibrous Drug Delivery Systems

Nanofibers have been used to deliver the antifungals into the site of superficial infections. Terbinafine hydrochloride has been incorporated inside the polycaprolactone (PCL)/gelatin nanofibers obtained from electrospinning technique. The obtained wound dressings were examined for their antifungal ability. They successfully hindered *T. mentagrophytes* and *Aspergillus fumigatus* growth (Fig. 5.4) and released the drug in a steady state in time (Paskiabi et al. 2017).

In another study, polyacrylonitrile (PAN) nanofibers were prepared as a eugenol delivery system. The eugenol-nanofibrous carriers hindered *C. albicans* and the authors suggested that it can be used for treatment of cutaneous mucocutaneous

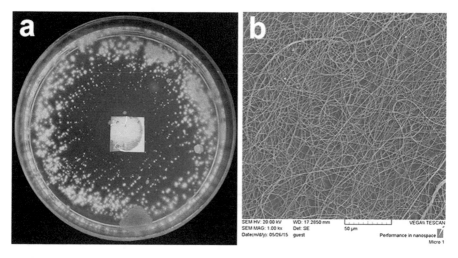

Fig. 5.4 (**a**) PCL/gelatin electrospun nanofibers containing terbinafine inhibited the growth of T. mentagrophytes. (**b**) SEM micrograph of PCL/gelatin electrospun nanofibers containing terbinafine

candidiasis (Semnani et al. 2018). Eugenol is a phenolic component of clove oil which has antifungal properties (Son et al. 1998; Devi et al. 2010).

Mofidfar et al. (2017) fabricated clotrimazole-loaded nanofibrous polymeric formulation. They first co-extracted a clotrimazole-contained PCL associated with poly(ethylene oxide) (PEO) and then removed PEO to obtain PCL-clotrimazole fibers. Antifungal activity was examined both in vitro and in vivo against *T. mentagrophytes*, *A. fumigatus*, and *C. albicans*. This formulation of clotrimazole maintained activity for longer times in comparison with electrospun meshes.

5.4   Concluding Remarks and Future Perspectives

One of the important barriers to treating superficial fungal infections is their resistance to common drugs. Oral medications also cause liver-related illnesses, because they enter the bloodstream before they affect the target tissue. According to the materials mentioned in this chapter, metal nanoparticles can be a good alternative to drugs used to treat superficial fungal infections. Silver and gold nanoparticles alone and sometimes in combination with other antibiotics have shown good antifungal effects against dermatophytes and other agents of superficial mycoses. One of the advantages of metal nanoparticles is the possibility of their synthesis in green ways. Nanoparticles have also been able to provide a good drug delivery agent to deliver antifungal drugs to the target tissue. Liposomal nanocomposites and other liposomal products, due to the nature of their lipophilicity, easily pass through the stratum layer and target the drug to the microorganism. Nanofiber coatings have been studied as a drug delivery tool to the target tissue with fungal infection. These structures are able to release the drug gradually in the target site and reduce the duration of the treatment by direct exposure to the aggressive microorganism. These findings promise new and more effective solutions to the treatment of superficial fungal infections, which can be very interesting, especially for cancer and autoimmune patients and recipients of immunosuppressive drugs.

References

Ahmad A, Wei Y, Syed F, Tahir K, Taj R, Khan A, Hameed M, Yuan Q (2016) Amphotericin B-conjugated biogenic silver nanoparticles as an innovative strategy for fungal infections. Microb Pathog 99:271–281

Ameen M (2010) Epidemiology of superficial fungal infections. Clin Dermatol 28:197–201

Asghari-Paskiabi F, Jahanshiri Z, Imani M, Shams-Ghahfarokhi M, Razzaghi-Abyaneh M (2016) In: Grumezescu AM (ed) Antifungal nanomaterials: synthesis, properties, and applications. Nanobiomaterials in antimicrobial therapy, vol 6. Elsevier, Oxford, pp 343–383

Asghari-Paskiabi F, Imani M, Razzaghi-Abyaneh M, Rafii-Tabar H (2018) *Fusarium oxysporum*, a bio-factory for nano selenium compounds: synthesis and characterization. Sci Iran 25:1857–1863

Asghari-Paskiabi F, Imani M, Rafii-Tabar H, Razzaghi-Abyaneh M (2019) Physicochemical properties, antifungal activity and cytotoxicity of selenium sulfide nanoparticles green synthesized by *Saccharomyces cerevisiae*. Biochem Biophys Res Commun 516:1078–1084

Benson HAE (2006) Transfersomes for transdermal drug delivery. Expert Opin Drug Deliv 3:727–737

Benson HAE (2009) Elastic liposomes for topical and transdermal drug delivery. Curr Drug Deliv 6:217–226

Bhalaria MK, Naik S, Misra AN (2009) Ethosomes: a novel delivery system for antifungal drugs in the treatment of topical fungal diseases. Indian J Exp Biol 47:368–375

Blume A, Jansen M, Ghyczy M, Gareiss J (1993) Interaction of phospholipid liposomes with lipid model mixtures for stratum corneum lipids. Int J Pharm 99:219–228

Campani V, Biondi M, Laura M, Cilurzo F, Franzé S, Pitaro M, De Rosa G (2016) Nanocarriers to enhance the accumulation of vitamin K1 into the skin. Pharm Res 33:893–908

Cevc G, Blume G (1992) Lipid vesicles penetrate into intact skin owing to the transdermal osmotic gradients and hydration force. Biochim Biophys Acta Biomembr 1104:226–232

Devi KP, Nisha SA, Sakthivel R, Pandian SK (2010) Eugenol (an essential oil of clove) acts as an antibacterial agent against *Salmonella typhi* by disrupting the cellular membrane. J Ethnopharmacol 130:107–115

Dias MFRG, Quaresma-Santos M, Bernardes-Filho F, Amorim AGF, Schechtman RC, Azulay DR (2013) Update on therapy for superficial mycoses: review article part I. An Bras Dermatol 88:764–774

Edwin B, Kannan I, Aarthi R, Sukumar RG, Prevathi RK, Shantha S (2017) Study on anti-fungal activity of silver nanoparticles obtained from *Lawsonia inermis* against *Candida albicans* and dermatophytes. Int J Adv Res Med Sci 1:19–22

Elmoslemany RM, Abdallah O, El-Khordagui LK, Khalafallah NM (2012) Propylene glycol liposomes as a topical delivery system for miconazole nitrate: comparison with conventional liposomes. AAPS Pharm Sci Tech 13:723–731

Elsherif NI, Shamma RN, Abdelbary G (2017) Terbinafine hydrochloride trans-ungual delivery via nanovesicular systems: in vitro characterization and ex vivo evaluation. AAPS Pharm Sci Tech 18:551–562

Gholami-Shabani MA, Akbarzadeh A, Norouzian D, Amini A, Gholami-Shabani Z, Imani A, Chiani M, Riazi G, Shams-Ghahfarokhi M, Razzaghi-Abyaneh M (2014) Antimicrobial activity and physical characterization of silver nanoparticles green synthesized using nitrate reductase from *Fusarium oxysporum*. Appl Biochem Biotechnol 172:4084–4098

Gholami-Shabani M, Imani A, Shams-Ghahfarokhi M, Gholami-Shabani Z, Pazooki A, Akbarzadeh A, Riazi G, Razzaghi-Abyaneh M (2016) Bioinspired synthesis, characterization and antifungal activity of enzyme-mediated gold nanoparticles using a fungal oxidoreductase. J Iran Chem Soc 13:2059–2068

Hamishehkar H, Rahimpour Y, Kouhsoltani M (2013) Niosomes as a propitious carrier for topical drug delivery. Expert Opin Drug Deliv 10:261–272

Hartsel S, Bolard J (1996) Amphotericin B: new life for an old drug. Trends Pharmacol Sci 17:445–449

Havlickova B, Czaika V, Friedrich M (2008) Epidemiological trends in skin mycoses worldwide. Mycoses 51:2–15

Hay R (2017) Superficial fungal infections. Medicine 45:707–710

Hussain A, Singh S, Sharma D, Webster T, Shafaat K, Faruk A (2017) Elastic liposomes as novel carriers: recent advances in drug delivery. Int J Nanomedicine 12:5087

Joshi PA, Bonde SR, Gaikwad SC, Gade AK, Abd-Elsalam K, Rai MK (2013) Comparative studies on synthesis of silver nanoparticles by *Fusarium oxysporum* and *Macrophomina phaseolina* and its efficacy against bacteria and *Malassezia furfur*. J Bionanosci 7:378–385

Kassem MAA, Esmat S, Bendas E, El-Komy M (2006) Efficacy of topical griseofulvin in treatment of tinea corporis. Mycoses 49:232–235

Kaushik N, Pujalte G, Reese S (2015) Superficial fungal infections. Primary Care Clin Office Pract 42:501–516

Kim K-J, Sung W, Moon S, Choi J, Kim JG, Lee DG (2008) Antifungal effect of silver nanoparticles on dermatophytes. J Microbiol Biotechnol 18:1482–1484

Kim K-J, Sung W, Suh BK, Moon S, Choi J-S, Kim JG, Lee DG (2009) Antifungal activity and mode of action of silver nano-particles on *Candida albicans*. Biometals 22:235–242

Kumar R, Shukla S, Pandey A, Srivastava S, Dikshit A (2015) Copper oxide nanoparticles: an antidermatophytic agent for *Trichophyton* spp. Nanotechnol Rev 4:401–409

Kumar L, Verma S, Singh K, Prasad DN, Jain AK (2016) Ethanol based vesicular carriers in transdermal drug delivery: nanoethosomes and transethosomes in focus. Nano World J 2:41–51

Lee J, Kim KJ, Sung WS, Kim JG, Lee DG (2010) The silver nanoparticle (nano-Ag): a new model for antifungal agents. Silver nanoparticles. InTech, Rijeka

Li C, Wang X, Chen F, Zhang C, Zhi X, Wang K, Cui D (2013) The antifungal activity of graphene oxide-silver nanocomposites. Biomaterials 34:3882–3890

Marcato PD, Durán M, Huber SC, Rai M, Melo PS, Alves OL, Duran N (2012) Biogenic silver nanoparticles and its antifungal activity as a new topical transungual drug. J Nano Res 20:99–107

Mofidfar M, Wang J, Long L, Hager C, Vareechon C, Pearlman E, Eric B, Ghannoum M, Wnek GE (2017) Polymeric nanofiber/antifungal formulations using a novel co-extrusion approach. AAPS Pharm Sci Tech 18:1917–1924

Mousavi SAA, Salari S, Hadizadeh S (2015) Evaluation of antifungal effect of silver nanoparticles against *Microsporum canis, Trichophyton mentagrophytes and Microsporum gypseum*. Iran J Biotechnol 13:38–43

Niemirowicz K, Bonita D, Tokajuk G, Głuszek K, Wilczewska AZ, Misztalewska I, Mystkowska J, Michalak G, Sodo A, Wątek M, Kiziewicz B, Góźdź S, Głuszek S, Bucki R (2016) Magnetic nanoparticles as a drug delivery system that enhance fungicidal activity of polyene antibiotics. Nanomed Nanotechnol Biol Med 12:2395–2404

Ouf SA, Mohamed AAH, El-Adly AA (2017) Enhancement of the antidermatophytic activity of silver nanoparticles by Q-switched Nd: YAG laser and monoclonal antibody conjugation. Med Mycol 55:495–506

Pandit J, Garg M, Jain NK (2014) Miconazole nitrate bearing ultraflexible liposomes for the treatment of fungal infection. J Liposome Res 24:163–169

Pannu J, McCarthy A, Martin A, Hamouda T, Ciotti S, Fothergill A, Sutcliffe J (2009) NB-002, a novel nanoemulsion with broad antifungal activity against dermatophytes, other filamentous fungi, and *Candida albicans*. Antimicrob Agents Chemother 53:3273–3279

Paskiabi FA, Bonakdar S, Shokrgozar MA, Imani M, Jahanshiri Z, Shams-Ghahfarokhi M, Razzaghi-Abyaneh M (2017) Terbinafine-loaded wound dressing for chronic superficial fungal infections. Mater Sci Eng C 73:130–136

Pereira L, Dias N, Carvalho J, Fernandes S, Santos C, Lima N (2014) Synthesis, characterization and antifungal activity of chemically and fungal-produced silver nanoparticles against *Trichophyton rubrum*. J Appl Microbiol 117:1601–1613

Rathna GS, Elavarasi A, Peninal S, Subramanian J, Mano G, Kalaiselvam M (2013) Extracellular biosynthesis of silver nanoparticles by endophytic fungus *Aspergillus terreus* and its antidermatophytic activity. Int J Pharmaceut Biol Arch 4:481–487

Razzaghi-Abyaneh M, Shams-Ghahfarokhi M, Rai M (2015) Medical mycology: current trends and future prospects, 1st edn. CRC, Boca Raton, FL

Rónavári A, Igaz N, Gopisetty M, Szerencsés B, Kovács D, Papp C, Vágvölgyi C, Boros IM, Kónya Z, Kiricsi M, Pfeiffer I (2018) Biosynthesized silver and gold nanoparticles are potent antimycotics against opportunistic pathogenic yeasts and dermatophytes. Int J Nanomedicine 13:695–704

Sadeghi G, Ebrahimi-Rad M, Mousavi SF, Shams-Ghahfarokhi M, Razzaghi-Abyaneh M (2018) Emergence of non-*Candida albicans* species: Epidemiology, phylogeny and fluconazole susceptibility profile. J Mycol Méd 28:51–58

Salehi Z, Shams-Ghahfarokhi M, Razzaghi-Abyaneh M (2018) Antifungal drug susceptibility profile of clinically important dermatophytes and determination of point mutations in terbinafine-resistant isolate. Eur J Clin Microbiol Infect Dis 37:1841–1846

Schwartz RA (2004) Superficial fungal infections. Lancet 364:1173–1182

Scorzoni L, de Paula e Silva AC, Marcos CM, Assato PA, de Melo WCMA, de Oliveira HC, Costa-Orlandi CB, Mendes-Giannini MJS, Fusco-Almeida AM (2017) Antifungal therapy: new advances in the understanding and treatment of mycosis. Front Microbiol 8:36–59

Seebacher C, Bouchara J-P, Mignon B (2008) Updates on the epidemiology of dermatophyte infections. Mycopathologia 166:335–352

Semnani K, Shams-Ghahfarokhi M, Afrashi M, Fakhrali A, Semnani D (2018) Antifungal activity of eugenol loaded electrospun pan nanofiber mats against *Candida albicans*. Curr Drug Deliv 15:860–866

Son KH, Kwon SY, Kim HP, Chang HW, Kang SS (1998) Constituents from *Syzygium aromaticum* Merr. et Perry. Nat Prod Sci 4:263–267

Song CK, Balakrishnan P, Shim C-K, Chung S-J, Chong S, Kim D-D (2012) A novel vesicular carrier, transethosome, for enhanced skin delivery of voriconazole: characterization and *in vitro/in vivo* evaluation. Colloids Surf B Biointerfaces 92:299–304

Sudhakar B, Ravi VJN, Ramana MKV (2014) Formulation, characterization and *ex vivo* studies of terbinafine hydrochloride liposomes for cutaneous delivery. Curr Drug Deliv 11:521–530

Thakkar M (2016) Opportunities and challenges for niosomes as drug delivery systems. Curr Drug Deliv 13:1275–1289

Tiwari N, Pandit R, Gaikwad S, Aniket G, Rai M (2016) Biosynthesis of zinc oxide nanoparticles by petals extract of *Rosa indica* L., its formulation as nail paint and evaluation of antifungal activity against fungi causing onychomycosis. IET Nanobiotechnol 11:205–211

Vandeputte P, Ferrari S, Coste TA (2012) Antifungal resistance and new strategies to control fungal infections. Int J Microbiol 2012:713687

Verma P, Pathak K (2012) Nanosized ethanolic vesicles loaded with econazole nitrate for the treatment of deep fungal infections through topical gel formulation. Nanomed Nanotechnol Biol Med 8:489–496

Verma S, Utreja P (2018) Vesicular nanocarrier based treatment of skin fungal infections: Potential and emerging trends in nanoscale pharmacotherapy. Asian J Pharmaceut Sci 4:1–13

Wypij M, Czarnecka J, Dahm H, Rai M, Golinska P (2017) Silver nanoparticles from *Pilimelia columellifera* subsp. *pallida* SL19 strain demonstrated antifungal activity against fungi causing superficial mycoses. J Basic Microbiol 57:793–800

Zamani S, Sadeghi G, Yazdinia F, Moosa H, Pazooki A, Ghafarinia Z, Abbasi M, Shams-Ghahfarokhi M, Razzaghi-Abyaneh M (2016) Epidemiological trends of dermatophytosis in Tehran, Iran: a five-year retrospective study. J Mycol Méd 26:351–358

Chapter 6
Role of Nanostructured Materials in the Treatment of Superficial Yeast Infections

Mahendra Rai and Alka Yadav

Abstract The rising fungal infections are a major cause of public health concern. With the advancements in the clinical field, the life span of the people all over the world has increased. But in the recent decades, the microbes have also developed resistance to a considerable number of traditional and modern drugs specially bacteria and fungi. Among the various virulent properties of microbes is their ability to form biofilm, which is directly related to its ability to cause infections and increase disease severity. Superficial skin infections caused by yeast mainly include oral candidiasis and vaginal candidiasis caused by *Candida albicans* and other non-albicans species. *Candida* can occur both as yeast and filamentous fungi. However, most of the *Candida* species have become resistant to traditionally available drugs like amphotericin B, fluconazole, itraconazole, etc. Nanoparticles combined with antifungal drugs have emerged as a drug delivery system to combat infections. Hence, this chapter deals with the superficial skin infections caused by yeast, different applications of nanotechnology, the role of nanoparticles in the treatment of infections and various nanoformulations developed as nanomedicine for the treatment of yeast infections.

Keywords Infections · Fungi · *Candida albicans* · Nanoparticles · Applications · Nanoformulations

6.1 Introduction

Fungal infections are a rising health concern which is mainly related to the developments in modern medicine to increase the life span of human life (Jain et al. 2010). A wide array of broad-spectrum antibiotics has made it possible to successfully treat

M. Rai
Nanobiotechnology Laboratory, Department of Biotechnology,
Amravati, Maharashtra, India

A. Yadav (✉)
Department of Biotechnology, Sant Gadge Baba Amravati University,
Amravati, Maharashtra, India

© Springer Nature Switzerland AG 2020
M. Rai (ed.), *Nanotechnology in Skin, Soft Tissue, and Bone Infections*,
https://doi.org/10.1007/978-3-030-35147-2_6

microbial infections fatal to existence resulting in expanded survival of patients (Voltan et al. 2017). Fungi occur in the form of yeast, mold, and dimorph. The skin infections caused due to fungi are categorized into superficial and deep infections (Santos et al. 2010). The superficial infections affect the epidermis, hairs, nails, and the mucous membrane. There are three most common types of superficial skin infections including dermatophytosis, *Tinea versicolor,* and candidiasis (Flores et al. 2009).

Candida species are the major yeast pathogens causing superficial fungal infections (Radhakrishnan et al. 2018). These infections occur in the form of oral thrush, diaper rash, vaginal yeast infection, etc. (Castillo et al. 2018). *C. albicans* is the main cause of candidiasis but other *Candida* species like *C. glabrata*, *C. parapsilosis*, *C.krusei*, and *C.tropicalis* are emerging as reasons for infections. Candidiasis is a common infection found all over the world. *C. albicans* is an opportunistic pathogen which exists both in yeast and fungal form. It's a commensal microbe found in gastrointestinal, respiratory, and genitourinary tract. It occurs predominantly in oral, genital, and cutaneous infections (Castillo et al. 2018).

The drugs used for the treatment of candidiasis include polyenes (amphotericin B and nystatin) with highest rate of success. The other drugs used for treatment include azoles (fluconazole and itraconazole), allylamines, and echinocandins (caspofungin, anidulafungin, and micafungin) (Castillo et al. 2018). However, the extensive and indiscriminate use of antifungal drugs has led to the appearance of more drug-resistant fungal species and lack of new drugs.

In this scenario, nanotechnology and nanoparticles have emerged as tools to overcome drug resistance. Nanoparticles system offers reduced toxicity, targeted tissue delivery, and increased bioavailability for the treatment of fungal infections (Ghosh 2019). Nanoparticles possess unique physicochemical and biological properties which makes them approving for several biomedical applications. Nanoparticles can be differentiated into organic, inorganic, or hybrid nanoparticles to highlight their advantages in diagnostics and therapeutics. Organic materials based nanomedicine utilizes biocompatible polymers like liposomes (carbohydrates, proteins, lipids, etc.) and are used in therapeutics due to controlled size, stability and drug entrapment and sustained drug release. Inorganic nanoparticles include transition metals (silver, gold, platinum, iron, cobalt, titanium, etc.) which possess unique optical, physical, and magnetic properties which make them multifunctional for biomedical applications (Bhardwaj and Kaushik 2017). A recent addition in the field of nanotechnology is the "nanocomposites." Nanocomposites combine the properties of two or more inorganic nanomaterials and can be efficiently used in drug delivery (Ramos et al. 2019).

Nanoformulations are a promising application of nanotechnology and are more advantageous compared to synthetic formulations due to high efficiency, minimum adverse effects and cost effectiveness. Novel dermatological and cosmetic preparations are introduced into the market everyday for the treatment of skin infections. However, chemical preservatives are used in these preparations to increase their shelf life. Introduction of nanoparticles in cosmetic formulations can increase their shelf life as well as stability. Nanoparticles like silver and zinc oxide possess significant antibacterial and antifungal properties. The incorporation of nanoparticles in cosmetic based products would replace conventional preservatives and also offer advantages like better penetration, UV protection, long lasting effects, etc. (Sonia et al. 2017).

In this chapter also we review the role of nanotechnology and nanoparticles in the treatment of superficial skin infections caused by yeast. Various nanoparticles and combination of nanoparticles with existing drugs show promise to treat microbial drug resistance. Nanomaterials like silver, gold, zinc oxide, and chitosan exhibit antimicrobial properties; nanoformulations prepared by harnessing these nanoparticles have also been discussed in the chapter.

6.2   Nanomaterials and Biomedical Applications of Nanotechnology

Nanotechnology and nanomaterials have shown significant advancement in medicine and health care system leading to a new terminology "Nanomedicine" (Bhardwaj and Kaushik 2017). Nanoparticles are solid colloidal particles varying in size from 1 to 100 nm. Nanoparticles due to their large surface area to volume ratio, low toxicity, biocompatibility, and chemical stability provide many biomedical applications (McNamara and Tofail 2016). The biomedical applications of nanomaterials include drug delivery, tissue engineering, biosensors, implants, etc. Enlisted are few biomedical applications of metal nanoparticles (Fig. 6.1):

- **Nanoparticles as drug delivery vehicles:** Research in nanomedicine is focusing on the use of nanoparticles as drug delivery vehicles for efficient delivery of drugs

Fig. 6.1 Schematic showing biomedical applications of nanoparticles

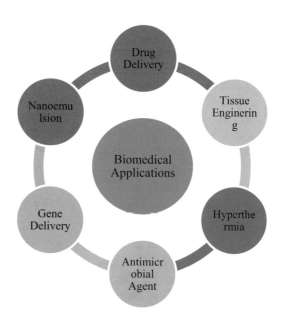

to the target site. Quantum dots, carbon nanotubes, chitosan, dendrimer, and polymer nanoparticles are widely investigated for their application in diagnostics. Inorganic hollow nanoparticles and nanotubes due to their generic transport ability and functionality have attracted interest in nanomedicine. Mesoporous silica nanoparticles offer application in loading and releasing large quantities of biomedical agents (Saji et al. 2010).

- **Tissue and implant engineering:** Due to their higher surface area to volume ratio, nanoparticles have found application in tissue and implant engineering. Titanium nanoparticles are considered to be most advantageous for bone replacement applications. Titanium depicts improved mechanical properties, high resistance to corrosion, low surface reactivity, and high biocompatibility in vitro and in vivo. Hence, titanium nanoparticles are highly used for dental and bone implants (Ramos et al. 2017).
- **Nanoparticles for gene delivery:** Gene therapy is a tool used for the treatment and/or prevention of genetic disorders by repairing the defective genes responsible for the ailment. Nanoparticles based non-viral vectors are used to transport plasmid DNA. Thus, nanomaterials based gene therapy could replace currently used viral vectors due to their potentially less nanosize (Muthu Lakshmi et al. 2017).
- **Antimicrobial Agents:** A major concern of the health care industry is the alarming rise in the phenomenon of pathogenic drug-resistant microbes. Silver nanoparticles depict bactericidal effects against both gram-positive and gram-negative micro-organisms (Lara et al. 2015). Also, it possesses anti-pathogenic effects against both planktonic and biofilm producing microbes. Thus, silver nanoparticles are used for various clinical purposes like antibacterial coats, coating medical devices, catheters, burn ointments, etc. (Burdusel et al. 2018).
- **Hyperthermia:** Hyperthermia is a technique in which heat is used to destroy malignant cells and tissues. In this process, the temperature of diseased cell is raised to 41–46°C to kill the malignant cells without damaging healthy cells (McNamara and Tofail 2016).
- **Nanoemulsions:** Nanoemulsions are heterogenous systems in which one phase is dispersed in another phase in the form of droplets in presence of an emulsifying agent. The physical and chemical properties of nanoemulsions are controlled by their composition, hence they are synthesized under strictly controlled conditions. Nanoemulsions are kinetically stable systems and possess several applications like drug delivery, antimicrobial agent, etc. (Ramos et al. 2019).

6.3   Role of Nanoparticles in the Treatment of Yeast Infections

A notable problem in the treatment of infections is the delivery of the drugs to the target site and also the growing number of antibiotic-resistant micro-organisms (Khadka et al. 2016). A major breakthrough in the medical field has been the reduc-

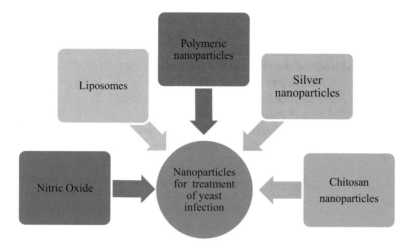

Fig. 6.2 Schematic of nanoparticles used for the treatment of yeast infections

tion of size from micrometer to nanometer. Thus, due to their small dimensions nanoparticles can target specific site of cells and tissues and deliver the drug where traditional drugs do not reach. Nanomaterials exhibit unique physical, chemical, and biological properties, which help in their enhanced use in the biomedical field (Ronavari et al. 2018). Nanomaterials like liposomes, polymeric nanoparticles, chitosan, dendrimers, silica, and other nanoparticles are used in medicine for diagnosis, treatment, and prevention of diseases (Fig. 6.2).

- **Liposomes**: Liposomes are a type of lipid formulations consisting of unilamellar or multilamellar layers of membrane lipids like phospholipids bounded by aqueous compartment. Liposomes carry hydrophilic drugs in the aqueous core and penetrate through the lipophilic membrane. Lipophilic drugs are inserted into the lipid bilayer increasing their solubility to the body fluids. Liposomes are biocompatible and biodegradable (Voltan et al. 2017).
- **Chitosan**: Chitosan has been widely used in topical formulations for ocular, mucosal, or skin applications due to its mucoadhesive and antimicrobial properties. Perinelli et al. (2018) reported synthesis of a mixed hydroxypropyl methylcellulose (HPMC)/chitosan (CS) hydrogel and evaluated its anticandidal activity against eight different albicans and non-albicans strains. Hydrogels containing 1% w/w chitosan depicted improved mucoadhesiveness and anticandidal activity against all tested *C. albicans* and non-albicans species. Thus, it was confirmed that the HPMC/CS mixed hydrogels are useful for the prevention and treatment of *Candida* infections
- **Nitric Oxide**: Nitric oxide regulates skin homeostasis by balancing circulation, UV-mediated melanogenesis, erythema, and wound healing. Thus, Macherla et al. (2012) developed nitric oxide releasing nanoparticles (NO-np) and studied its efficacy against burn infections. For the study a murine burn model was used and the antifungal activity of NO-np was checked against *C. albicans* in vivo.

The NO-np depicted efficiency against the yeast and filamentous form of *C. albicans* most likely by arresting its growth and morphogenesis. Also, the NO-np distinctly fastened wound healing in cutaneous burn infections and in the histopathological study of the affected tissues it was observed that the NO-np modified leukocyte infiltration, reduced fungal burden, and collagen degradation. Thus, the authors concluded that NO-np can be used ably as an antifungal agent for wound healing and burn infections.

- **Silver nanoparticles**: Silver nanoparticles are known for their enhanced antimicrobial activity against numerous drug-resistant microbes (Keuk-Jun et al. 2008). Silver nanoparticles efficiently kill the microbes without causing any host toxicity. Radhakrishnan et al. (2018) reported silver nanoparticles induced toxicity against *C. albicans*. The silver nanoparticles (AgNPs) were synthesized using chemical reduction method and characterized. The antifungal activity of the AgNPs was checked using broth microdilution and spot assay. In the study, spherical AgNPs were synthesized with mean size 10–30 nm and depicted minimum inhibitory concentration at 40 µg/mL. The results also revealed that AgNPs induced dose-dependent intracellular ROS (Reactive Oxygen Species) which exerted antifungal effects. The AgNPs distorted the surface morphology, cellular structure, membrane fluidity, ergosterol content, and fatty acid composition specially of oleic acid.

- **Polymeric Nanoparticles**: Natural or synthetic polymers are used for the synthesis of polymeric nanoparticles (Levya-Gomez et al. 2018). Natural polymers like collagen, albumin, gelatin, etc. and polysaccharides like alginate, agarose, hyaluronic acid are biodegradable in vivo, hence they are used to a lesser extent. Synthetic preformed polymers are more preferred in the pharmaceutical field due to their biocompatibility. Choice of the polymer depends on the properties of the system, targeted drug release, biocompatibility, etc. Polyethylene glycol (PEG) is the most widely used polymer in the drug delivery field (Levya-Gomez et al. 2018).

- **Other Nanoparticles**: Gold nanoparticles possess unique properties compared to other inorganic nanomaterials. Khan et al. (2012) reported a novel gold nanoparticles-enhanced photodynamic therapy of methylene blue (GNP-MB) against *C. albicans* biofilm. The Scanning Electron Microscopy (SEM) and Transmission Electron Microscopy (TEM) images reported the damaging effects of the bioconjugate on the *C. albicans* biofilm. The GNP-MB conjugate distorted the cell wall integrity, nuclear integration, and metabolic viability. The fluorescence spectroscopic study confirmed type I toxicity against the biofilm. Thus, the GNP-MB conjugate could be a novel approach to control infections related to candidiasis.

Graphene nanoplatelets conjugated with zinc oxide nanorods (ZNGs) depict promising activity against human pathogen *C. albicans* (Ficociello et al. 2018). For the study, the biocomposite nanomaterial was synthesized using the hydrothermal method. The antifungal study showed noteworthy reduction in fungal cells. The reactive oxygen species (ROS) formation was hypothesized to be responsible for the death of fungal cells. The toxicity study of the nanomaterial was checked against human keratinocyte cell line HaCaT and it was concluded that the ZNGs were no-toxic in their aggregation state. Hence, ZNGs are considered to be used as an antifungal agent due to high compatibility with human cells.

6.4 Nanoformulations

Nanoformulations based on traditionally available drugs have attracted interest in recent times for drug delivery applications. Due to their distinctive properties, nanoformulations enhance the properties of conventional drugs. Liposomes, dendrimers, polymeric nanoparticles, magnetic nanoparticles, and micelles are some of the nanoformulations that are gaining impotence in medical field for improved drug formulation (Jeevanandam et al. 2016; Niemirowicz and Bucki 2017).

Nanostructure layered double hydroxides have received considerable attention for their application in slow and controlled release of drug formulations. Perera et al. (2015) reported encapsulation of citric acid into an Mg-Al-layered double hydroxide (LDH) to formulate a slow release topical skin formulation containing cocoa butter using one step co-precipitation reaction technique. The nanoformulation was characterized using XRD and FTIR, the results of which showed the change in the electron density around the carboxylate groups of the citrate ion providing evidence for formation of encapsulated hybrid composite. In the study, both the citrate LDH and the cream depicted prolonged slow release up to 8 h in aqueous medium. Also, the nanoformulated cream was checked for antifungal activity against *C. albicans*, *C. glabrata*, and *C. tropicalis*. The formulated cream demonstrated improved activity and slow release up to 48 h against *C. albicans* and *C. glabrata* but not for *C. tropicalis*.

Raghuvanshi et al. (2017) studied the therapeutic effect of nano-gold nanoparticles synthesized biologically using *Woodfordia fruticosa* (WfAuNPs) and reported its microbial adhesion and wound healing potential on Wistar albino rats. The biosynthesized WfAuNPs were characterized using UV-vis spectroscopy, XRD, FTIR, dynamic light scattering (DLS), zeta potential, Field Emission Scanning Electron Microscopy (FE-SEM), and High Resolution Transmission Electron Microscopy (HR-TEM). The UV-vis spectra of WfAuNPs were recorded at 524 nm and the nanoparticles were observed to be crystalline in nature in the XRD study. The WfAuNPs exhibited high negative surface zeta potential value (-29.9) and stability. The biogenically synthesized WfAuNPs in the size range of 10–20 nm were used to develop 1%Carbopol®934 based nanoformulation (WfAuNPs-Carbopol®934) and evaluated for viscosity and spreadability measurements. The wound healing capacity of the nanoformulation was tested up to 12 days by performing wound contraction (%), epithelialization, and histopathological studies on Wistar albino rats. The results of the study depicted rapid aggregation of collagen fibrils, granular tissue formation, and rejuvenation of epithelial lining leading to fast healing and closure of wounds compared to marketed drug (5% povidone iodine). The microbial adhesion leading to biofilm formation was checked against *C. albicans* and *Cryptococcus neoformans*.

In the study, it was confirmed that the nanoformulation was more effective than the current marketed formulations.

Niemirowicz et al. (2017) formulated magnetic nanoparticles coated with cathelicidin LL-37 and ceragenin CSA-13 and checked their candidacidal activity. For the study, LL-37 peptide, ceragenin-13 and its magnetic derivatives (MNP@LL-37, MNP@CSA-13) were checked for their fungicidal activity against clinical and laboratory strains of *C. albicans*, *C. glabrata*, and *C. tropicalis*. The authors reported that the incubation of fungal cells with MNP inactivated the catalase Cta 1 and disturbed the oxidation reduction balance. Also, the MNPs coated with LL-37 and CSA-13 increased generation of ROS, destruction of fungal cell wall integrity enhanced MNP internalization and exertion of oxidative damage.

Nanocosmetics is a recent application of nanotechnology. Sonia et al. (2017) exploited colloidal zinc oxide nanoparticles (ZnONps) as a potential biomaterial for formulation of a topical cold cream. For the study, ZnONps were synthesized using the *Adhatoda vasica* leaf extract and characterized. The ZnONps were found to be of 10–12 nm particle size with hexagonal structure. The zeta potential of the ZnONps was measured at −24.6 mV confirming the stability of the nanoparticles. The antibacterial and antifungal activity of the ZnONps were calculated by measuring the zone of inhibition and it was found to be 08.667 ± 0.282 to 21.666 ± 0.447 (mm), 09.000 ± 0.177 to 19.000 ± 0.307 (mm). The IC50 value exerted from the antioxidant activity of ZnONps was observed to be 139.27 µg/mL. The microbicidal and antioxidant properties of the cold cream infused with ZnONps were tested against clinical skin pathogens and depicted significant inhibitory activity against *Candida* species.

Raj et al. (2018) designed nano zinc oxide (ZnO NP) formulations based on poly methyl methacrylate (PMMA) matrix using facile ex situ compression molding technique. The nanoformulations were tested for biocompatibility and mechanical properties; it was observed that 75% of the fibroblasts were alive and also the mechanical properties were enhanced by addition of 1wt% ZnO NP. The ZnO NP formulation depicted potential biofilm-resisting effects against *C. albicans* and *Streptococcus* mutans. This nanoformulation was found to be suitable for biomedical applications like bone replacement, skin/tissue engineering, implants, etc.

Amphotericin B (AmB) is a broad-spectrum antifungal drug used for the treatment of fungal infections. However, its wide spectrum use is limited due to severe side effects and toxicity, especially nephrotoxicity. Marcano et al. (2018) formulated chitosan coated poly (Ɛ-caprolactone) nanoparticles for oral delivery of AmB, thus reducing its toxicity. The nanoparticles were developed using the nanoprecipitation technique and characterized using parameters like particle size, polydispersity, zeta potential, morphology, in vitro AmB release, molecular aggregation, cytotoxicity, and in vitro antifungal activity. The nanoparticles were observed to be of mean size 318 ± 35 nm, zeta potential of $+36.2 \pm 1.8$ mV due to chitosan coating and 69% of AmB encapsulation. The release of nanoparticles in gastrointestinal fluids depicted good stability of chitosan-coated nanoparticles. The cytotoxicity study of nanoparticles over erythrocytes and Vero cell lines showed that nanoencapsulation efficiently reduced AmB related cytotoxicity. Also, the antifungal activity of chitosan-coated nanoparticles was five times higher compared to free AmB against *C. parapsilosis*. Thus, the nanoformulation was considered to be a potent carrier for oral AmB delivery.

Miltefosine (MFS) is used as an alternative antifungal agent, but it presents various side effects. Thus, Spadari et al. (2019) designed miltefosine loaded alginate nanoparticles (MFS.Alg) to reduce toxicity of miltefosine and use it as an antifungal agent against candidiasis and cryptococcosis. Alginate nanoparticles were synthesized using external emulsification/gelation method. The alginate obtained ranged in size from 279.1 ± 56.7 nm with a polydispersity index of 0.42 ± 0.15 and a zeta potential of −39.7 ± 5.2 mV. The encapsulation efficiency of MFS was found to be 81.70 ± 6.64% and its release from the nanoparticles was observed to be in a sustained manner. The MFS.Alg nanoparticles were checked for their antifungal activity in vitro and in vivo against larval models of *G. mellonella* infected with *Candida albicans* (SC5314 and IAL-40), *Cryptococcus neoformans* H99, and *Cryptococcus gattii* ATCC 56990. The MFS.Alg nanoparticles depicted no hemolytic effect and toxicity in *G. mellonella* larvae. Also, MFS.Alg nanoparticles extended the survival time of larvae infected with *C. albicans* and *C. gattii*. The CFU (colony forming unit) study of the nanoparticles revealed that the MFS.Alg nanoformulation reduced the fungal burden.

Candida tropicalis is one of the most virulent and drug-resistant microbe among the *Candida* species. Thus, an alternative antimicrobial therapy is needed to destroy the *C. tropicalis* infection. Hsieh et al. (2019) formulated cationic chitosan/tripolyphosphate nanoparticles to encapsulate phthalocyanine (FNP) (Fig. 6.3).

Phthalocyanine is similar to porphyrin and used as photosensitizer. The encapsulation increased fourfold accessibility of FePC to *C. tropicalis* cells. Also, in the study FNP-PDT inhibited the growth of *C. tropicalis* but was not highly toxic.

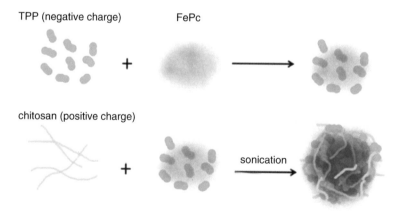

Fig. 6.3 Diagrammatic presentation of the fabrication of phthalocyanine encapsulated chitosan/TPP nanoparticles (FNP) from chitosan, tripolyphosphate (TPP), and phthalocyanine-4,4′,4″,4‴-tetrasulfonic acid (FePC) (Hsieh et al. 2019)

However, PDT as an antifungal agent, flucytosine killed *C. tropicalis* cells but could not eliminate the pseudohyphae. But when applied together FNP-PDT and flucytosine significantly restrained the growth of *C. tropicalis*.

6.5 Conclusion

The rising case of developing antibiotic resistance in many micro-organisms has encouraged researchers to explore novel approaches to combat infections and improve human life. Yeast infections are complex to treat due to the formation of biofilm. In this scenario, nanotechnology and nanoparticles have emerged as alternative therapy to kill drug-resistant *Candida* cells and reduce biofilm-associated virulence. Nanoparticles in association with traditionally available drugs have shown improved antifungal properties and faster wound healing. Also, the nanoformulations are more target specific due to their multifunctional properties. However, despite the significant advancements a control over size, stability, and functionality of nanoparticles need to be considered in the formulation and functionality of novel next-generation nanomaterials.

References

Bhardwaj V, Kaushik A (2017) Biomedical applications of nanotechnology and nanomaterials. Micromachines 8:298

Burdusel AC, Gherasim O, Grumezescu AM, Mogoanta L, Ficai A, Andronescu E (2018) Biomedical applications of silver nanoparticles: an up-to-date review. Nanomaterials 8:681

Castillo HAP, Castellanos LNM, Chamorro RM, Martinez RR, Borunda EO (2018) In: Sandai D (ed) Nanoparticles as new therapeutic agent against *Candida albicans*. IntechOpen, London. https://doi.org/10.5772/intechopen.80379

Ficociello G, De Caris MG, Trillo G, Cavallini D, Sarto MS, Uccelletti D, Mancini P (2018) Anti-candidal activity and *in vitro* cytotoxicity assessment of graphene nanoplatelets decorated with zinc oxide nanorods. Nanomaterials 8:752

Flores JM, Castillo VB, Franco FC, Huata AB (2009) Superficial fungal infections: clinical and epimediological study in adolescents from marginal districts Lima and Callao, Peru. J Infect Dev Ctries 3(4):313–317

Ghosh S (2019) Green synthesis of nanoparticles and fungal infection. https://doi.org/10.1016/B978-0-08-102579-6.00004-6

Hsieh YH, Chuang WC, Yu KH, Jheng CP, Lee CI (2019) Sequential photodynamic therapy with Phthalocyanine encapsulated chitosan-tripolyphospahte nanoparticles and flucytosine treatment against *Candia tropicalis*. Pharmaceutics 11(16):1–11

Jain A, Jain S, Rawat S (2010) Emerging fungal infections among children: a review on its clinical manifestations, diagnosis, and prevention. J Pharm Bioallied Sci 2(4):314–320

Jeevanandam J, Chan YS, Danquah MK (2016) Nano-formulations of drugs: recent developments, impact and challenges. Biochimie 128-129:99–112

Keuk-Jun K, Sung SW, Moon SK, Choi JS, Kim JC, Lee DG (2008) Antifungal effect of silver nanoparticles on dermatophytes. J Microbiol Biotechnol 18(8):1482–1484

Khadka S, Sherchand JB, Pokharel DB, Pokhrel BM, Mishra SK, Dhital S, Rijal B (2016) Clinicomycological characterization of superficial mycoses from a tertiary care hospital in Nepal. Dermatol Res Pract 9509705:1–8

Khan S, Alam F, Azam A, Khan AU (2012) Gold nanoparticles enhance methylene blue-induced photodynamic therapy: a novel therapeutic approach to inhibit *Candida albicans* biofilm. Int J Nanomedicine 7:3245–3257

Lara HH, Romero-Urbina DG, Pierce C, Lopez-Ribot JL, Arellano-Jimenez MJ, Jose-Yacaman M (2015) Effect of silver nanoparticles on *Candida albicans* biofilms: an ultrastructural study. J Nanobiotechnol 13:91

Levya-Gomez G, Pinon-Segundo E, Mendoza-Munoz N, Zambrano-Zaragoza ML, Mendoza-Elvira S, Quintanar-Guerrero D (2018) Approaches in polymeric nanoparticles for vaginal drug delivery: a review of the state of the art. Int J Mol Sci 19:1549

Macherla C, Sanchez DA, Ahmadi MS, Vellozzi EM, Friedman AJ, Nosanchuk JD, Martinez LR (2012) Nitric oxide releasing nanoparticles for treatment of *Candida albicans* burn infections. Front Microbiol 3:193

Marcano RGJV, Tominaga TT, Khalil NM, Pedroso LS, Mainardes RM (2018) Chitosan functionalized poly (Ɛ-caprolactone) nanoparticles for Amphotericin-B delivery. Carbohydr Polym 202:345–354

McNamara K, Tofail SAM (2016) Nanoparticles in biomedical applications. Adv Phys X 2(1):54–88

Muthu Lakshmi NV, Poojitha C, Swarajyalakshmi B (2017) Applications of nanotechnology in medical field. Int J Adv Sci Technol Eng Manage Sci 3(3):5–11

Niemirowicz K, Bucki R (2017) Enhancing the fungicidal activity of antibiotics: are magnetic nanoparticles the key? Nanomedicine 12(15):1747–1749

Niemirowicz K, Durnas B, Tokajuk G, Piktel E, Michalak G, Gu X, Kulakowska A, Savage PB, Bucki R (2017) Formulation and Candidacidal activity of magnetic nanoparticles coated with cathelicidin LL-37 and ceragenin CSA-13. Sci Rep 7:4610–4622

Perera J, Weerasekera M, Kottegoda N (2015) Slow release anti-fungal skin formulations based on citric acid intercalated layered double hydroxides nanohybrids. Chem Cent J 9:27

Perinelli DR, Campana R, Skouras A, Bonacucina G, Cespi M, Mastrotto F, Baffone W, Casettari L (2018) Chitosan loaded into a hydrogel delivery system as a strategy to treat vaginal co-infection. Pharmaceutics 10:23

Radhakrishnan SV, Mudiam MKR, Kumar M, Dwivedi SP, Singh SP, Prasad T (2018) Silver nanoparticles induced alterations in multiple cellular targets, which are critical for drug susceptibilities and pathogenicity in fungal pathogen (*Candida albicans*). Int J Nanomedicine 13:2647–2663

Raghuvanshi N, Kumari P, Srivastava AK, Vashisth P, Yadav TC, Prasad R, Pruthi V (2017) Synergistic effects of *Woodfordia fruticosa* gold nanoparticles in preventing microbial adhesion and accelerating wound healing in Wistar albino rats *in vivo*. Mater Sci Eng C 80:252–262

Raj I, Mozetic M, Jayachandran VP, Jose J, Thomas S, Kalarikkal N (2018) Fracture resistant, antibiofilm adherent, self assembled PMMA/ZnO nanoformulations for biomedical applications: physico-chemical and biological perspectives of nano reinforcement. Nanotechnology 29:305704

Ramos AP, Cruz MAE, Tovani CB, Ciancaglini P (2017) Biomedical applications of nanotechnology. Biophys Rev 9:79–89

Ramos MADS, Da Silva PB, Sposito L, Bonifacio BV, Rodero CF, Dos Santos KC, Chorilli M, Bauab TM (2019) Nanotechnology based drug delivery systems for control of microbial biofilms: a review. Int J Nanomedicine 13:1179–1213

Ronavari A, Igaz N, Gopisetty MK, Szerencses B, Kovacs D, Papp C, Vagvolgyi C, Boros IM, Konya Z, Kiricsi M, Pfeiffer I (2018) Biosynthesized silver and gold nanoparticles are potent antimycotics against opportunistic pathogenic yeasts and dermatophytes. Int J Nanomedicine 13:695–703

Saji VS, Choe HC, Yeung KWK (2010) Nanotechnology in biomedical applications: a review. Int J Nanotechnol Biomater 3(2):119–139

Santos MM, Amaral S, Harmen SP, Joseph HM, Fernandes JL, Counahan ML (2010) The prevalence of common skin infections in four districts Timor-Leste: a cross sectional survey. BMC
  Infect Dis 10:61–67
Sonia S, Linda JKH, Ruckmani K, Sivakumar M (2017) Antimicrobial and antioxidant potentials
  of biosynthesized colloidal zinc oxide nanoparticles for a fortified cold cream formulation: a
  potent nanocosmeceutical application. Mater Sci Eng C 79:581–589
Spadari CC, da Silva de Bastiani FWM, Lopes LB, Ishida K (2019) Alginate nanoparticles as
  non-toxic delivery system for miltefosine in the treatment of candidiasis and cryptococcosis.
  Int J Nanomedicine 14:5187–5199
Voltan AR, Quindos G, Alarcon KPM, Fusco-Almeida AM, Mendes-Giannini MJS, Chorilli M
  (2017) Fungal diseases: could nanostructured drug delivery systems be a novel paradigm for
  therapy. Int J Nanomedicine 11:3715–3730

Chapter 7
Essential Oil Encapsulated in Nanoparticles for Treatment of Skin Infections

Hercília Maria Lins Rolim and Thais Cruz Ramalho

Abstract Skin infections are usually caused by bacteria (*Staphylococcus* and *Streptococcus*), fungi, or viruses. The treatment is essential to maintain tissue function and aesthetics. The use of essential oils as antimicrobial agents is studied as a viable option in the healing. Nano-encapsulation increases the physical stability of essential oils, enhances bioactivity, reduce toxicity, decreases volatility, and protects it from environmental interactions. Recent studies have shown that nanoparticles containing essential oils have significant antimicrobial potential against multidrug-resistant pathogens. The aim of this chapter is to discuss various studies on essential oils in combination with nanoparticles for the treatment of cutaneous infections.

Keywords Essential oils · Nanotechnology · Cutaneous infections · Antimicrobial potential

7.1 Introduction

Cutaneous infections or skin infections are usually caused by bacteria, fungi, or viruses. Many bacterial species colonize the skin as normal flora. *Staphylococcus* and *Streptococcus* are uncommon bacterial flora; however, these are the most common cause of bacterial skin infections, being considered as an aesthetic problem. Predisposing factors for infection include previous skin diseases, skin injury, poor hygiene, or low host immunity (Shortridge and Flamm 2019). The cutaneous fungal infections usually involve a number of fungi such as different species of dermatophytes including *Epidermophyton* sp., *Microsporum* spp. and *Trichophyton* spp., filamentous non-dermatophytic fungi, and infections caused by yeasts. The dermatophytic fungi are also called ringworm fungi or tinea infections. These are nonin-

H. M. L. Rolim (✉) · T. C. Ramalho
Laboratory of Pharmaceutical Nanosystems—NANOSFAR, Postgraduate Program in
Pharmaceutical Sciences, Federal University of Piauí, Teresina, Piauí, Brazil

© Springer Nature Switzerland AG 2020
M. Rai (ed.), *Nanotechnology in Skin, Soft Tissue, and Bone Infections*,
https://doi.org/10.1007/978-3-030-35147-2_7

vasive infections and are responsible for causing diseases of hair, skin, and nails. The yeasts such as various species of *Candida* cause candidiasis.

When the skin is injured, bacteria can seep into underlying tissues, potentially causing life-threatening infections. Thus, the treatment of skin wounds is essential to maintain tissue function and aesthetics (Carbone et al. 2019). The use of encapsulated essential oils (EOs) as antimicrobial agents is studied as viable options in the healing process through the bactericidal or bacteriostatic action of wounds and infections. Due to their volatile and lipophilic nature, oils are nanocapsulated to reverse these limitations (Ghodrati et al. 2019; Kaul et al. 2018).

The use of nanotechnology in the treatment of skin infections is becoming an important driving force in enhancing the antimicrobial potential of essential oils. In the current scenario, oil encapsulation occurs in different nanosystems, for example, liposomes, lipid nanoparticles, silver nanoparticles, and nanoemulsion, as promising drug delivery systems to treat skin disorders (Balasubramani et al. 2018; Thakur et al. 2018).

Nano-encapsulation increases the physical stability of essential oils, enhances bioactivity, reduces toxicity, decreases volatility, and protects it from environmental interactions (e.g., light, oxygen, moisture, pH) and also improves patient compliance (Hasani et al. 2018). In this context, oils that have antimicrobial activity when used in combination with other antimicrobial agents or nanocarriers, such as nanoparticles, may increase antimicrobial potential against various types of pathogens and different mechanisms of action. Therefore, this complementation between antimicrobials suggests a promising strategy for combating pathogens resistant to multiple existing topical drugs (Soulaimani et al. 2019; Ong et al. 2019).

The aim of this chapter is to discuss various studies antimicrobial activity of essential oils in combination with nanoparticles for the treatment of skin infections.

7.2 Nanoparticles Encapsulated with Essential Oils

Recent studies have shown that nanoparticles containing essential oils have significant antimicrobial potential against multidrug-resistant pathogens, as it allows the controlled and sustained release of the active for wound healing.

Silver nanoparticles are widely used in studies because of their small size and large surface area, providing better contact and internalization into microbial cells due to increased bioactivity and bioavailability of Ag + (Niska et al. 2018). In addition, it shows antimicrobial effects against various microorganisms, including antibiotic-resistant strains (Freire et al. 2018).

Studies with encapsulated essential oils in nanoparticles with antibacterial and antifungal activity are shown in Table 7.1.

For example, Abdellatif and Alkarib (2018) developed liposome-encapsulated silver nanoparticles (AgNPs) and tea tree oil (TTO) topical formulation, obtained from *Melaleuca alternifolia* (Myrtaceae). The AgNPs was synthesized by green synthesis method using leaves aqueous extract, and the TTO was obtained by steam

Table 7.1 Antimicrobial activity of essential oil containing nanoparticles

Source of essential oils/EOs constituents	Microbes inhibited	Nanoparticle type	References
Thymus boissieri, T. longicaulis, T. ocheus, T. leucospermus	Gram-positive and Gram-negative bacteria and human pathogenic fungi	Phosphatidylcholine and cholesterol	Gortzi et al. (2006)
Origanum dictamnus	Gram-positive and Gram-negative bacteria and fungus (*Listeria monocytogenes*)	Lipid	Gortzi et al. (2007)
Vegetable oil	*Staphylococcus aureus, E. coli*	Silver	Kumar et al. (2008)
Zanthoxylum tingoassuiba	*S. aureus*, Dermatophytes	Phosphatidylcholine	Detoni et al. (2009)
Origanum dictamnus	Gram-positive and Gram-negative bacteria and human pathogenic fungi	Phosphatidylcholine-based liposomes	Liolios et al. (2009)
Rosmarinus officinalis	*Candida albicans, C. tropicalis*	Magnetic	Chifiriuc et al. (2012)
Eugenia caryophyllata	Fungi	Magnetite/oleic acid core/shell NP	Grumezescu et al. (2012)
Syzygium aromaticum	*E. coli, S. aureus, Salmonella typhi, Pseudomonas aeruginosa, Bacillus cereus, Listeria monocytogenes*	Eugenol	Hamed et al. (2012)
Oreganum spp.	Antimicrobial	Chitosan	Hosseini et al. (2013)
Artemisia argyi	*S. aureus, E. coli*	Hydroxyapatite	Hu et al. (2013)
Oreganum spp.	*S. aureus, Listeria monocytogenes*	Silver and zinc oxide	Khalaf et al. (2013)
Anethum graveolens, Salvia officinalis	*C. albicans*	Magnetic	Anghel et al. (2013)
Prunus dulcis	*C. albicans*	Solid lipid	Cerreto et al. (2013)
Lippia sidoides	Fungicide and bactericide	Alginate/cashew gum	De Oliveira et al. (2014)
Oreganum spp.	*S. aureus, Salmonella typhimurium, Listeria monocytogenes, E. coli*	Zinc oxide and silver	Morsy et al. (2014)
Cananga odorata, Pogostemon cablin, Vanilla planifólia	*S. aureus, Klebsiella pneumoniae*	Magnetic	Bilcu et al. (2014)
Cinnamomum cassia	*Candida krusei, C. albicans, C. glabrata*	Silver	Szweda et al. (2015)
Copaifera spp.	*Candida krusei, C. parapsilosis, Trichophyton rubrum, Microsporum canis*	Solid lipid	Svetlichny et al. (2015)

(continued)

Table 7.1 (continued)

Source of essential oils/EOs constituents	Microbes inhibited	Nanoparticle type	References
Melaleuca alternifolia	*Pseudomonas aeruginosa*	Solid lipid	Comin et al. (2016)
Zataria multiflora	*Aspergillus ochraceus, Aspergillus niger, Aspergillus flavus, Alternaria solani, Rhizoctonia solani,* and *Rhizopus stolonifer*	Solid lipid	Nasseri et al. (2016)
Origanum vulgare	Gram-positive and Gram-negative bacteria	Silver	Scandorieiro et al. (2016)
Zataria multiflora	*Staphylococcus epidermidis* and *S. aureus*	Silver	Sheikholeslami et al. (2016)
Melaleuca alternifolia	*Candida* species	Solid lipid	Souza et al. (2017)
Melaleuca alternifólia (Myrtaceae)	*Staphylococcus aureus,* methicillin-resistant *Staphylococcus aureus, S. epidermidis, Streptococcus pyogenes, Klebsiella pneumoniae, Pseudomonas aeruginosa, Trichophyton mentagrophytes, C. albicans*	Silver	Abdellatif and Alkarib (2018)
Eugenia caryophyllata	*Salmonella typhi, Pseudomonas aeruginosa, Staphylococcus aureus,* and *Candida albicans*	Solid lipid	Fazly Bazzaz et al. (2018)
Eucalyptus or rosemary	*Staphylococcus aureus* and *Streptococcus pyogenes*	Solid lipid	Saporito et al. (2018)
Peppermint	*Staphylococcus aureus, E. faecium, Escherichia coli, P. aeruginosa,* and *Candida parapsilosis*	Hydroxyapatite	Badea et al. (2019)
Coriandrum sativum	*Aspergillus niger, A. fumigatus, A. sydowii, A. repens, A. versicolor, A. luchuensis, Alternaria alternata, Penicillium italicum, P. chrysogenum, P. spinulosum, Mycelia sterilia, Cladosporium herbarum, Fusarium poae,* and *F. oxysporum*	Chitosan	Das et al. (2019)
Rosemary	*Staphylococcus epidermidis, S. aureus, Listeria monocytogenes, Escherichia coli,* and *Pseudomonas aeruginosa*	Solid lipid	Khezri et al. (2019)

(continued)

Table 7.1 (continued)

Source of essential oils/EOs constituents	Microbes inhibited	Nanoparticle type	References
Peppermint	*Escherichia coli, Salmonella typhimurium, Pseudomonas aeruginosa, S. aureus, Staphylococcus epidermidis, Bacillus anthracis, Staphylococcus pneumonia,* and *Listeria monocytogenes*	Solid lipid	Ghodrati et al. (2019)
Mediterranean (*Rosmarinus officinalis, Lavandula x intermedia* "Sumian," *Origanum vulgare* subsp. *hirtum*)	*Candida albicans, C. krusei,* and *C. parapsilosis*	Solid lipid	Carbone et al. (2019)
Melaleuca alternifolia	*Staphylococcus aureus, Staphylococcus epidermidis, Streptococcus pyogenes, Klebsiella pneumoniae, Pseudomonas aeruginosa, Trichophyton mentagrophytes, Candida albicans*	Silver	Ramadan et al. (2019)
Origanum vulgare	*Alternaria alternata*	Chitosan	Yilmaz et al. (2019)

hydro-distillation of the plant leaves. AgNPs and TTO have been tested isolated and in liposome encapsulated against selected skin-infecting microbes: *Staphylococcus aureus, methicillin-resistant Staphylococcus aureus, Staphylococcus epidermidis, Streptococcus pyogenes, Klebsiella pneumoniae, Pseudomonas aeruginosa, Trichophyton mentagrophytes, Candida albicans* (Table 7.1), herpes simplex virus type 1 (HSV-1), and herpes simplex virus type 2 (HSV- 2). In vitro results showed that both TTO and AgNPs possess good antimicrobial properties against tested strains, producing marked inhibition zones (14.8–24.7 mm). However, AgNPs and TTO liposome-encapsulated formulation showed better antimicrobial activities with inhibition zones (21.3–26.4 mm). Tests against HSV-1 and HSV-2 showed that AgNPs and TTO liposome-encapsulated form had the strongest antiviral activity, causing 52.0% and 55.1% reduction of the cytopathic effect for HSV-1 and HSV-2, respectively. These results showed the potential of using AgNPs and TTO in liposome-encapsulated formulation as a promising delivery system against skin infections caused by the tested strains.

Similar to the previous study, Ramadan et al. (2019) evaluated the antimicrobial efficacy of *Melaleuca alternifolia* containing tea tree oil (TTO) and silver nanoparticles (AgNPs) against skin-infecting microbe: *Staphylococcus aureus,* methicillin-resistant *Staphylococcus aureus, Staphylococcus epidermidis, Streptococcus pyogenes, Klebsiella pneumoniae, Pseudomonas aeruginosa, Trichophyton menta-*

grophytes, Candida albicans, herpes simplex virus type 1 (HSV-1), and herpes simplex virus type 2 (HSV-2). The results of transmission electron microscopy (TEM) showed that AgNPs are homogenous and spherical with an average size of 11.56 nm. TEM micrograph showed aggregation of AgNPs around and within bacterial cells (*S. aureus*), with loss of normal cell structure indicating biocidal action. Thus, in the bioassay showed that both TTO and AgNPs possess potent antimicrobial properties against tested strains, producing marked inhibition zones (14.8–24.7 mm). The tests against HSV-1 and HSV-2 showed that AgNPs had the strongest antiviral activity, with 44.0% and 45.04% reduction of the cytopathic effect for HSV-1 and HSV-2, respectively. In conclusion, TTO and AgNPs possess good antimicrobial activities against the selected skin pathogens, and could be an alternative for treating skin infections.

Candida infection has been associated with resistance to the antimicrobial therapy and the ability of microorganism to form biofilms, in immunosuppressed patients. The present study aimed to evaluate in vitro antibiofilm activity of TTO (*Melaleuca alternifolia* containing tea tree oil) nanoparticles against many *Candida* species. The TTO nanoparticles at pH 6.3 showed mean diameter of 158.2 ± 2 nm, polydispersion index (PDI) of 0.213 ± 0.017, and zeta potential of -8.69 ± 0.80 mV. Besides that, the TTO and its nanoparticles had a significant reduction of biofilm formed by all *Candida* species (Souza et al. 2017).

Sheikholeslami et al. (2016) investigated the antibacterial activity of silver nanoparticles (AgNPs) and in combination with *Zataria multiflora* essential oil and methanolic extract on some photogenic bacteria. To determine the minimum inhibitory concentrations (MICs) and fractional inhibitory concentrations (FICs) of plant essential oil, methanolic extract, and silver nanoparticles against bacteria, the broth microdilution method and check board microtiter assays were used. The results showed that the MIC and minimal bacterial concentration (MBC) values of AgNPs against all strains were in the range of 15.625–500 µg/mL, and values for the essential oil and plant extract were in the range of 1.56–100 mg/mL. Silver nanoparticles were observed to have additive effects with essential oil against *Staphylococcus epidermidis* and *S. aureus*.

Fazly Bazzaz et al. (2018) prepared solid lipid nanoparticles containing *Eugenia caryophyllata* essential oil (SLN-EO) by high-shear homogenization and ultrasound methods. The formulations were chosen and tested to investigate the antimicrobial activity against *Salmonella typhi, Pseudomonas aeruginosa, Staphylococcus aureus,* and *Candida albicans*. For this, minimum inhibitory concentration (MIC), minimal bacterial concentration (MBC), and time-kill curves were determined. The encapsulation efficacy of EO was approximately 70%. MIC and MBC values of SLN-EO were lower than those of the oil alone. The time-kill studies showed that SLN-EO was either equivalent to or better than essential oil (*P*-value <005). The results highlighted the effectiveness of SLN formulations against human pathogens.

In a study, Ghodrati et al. (2019) evaluated the in vitro efficiency of peppermint essential oil (PEO) loaded into nanostructured lipid carriers (PEO-NLC) against bacteria and also in vivo infected wound healing in mice model. The PEO-NLC was prepared using hot melt homogenization technique. In the in vitro study, PEO and

PEO-NLC were tested against *Escherichia coli, Salmonella typhimurium, Pseudomonas aeruginosa, Staphylococcus aureus, Staphylococcus epidermidis, Bacillus anthracis, Staphylococcus pneumonia*, and *Listeria monocytogenes*. Two full-thickness wounds with the size of 5 mm were induced in each mouse and inoculated with *Pseudomonas aeruginosa* and *Staphylococcus aureus* to conduct the in vivo study. The animals were divided into four groups as control, Mupirocin®, PEO, and PEO-NLC and were performed wound contraction, bacterial count, histological examinations, and molecular analyses. Particle size analyses showed that all PEO-NLC were in the range from 40 to 250 nm with narrow PDI ~0.4 and the ZP value from −10 to −15 mV. Scanning Electron Microscopy (SEM) analysis indicated that the particles had a smooth surface, spherical, and uniformly distributed around. In vitro analysis showed that both PEO and PEO-NLC have antibacterial activities against *S. epidermidis, S. aureus, L. monocytogenes, E. coli*, and *P. aeruginosa* species. In the in vivo test, wound contraction rate, fibroblast infiltration, collagen deposition, and re-epithelialization were increased in PEO and PEO-NLC-treated animals compared to the control group. These results show the efficacy of PEO-NLC in order to treat an infected wound model and provide an option for producing topical formulations.

Some fungal and bacterial species are resistant to the usual antimicrobials, which represent a major challenge for the treatment of skin infections. Essential oils, obtained from natural source, are being widely used to increase the effectiveness of medicines in this disease. Carbone et al. (2019) developed Mediterranean essential oil (*Rosmarinus officinalis, Lavandula* × *intermedia* "Sumian," *Origanum vulgare* subsp. *hirtum*) lipid nanoparticles for clotrimazole delivery, exploring the potential synergistic effects against *Candida* spp. The nanoparticles showed small sized (<100 nm) with a broad size distribution (PDI < 0.15) and long term. In vitro biosafety results on HaCaT (normal cell line) and A431 (tumoral cell line), the authors selected *Lavandula* and *Rosmarinus* as anti-proliferative agents to use as co-adjuvants in the treatment of non-tumoral proliferative dermal diseases. In the calorimetric studies on biomembrane models, presented as a result the confirmation of the antimicrobial activity of the selected oils due to their interaction with membrane permeabilization. In vitro studies against *Candida albicans, Candida krusei,* and *Candida parapsilosis* showed enhancement of the antifungal activity of clotrimazole-loaded nanoparticles prepared with *Lavandula* or *Rosmarinus*. Therefore, nano-structured lipid carriers (NLC) containing Mediterranean essential oils represent a strategy to improve drug effectiveness against topical candidiasis.

In another study, Khezri et al. (2019) used encapsulated rosemary essential oil (REO) into nanostructured lipid carriers (NLCs) for determination of in vitro antibacterial activity and in vivo infected wound healing in the animal model. REO-NLCs morphology, size, and in vitro antibacterial activity were studied. Two full-thickness wound (each 6 mm) were made on the back of each mouse and then was infected with a solution containing 107 CFU *Staphylococcus aureus* and *Pseudomonas aeruginosa*. Animals were divided into four groups: control, Mupirocin®, and two treated groups with a gel containing REO and REO-NLCs. Therefore, bacterial count and histological assessment were performed. REO-NLCs showed antibacterial activity against *Staphylococcus epidermidis, Staphylococcus aureus, Listeria monocytogenes, Escherichia coli,* and *Pseudomonas aeruginosa.* Besides that, while REO-NLCs could reduce the rate of tissue bacterial colonization and wound size, they increased the vascularization, fibroblast infiltration, re-epithelialization, and collagen production. The authors finding revealed that the REO-NLCs have antibacterial properties and accelerated infected wound healing, which confirms their potential clinical uses for the treatment of infected wounds.

Saporito et al. (2018) developed of lipid nanoparticles (solid lipid nanoparticles and nanostructured lipid carriers [NLC]), which were loaded with eucalyptus or rosemary essential oils and evaluated as antimicrobials to enhance healing of skin wounds. Lipid nanoparticles were prepared with natural lipids: cocoa butter, as solid lipid, and olive oil or sesame oil, as liquid lipids. Lecithin was used as surfactant to stabilize nanoparticles and prevent their aggregation. The formulations were prepared by high-shear homogenization followed by ultrasound. Antimicrobial activity of nanoparticles was evaluated against *Staphylococcus aureus* and *Streptococcus pyogenes.* The capability of nanoparticles to promote wound healing in vivo was observed on a rat burn model. NLC formed from olive oil and loaded with eucalyptus oil showed appropriate physical–chemical properties, cytocompatibility, good bioadhesion, in vitro proliferation enhancement, wound healing toward fibroblastos, and antimicrobial properties. The in vivo results showed the capability of these NLC to enhance the healing process. Olive oil presented synergic effect with eucalyptus oil with respect to antimicrobial activity and wound repair process.

7.3　Conclusion and Future Perspectives

The search for new therapies to solve old problems related to efficacy of antimicrobials is essential. Unfortunately, one of the biggest challenges is the resistance of pathogens to conventional treatments. Research on essential oils has been shown to be effective, especially involving antimicrobial activities and in the nanocapsulated form recommended to ensure controlled and sustained release of the antimicrobial drugs.

Advances in nanotechnology show the use of nanoparticles to encapsulate essential oils as a way of increasing chemical stability and solubility, minimizing evaporation and degradation of their components. In addition, the use of nanoparticles allows controlled and sustained release of actives to enhance the effect of wound healing pharmaceutical formulations and efficacy against resistant pathogens. The perspective is that essential oils incorporated into nanosystem with antimicrobial activities can be used, especially for wound healing and efficacy against resistant pathogens, reducing many of the skin infection problems.

References

Abdellatif AO, Alkarib SY (2018) Development and formulation of liposome encapsulated silver nanoparticles and tea tree oil for skin infections. J Med Microbiol Diagn 7:64–73

Anghel I, Holban AM, Andronescu E, Grumezescu AM, Chifiriuc MC (2013) Efficient surface functionalization of wound dressings by a phytoactive nanocoating refractory to *Candida albicans* biofilm development. Biointerphases 8:12

Badea ML, Iconaru SL, Groza A, Chifiriuc MC, Beuran M, Predoi D (2019) Peppermint essential oil-doped hydroxyapatite nanoparticles with antimicrobial properties. Molecules 24:1–13

Balasubramani S, Moola AK, Vivek K, Kumari BDR (2018) Formulation of nanoemulsion from leaves essential oil of *Ocimum basilicum* L. and its antibacterial, antioxidant and larvicidal activities (*Culex quinquefasciatus*). Microb Pathog 125:475–485

Bilcu M, Grumezescu AM, Oprea AE, Popescu RC, Mogoşanu GD, Hristu R, Stanciu GA, Mihailescu DF, Lazar V, Bezirtzoglou E, Chifiriuc MC (2014) Efficiency of vanilla, patchouli and ylang–ylang essential oils stabilized by iron oxide@C14 nanostructures against bacterial adherence and biofilms formed by *Staphylococcus aureus* and *Klebsiella pneumoniae* clinical strains. Molecules 19:17943–17956

Carbone C, Teixeira MC, Sousa MC, Martins-Gomes C, Silva AM, Souto EMB, Musumeci T (2019) Clotrimazole-loaded mediterranean essential oils NLC: a synergic treatment of *Candida* skin infections. Pharmaceutics 11:231–243

Cerreto F, Paolicelli P, Cesa S, Abu Amara HM, D'Auria FD, Simonetti G, Casadei MA (2013) Solid lipid nanoparticles as effective reservoir systems for long-term preservation of multidose formulations. AAPS J 14:847–853

Chifiriuc C, Grumezescu V, Grumezescu AM, Saviuc C, Lazar V, Andronescu E (2012) Hybrid magnetite nanoparticles/*Rosmarinus officinalis* essential oil nanobiosystem with antibiofilm activity. Nanoscale Res Lett 7:209

Comin VM, Lopes LQS, Quatrin PM, Souza ME, Bonez PC, Pintos FG, Raffin RP, Vaucher RA, Martinez DST, Santos RCV (2016) Influence of *Melaleuca alternifolia* oil nanoparticles on aspects of *Pseudomonas aeruginosa* biofilm. Microb Pathog 93:120–125

Das S, Singh VK, Dwivedy AK, Chaudhari AK, Upadhyay N, Singh P, Sharma S, Dudey (2019) Encapsulation in chitosan-based nanomatrix as an efficient green technology to boost the antimicrobial, antioxidant and *in situ* efficacy of *Coriandrum sativum* essential oil. Int J Biol Macromol 133:294–305

De Oliveira EF, Paula HCB, De Paula RCM (2014) Alginate/cashew gum nanoparticles for essential oil encapsulation. Colloids Surf B Biointerfaces 113:146–151

Detoni CB, Cabral-Albuquerque EC, Hohlemweger SV, Sampaio C, Barros TF, Velozo ES (2009) Essential oil from *Zanthoxylum tingoassuiba* loaded into multilamellar liposomes useful as antimicrobial agents. J Microencapsul 26:684–691

Fazly Bazzaz BS, Khameneh B, Namazi N, Iranshahi N, Davoodi D, Golmohammadzadeh (2018) Solid lipid nanoparticles carrying *Eugenia caryophyllata* essential oil: the novel nanoparticulate systems with broad-spectrum antimicrobial activity. Lett Appl Microbiol 66:506–513

Freire NB, Pires LCSR, Oliveira HP, Costa MM (2018) Antimicrobial and antibiofilm activity of silver nanoparticles against *Aeromonas* spp. isolated from aquatic organisms. Pesq Vet Bras 38:244–249

Ghodrati M, Farahpour MR, Hamishehkar H (2019) Encapsulation of *Peppermint* essential oil in nanostructured lipid carriers: *in-vitro* antibacterial activity and accelerative effect on infected wound healing. Colloids Surf A Physicochem Eng Asp 564:162–169

Gortzi O, Lalas S, Chinou I, Tsaknis J (2006) Reevaluation of antimicrobial and antioxidant activity of *Thymus* sp. extracts before and after encapsulation in liposomes. J Food Prot 69:2998–3005

Gortzi O, Lalas S, Chinou I, Tsaknis J (2007) Evaluation of the antimicrobial and antioxidant activities of *Origanum dictamnus* extracts before and after encapsulation in liposomes. Molecules 12:932–945

Grumezescu AM, Chifiriuc MC, Saviuc C, Grumezescu V, Hristu R, Mihaiescu DE, Stanciu GA, Andronescu E (2012) Hybrid nanomaterial for stabilizing the antibiofilm activity of *Eugenia caryophyllata* essential oil. IEEE T Nano Bio Sci 11:360–365

Hamed SF, Sadek Z, Edris A (2012) Antioxidant and antimicrobial activities of clove bud essential oil and eugenol nanoparticles in alcohol-free microemulsion. J Oleo Sci 61:641–648

Hasani S, Ojagh SM, Ghorbani M (2018) Nanoencapsulation of lemon essential oil in chitosan-Hicap system. Part 1: study on its physical and structural characteristics. Int J Biol Macromol 115:143–151

Hosseini SF, Zandi M, Rezaei M, Farahmandghavi F (2013) Two-step method for encapsulation of oregano essential oil in chitosan nanoparticles: preparation, characterization and in vitro release study. Carbohydr Polym 95:50–56

Hu Y, Yang Y, Ning Y, Wang C, Tong Z (2013) Facile preparation of *Artemisia argyi* oil-loaded antibacterial microcapsules by hydroxyapatite-stabilizedpickering emulsion templating. Colloids Surf B Biointerfaces 112:96–102

Kaul S, Gulati N, Verma D, Mukherjee S, Nagaich U (2018) Role of nanotechnology in cosmeceuticals: a review of recent advances. J Pharm 1:19

Khalaf HH, Sharoba AM, El-Tanahi HH, Morsy MK (2013) Stability of antimicrobial activity of pullulan edible films incorporated with nanoparticles and essential oils and their impact on Turkey deli meat quality. J Food Dairy Sci Mansoura Univ 4:557–573

Khezri K, Farahpour MR, Rad SM (2019) Accelerated infected wound healing by topical application of encapsulated rosemary essential oil into nanostructured lipid carriers. Artif Cell Nanomed Biotechnol 47:980–988

Kumar A, Vemula PK, Ajayan PM, John G (2008) Silver nanoparticle embedded antimicrobial paints based on vegetable oil. Nat Mater 7:236–241

Liolios CC, Gortzi O, Lalas S, Tsaknis J, Chinou I (2009) Liposomal incorporation of carvacrol and thymol isolated from the essential oil of *Origanum dictamnus* L: and in vitro antimicrobial activity. Food Chem 112:77–783

Morsy MK, Khalaf HH, Sharoba AM, El-Tanahi HH, Cutter CN (2014) Incorporation of essential oils and nanoparticles in pullulan films to control foodborne pathogens on meat and poultry products. J Food Sci 79:675–684

Nasseri M, Golmohammadzadeh S, Arouiee H, Jaafari MR, Neamati H (2016) Antifungal activity of *Zataria multiflora* essencial oil-loaded solid lipid nanoparticles *in vitro* condition. Iran J Basic Med Sci 19:1231–1237

Niska K, Zielina E, Radomski MW, Inkielewicz-Stepniak I (2018) Metal nanoparticles in dermatology and cosmetology: interactions with human skin cells. Chem Biol Interact 295:38–51

Ong TH, Chitra E, Ramamurthy S, Ling CCS, Ambu SP, Davamani F (2019) Cationic chitosan-propolis nanoparticles alter the zeta potential of *S. epidermidis*, inhibit biofilm formation by modulating gene expression and exhibit synergism with antibiotics. PLoS One 14:1–13

Ramadan MA, Shawkey AE, Mohamed AR, Abdellatif AO (2019) Promising antimicrobial activities of oil and silver nanoparticles obtained from *Melaleuca alternifolia* leaves against selected skin-infecting pathogens. J Herb Med 100289

Saporito F, Sandri G, Benferoni MV, Rossi S, Boselli C, Cornaglia IA, Mannucci B, Grisoli P, Vigani B, Ferrari F (2018) Essencial oil-loaded lipid nanoparticles for wound healing. Int J Nanomedicine 12:175–186

Scandorieiro S, Camargo LC, Lancheros CAC, Yamada-Ogatta SF, Nakamura CV, Oliveira AG, Andrade CGTJ, Duran N, Nakazato G, Kobayashi RKT (2016) Synergistic and additive effect of oregano essential oil and biological silver nanoparticles against multidrug-resistant bacterial strains. Front Microbiol 7:760

Sheikholeslami S, Mousavi SE, Ashtiani HRA, Doust SRH, Rezayat SM (2016) Antibacterial activity of silver nanoparticles and their combination with *Zataria multiflora* essential oil and methanol extract. Jundishapur J Microbiol 9:360–370

Shortridge D, Flamm RK (2019) Comparative *in vitro* activites of new antibiotics for the treatment of skin infections. Clin Infect Dis 68:200–2005

Soulaimani B, Nafis A, Kasrati A, Rochdi A, Mezrioui NE, Abbad A, Hassani L (2019) Chemical composition, antimicrobial activity and synergistic potencial of essential oil from endemic *Lavandula maroccana* (Mill.). S Afr J Bot 125:202–206

Souza ME, Lopes LQS, Bonez PC, Gundel A, Martinez DST, Sagrillo MR, Giongo JL, Vaucher RA, Raffin RP, Boligon AA, Santos RCV (2017) *Melaleuca alternifolia* nanoparticles against *Candida* species biofilms. Microb Pathog 104:125–132

Svetlichny G, Külkamp-Guerreiro IC, Cunha SL, Silva FE, Bueno K, Pohlmann AR, Fuentefria AM, Guterres SS (2015) Solid lipid nanoparticles containing copaiba oil and allantoin: development and role of nanoencapsulation on the antifungal activity. Pharmazie 70:155–164

Szweda P, Gucwa K, Kurzyk E, Romanowska E, Dzier K, Fangrat Z, Zielinska-Jurek A, Kus PM, Milewski S (2015) Essential oils, silver nanoparticles and propolis as alternative agents against fluconazole resistant *Candida albicans, Candida glabrata* and *Candida krusei* clinical isolates. Indian J Microbiol 55:175–183

Thakur K, Sharma G, Singh B, Chhibber S, Katare OP (2018) Current state of nanomedicines in the treatment of topical infectious disorders. Recent Pat Antiinfect Drug Discov 13:127–150

Yilmaz MT, Yilmaz A, Akman PK, Bozkurt F, Dertli E, Basahel A, Al-Sasi B, Taylan O, Sagdic O (2019) Electrospraying method for fabrication of essential oil loaded-chitosan nanoparticle delivery systems characterized by molecular, thermal, morphological and antifungal properties. Innov Food Sci Emerg Technol 52:166–178

Part II
Soft Tissue Infections

Chapter 8
Nanotechnological Approaches to Manage Diabetic Foot Ulcer

Aswathy Jayakumar and E. K. Radhakrishnan

Abstract Diabetic foot ulcers (DFUs) are chronic, non-healing complications associated with diabetes mellitus and these account for morbidity, mortality, poor psychosocial adjustment, and health care expenditures. The major risk factors which prevent the healing process of DFUs are diabetic neuropathy, peripheral vascular diseases, and abnormal immune responses. The chronic nature of DFU imposes an immense challenge to conventional treatments and has led to the emergence of nanotechnology-based therapeutics. The unique biological, chemical, and physical properties of nanomaterials make them to have significant applications to treat chronic diabetic ulcers. The current chapter is designed to discuss the nanotechnological approaches in treating chronic diabetic foot ulcers and its healing. The chapter specifically includes pathology of DFUs, standard of care, and the various nanomaterials with promises for chronic wound healing.

Keywords Diabetic foot ulcer · Pathology · Treatments and nanotechnology

8.1 Introduction

Diabetic foot ulcers (DFUs) are the major complications associated with diabetes mellitus and can be defined as the ulcerations of the diabetic foot associated with neuropathy or peripheral arterial diseases of lower limb, cytokine/chemokine activity that leads to morbidity, mortality, and hospitalizations. About 19–34% of patients with diabetes are expected to be affected with DFUs. The occurrence of DFUs is expected to be more frequent in aged patients. About 60–80% of DFUs will heal, 10–15% remains active, and 5–24% will lead to limb amputations (Everett and Mathioudakis 2018). The major risk factors concerned in the development of DFUs are older aging, infections, poor glycemic control, diabetic neuropathy, smoking habit, peripheral vascular diseases, ischemia, previous foot ulcer, amputation, and

A. Jayakumar · E. K. Radhakrishnan (✉)
School of Biosciences, Mahatma Gandhi University, Kottayam, Kerala, India
e-mail: radhakrishnanek@mgu.ac.in

© Springer Nature Switzerland AG 2020
M. Rai (ed.), *Nanotechnology in Skin, Soft Tissue, and Bone Infections*,
https://doi.org/10.1007/978-3-030-35147-2_8

the reduced personal care. DFUs are painless due to the lower concentration of sensory neuron and lead to decreased pressure, heat, and pain sensation. In addition to neuropathy and imbalance in biochemical function, diabetic patients are generally in a hypercoagulable condition with decreased fibrinolysis which can lead to vascular injury. Impaired angiogenesis leads to decreased flow of blood, impaired inflammation, leukocyte chemotaxis restriction, and thereby altered the pathogen elimination.

Non-migratory epidermis, unresolved inflammation, impaired fibroblast function, ECM deposition, decreased angiogenesis, increase in metalloproteinases level, and polymicrobial infections are characteristic features of chronic wounds. Several treatment approaches have been adopted to treat diabetic foot ulceration and include the use of various topical and systemic compounds. Many of the treatment methods are challenged by the emergence of multidrug-resistant bacteria and the non-healing wounds. The complications with chronic ulcerations and the failure of other conventional treatments paved the way for the emergence of nanotechnology-based therapeutic agents.

Nanotechnology-based treatment strategies play an important role in the diagnosis, repair, and control of human diseases at cellular level. Nowadays, several nanoparticles are proposed for treating chronic infections and for wound healing. Most of them are under research and some are under clinical trials. Hence, this chapter has been designed to discuss about the recent progress in nanotechnological methods for diabetic foot ulcer healing.

8.2   Pathology of Diabetic Foot Ulcer

Approximately 405.6 million adults are affected with type 2 diabetes around the world and are predicted to reach more than 510.8 million by 2030 (Basu et al. 2019). Mainly, type 2 diabetes is characterized by the resistance to insulin and its declined glycemic control The major diabetic complications include retinopathy, impaired wound healing, ischemia, kidney failure, and peripheral neuropathy which can lead to the formation of chronic diabetic foot ulcer (Mavrogenis et al. 2018).

About 15–25% of diabetic patients can develop foot ulcers which eventually lead to amputation (Behl et al. 2019). Woefully, the survival rate after amputation is only up to 3 years due to the chronic infection and vascular damage. The major reason behind is that the person with DFU does not pass through the normal wound healing stages such as inflammation, re-epithelialization, and wound remodeling (Fig. 8.1). In addition, they proceed through chronic inflammatory stages which are characterized by cellular and cytokine deregulation.

Due to the phenotypic changes, the macrophages, fibroblast, and keratinocytes in diabetic wounds fail to react with inflammatory cytokines and growth factors. These inflammatory macrophages persist and overexpress pro-inflammatory cytokines (IL6 and TNF-α) and reactive oxygen species. The overexpression of these leads to the activation of inflammatory macrophages which reduces the inflammatory signals and promotes the production of proliferative factors/inflammatory proteins. This

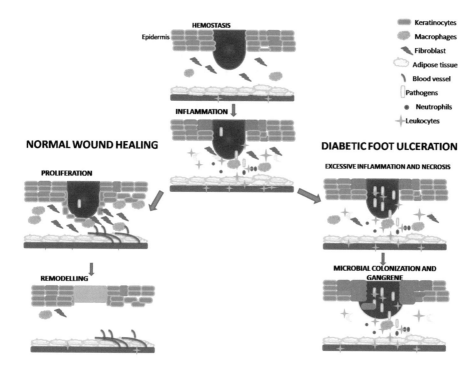

Fig. 8.1 Schematic representation of diabetic foot ulceration

results in the apoptosis of fibroblast, degradation of collagen, and decreased angiogenesis. Also, the dysfunctional fibroblast loses its ability to exert tension on extracellular matrix for contracting the wound. The wound fibroblast overexpress matrix metalloproteinases (MMP-2, MMP-8 and MMP-9) that degrade the collagen which is followed by the prevention of tissue reconstruction.

The most common pathogens associated with DFU infections include Gram-positive *Staphylococcus aureus* and *Staphylococcus epidermidis* and the common Gram-negative includes *Escherichia coli*, *Klebsiella pneumoniae*, *Proteus* sp., and *Pseudomonas aeruginosa*. The appropriate recognition of infections during DFUs and the proper antibiotic treatments can improve better healing of wounds (Pereira et al. 2017). However, the presence of multidrug-resistant pathogenic bacteria with biofilm formation can elevate the severity of chronic infections.

8.3 Evaluation and Standard of Care: Diabetic Foot Ulcer

The effectiveness of DFU treatment depends on patient's medical history, dermatological, musculoskeletal, vascular, and neurological status. Medical history should contain past blood glucose values, vascular symptoms, smoking habit, cholesterol index (HDL and LDL), previous ulcer or amputations, comorbidities, surgeries and angioplasties, renal and retinal functions, and reports of liver and pancreas function tests if any. Physical evaluation includes size, depth, color, position, neuropathy, ischemia, necrosis, infection, exposed bone, and status of exudates from DFU. Surgical debridement, wound dressing, wound off loading, vascular assessment, treatment of infection, and glycemic control are the basic and active treatments associated with DFU. Nowadays, it is strongly recommended that DFUs patients should be evaluated by multidisciplinary teams. Several studies reported the efficiency of multidisciplinary care in declining the amputation rates, wound healing time, and infections. They must be referred by general, vascular, orthopedic surgeon, podiatrist, diabetes specialist, and physical therapist. In addition to the basic and multidisciplinary care, adjuvant therapies have a major role in DFU treatment (Alexiadou and Doupis 2012).

In adjuvant therapy, a wide range of agents are reported. This category involves dressing and topical products, non-surgical debridement agents, acellular byproducts, oxygen therapies, human growth factors, oxygen therapies, systemic therapies, energy-based therapies (electrical stimulation, laser therapy, shock wave therapy phototherapy, and electromagnetic therapy), negative pressure wound therapy, skin grafts, and bioengineered skin. But there is a great need to assess the efficiencies of these therapies by clinical contest and further analysis. In addition to these, other strategies involve the use of therapeutic shoes to prevent or avoid the recurrence of DFU-related consequences. The current scenario is the development of mobile phone applications to monitor and remind about the self-care. Such an application is MyFootCare that engages people with DFU through progress monitoring about the size of DFU and reminds in self-care by taking photos of foot (Ploderer et al. 2018). Above all, personal care is the most suitable way to care diabetic foot (Fig. 8.2).

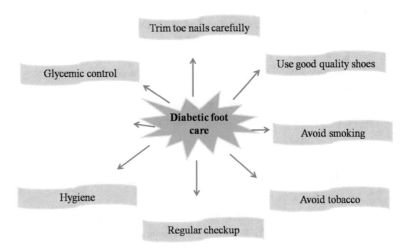

Fig. 8.2 Diabetic foot care strategies

8.4 Nanotechnology and DFUs

The chronic nature of DFUs and the associated complications have led to the emergence of nanotechnology-based therapeutic inventions. The unique chemical, physical, and biological properties of nanoparticles have gained special attention, and many of them are currently under investigation. They play a crucial role in diagnosing, controlling, and reducing the risk factors associated with DFUs. The properties of biomaterials, size, stability, functionalization, and charge are the factors that influence the functioning of nanoparticles. Some of the nanoparticles used in treatment and under research include metallic nanoparticles (silver nanoparticles, zinc oxide nanoparticles, gold nanoparticles, copper nanoparticles, aluminum nanoparticles, titanium dioxide nanoparticles), cerium nanoparticles, nitric oxide-based nanoparticles, polymeric nanoparticles, lipid-based nanoparticles, and peptide-based nanoparticles (Fig. 8.3).

These nanoparticles have promising antimicrobial mechanisms which generate reactive oxygen species that alters the microbial replication and also enhance wound healing process. Most of these nanoparticles are administered topically to minimize the risks associated oral administration or others (Fig. 8.4). Several studies proved the efficiency of topical administration of active nanoparticles in healing wound than systemic administration (Table 8.1).

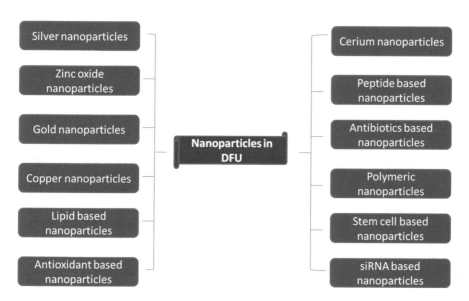

Fig. 8.3 Nanoparticles used in diabetic foot ulcer

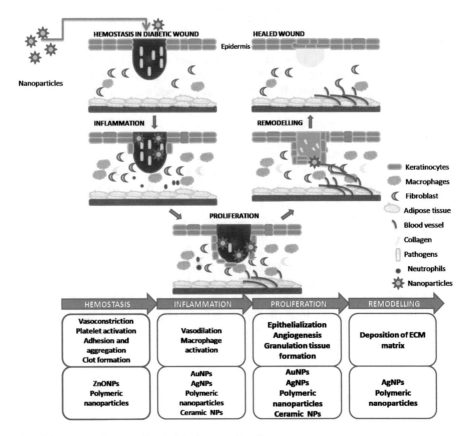

Fig. 8.4 Nanoparticles mediated diabetic wound healing

8.4.1 Silver Nanoparticles (AgNPs)

Silver nanoparticles are well known for their antibacterial activity against multidrug-resistant biofilm-forming bacterial pathogens through the blockage of respiratory pathways and the alteration of DNA and cell wall. They assist in differentiation of fibroblast into myofibroblasts that effectively promote the contractility of wound and accelerates the healing of wound. Also AgNPs do not negatively affect the proliferation of keratinocytes and fibroblasts, even for a prolonged time. During several in vivo studies, it showed reduction in inflammatory cytokines, oxidative stress and the promotion of wound healing were reported (Singla et al. 2017; Rigo et al. 2013). Topical administration of AgNPs on DFUs has reported to result in the closure of injury with re-epithelialization and normalization of pigmentation. Green synthesized AgNPs are demonstrated to be active against multidrug-resistant biofilm-forming *S. epidermidis* (Thomas et al. 2014). Topical administration of AgNPs have also reported to result in the wound healing of Wagner classification degrees II and III DFUs (Chen et al. 2015). Polycaprolactone incorporated with AgNPs has

Table 8.1 Different nanoparticles applied in diabetic wound healing

Nanoparticles	Application	Mechanism of action	Reference
Silver nanoparticles	Topical administration	Antibacterial, re-epithelialization, and closure of DFU	Singla et al. (2017)
	Topical administration	Healed Wagner classification degrees II and III DFU	Chen et al. (2015)
	Interaction with insulin	Inhibition of pro-inflammatory cytokines and remodeling of diabetic wound	Kaur et al. (2018)
Gold nanoparticles	Topical administration	Antioxidant, antibacterial, increased re-epithelialization, granulation, ECM deposition, and collagen fiber	Naraginti et al. (2016)
	Functionalized with calreticulin	Promotes clonogenicity of fibroblasts	Hernández Martínez et al. (2019)
Cerium nanoparticles	Conjugated with microRNA-146a	Antimicrobial, antioxidant, enhanced diabetic wound healing	Zgheib et al. (2018)
	Topical administration	Antibacterial, treatment of neuropathic DFUs with reduced oxidative damage	Nazarii et al. (2018)
	Topical application	Healing of neuropathic diabetic foot ulcer	Kobyliak et al. (2019)
Copper nanoparticles	Incorporated with folic acid	Induced angiogenesis, collagen deposition, and wound closure	Xiao et al. (2018)
Peptide-based nanoparticles	PGLA nanoparticles incorporated with rhEGF	Closure of diabetic wound	Chu et al. (2010)
	Fibrin scaffold with VEGF and bFGF-loaded NPs	Complete re-epithelialization, enhanced granulation, and collagen deposition	Losi et al. (2013)
Nitric oxide-based NPs	Topical administration	Reduced inflammatory cells, increased fibroblast, and collagen content	Blecher et al. (2012)
	In vivo	Increased anti-inflammatory cytokines, and growth factors (TGF-β)	Leu et al. (2012)
	In vivo	Proliferation and migration of fibroblasts, increased collagen content	Han et al. (2012)
Lipid-based nanoparticles	Delivery of rhEGF	Reduced wound area, neovascularization, and re-epithelialization	Gainza et al. (2014)
	Incorporation with siTNF-α	Down regulate the expression of TNF-α and MCP-1 and accelerated closure of DFUs	Kasiewicz and Whitehead (2016)
	In vivo and in vitro	Proliferation of fibroblast and enhanced wound healing	Saporito et al. (2018)

(continued)

Table 8.1 (continued)

Nanoparticles	Application	Mechanism of action	Reference
Lipid nanostructure	Incorporation with phenytoin	Healing of neuropathic diabetic foot ulcer	Motawea et al. (2019)
siRNA-loaded nanoparticles		Down regulation of MCP-1	Kasiewicz and Whitehead (2016)
Polymeric nanoparticles Natural polymers			
Chitosan nanoparticles	Incorporated to collagen alginate scaffold	Complete epithelialization and thick granulation tissue formed	Karri et al. (2016)
Synthetic polymers			
PLGA nanoparticles	In vivo and in vitro	Re-epithelialization, improved granulation tissue formation, and angiogenesis	Gainza et al. (2014)
	Incorporated with VEGF In vivo and in vitro	Enhanced granulation tissue formation, collagen content, and angiogenesis	Chereddy et al. (2015)
	Curcumin loaded	Re-epithelialization, improved granulation tissue formation with down regulation of inflammatory response	Chereddy et al. (2013)

also been reported as antimicrobial agent against wound infection (Thomas et al. 2015). The interaction of insulin with AgNPs (nano insulin formulation) has described to inhibit pro-inflammatory cytokines and remodeling of diabetic wound (Kaur et al. 2018).

8.4.2 Zinc Oxide Nanoparticles (ZnONPs)

The intrinsic antibacterial properties, anti-inflammatory and accelerated wound healing abilities make ZnONPs to be suitable for chronic wound treatments. In addition, they are biocompatible and non-toxic to humans and are listed as Generally Recognized As Safe (GRAS) category by FDA. Kumar et al. (2012) reported the ZnONPs incorporated micro porous chitosan hydrogel bandage to have the ability to absorb wound exudates, influence hemostasis, re-epithelialization, and collagen deposition. Green synthesized ZnONPs have reported to be active against multidrug pathogens infecting DFUs (Steffy et al. 2018). Recently, greenly synthesized ZnONPs from *Aristolochia indica* have been shown to inhibit the growth of multidrug-resistant organisms from pus samples of DFU patients (Steffy et al. 2018).

8.4.3 Gold Nanoparticles (AuNPs)

AuNPs are biologically active materials which have potential medical applications in tissue regeneration, wound healing, and drug delivery. They inhibit lipid peroxidation and prevent reactive oxygen species and hence have the ability to reinstate the antioxidant imbalances. The wound healing efficiency of AuNPs is operated at the phase of hemostasis and inflammation which is highly beneficial to DFUs. Several studies have reported the anti-oxidative and anti-hyperglycemic potential of AuNPs. The topical application of AuNPs at the wound site has also described to have better healing effect in Wistar rats due to the increased re-epithelialization, granulation, and increased ECM deposition along with the increase in collagen fiber content (Naraginti et al. 2016). These have been reported to induce cell death in multidrug-resistant bacteria by reactive oxygen species independent mechanisms. The conjugation of AuNPs with polymers, stem cells/ antibiotics, pathogen-specific antibodies, and photosensitizing molecules are gaining more attention as these improve the hemostasis and increased wound healing activity along with enhanced antimicrobial activity. The study conducted by Gu et al. (2003) has reported the vancomycin-conjugated gold nanoparticles to have 50-fold increased activity against vancomycin-resistant enterococci. AuNPS when conjugated with photosensitizer had also shown to have better antifungal activity against *Candida albicans* present at the wound site of mice (Sherwani et al. 2015). Gold nanocomposite functionalized with calreticulin was found to promote clonogenicity of fibroblasts, keratinocytes, and accelerates the migration of fibroblasts (Hernández Martínez et al. 2019).

8.4.4 Copper-Based Nanoparticles

Copper is an essential element that is involved in all metabolic processes and is considered as safe to humans. Copper-based nanoparticles can promote wound healing by enhancing angiogenesis, re-epithelialization, matrix remodeling, and stabilization of collagen content. Copper-based metal organic framework nanoparticles incorporated with folic acid have been shown to induce angiogenesis, collagen deposition, and increased wound closure in diabetic mice (Xiao et al. 2018).

8.4.5 Cerium Oxide Nanoparticles (CeO$_2$ NPs)

CeO$_2$ is considered as one of the most important options to be utilized for the treatment of DFU. Instead of bacteriostatic activity, they have antioxidant and auto-regenerative abilities along with non-toxicity to neutrophils and macrophages. The free radical scavenging nature and rescuing of cells from oxidative stress-induced cell death make CeO_2 NPs to be exploited in healing of DFUs. CeO_2 NPs when conjugated with microRNA-146a enhanced the diabetic wound healing without impairing the biomechanical properties of the skin post healing (Zgheib et al. 2018). Nazarii et al. (2018) have reported the topical administration of CeO_2 NPs to be effective in healing neuropathic DFUs with reduced oxidative damage along with bacteriostatic activity. The topical application of cerium dioxide nanoparticles having antibacterial, antioxidant and anti-inflammatory can be used for the treatment of neuropathic diabetic foot ulcer (Kobyliak et al. 2019).

8.4.6 Polymeric Nanoparticles

Polymers are generally employed in wound dressings or as drug delivering systems due to its hydrophilic nature. The wound healing properties of polymers are because of its moisture absorption capacity and water vapor transmission that allow the maintenance of moist environment in wound along with the collection of wound exudates. Both natural and synthetic polymers and the combination of natural and synthetic polymers are investigated for wound healing and antimicrobial mechanisms. Poly-lactic-co-glycolic acid (PLGA) nanoparticles, polycaprolactone (PCL), and polyethylene glycol (PEG) are the main synthetic polymers that have been used for the development of nanoformulation for chronic wounds. Among them, PLGA is one of the FDA-approved effective drug-eluting nanoparticles and scaffold used in medical field. PLGA has been reported to induce angiogenesis, but with decreased wound healing time and with the protection against muscle atrophy in ischemic wounds. Chereddy et al. (2013) have reported the PLGA nanoformulation incorporated with curcumin to have the ability to down regulate the expression of glutathionine peroxidase and NF-κβ along with acceleration of granulation tissue formation and re-epithelialization. PGLA loaded with peptide LL37 has also been reported to enhance angiogenesis along with accelerated healing and antimicrobial activity (Chereddy et al. 2014). PLGA incorporated with curcumin nanoparticles also showed enhanced wound healing, antioxidant and anti-inflammatory properties (Chereddy et al. 2013).

Topical administration of PCL nanoparticles embedded with enoxaparin capped chitosan showed improved wound healing and skin penetration (Huber et al. 2012). Chitosan is a biopolymer with the advantage of biocompatibility, biodegradability, and non-immunogenicity. In addition to the antimicrobial properties, it can also mediate the release of growth factors and promote the differentiation of stem cells. Collagen alginate scaffolds incorporated with curcumin-loaded chitosan nanoparticles have induced complete epithelialization and thick granulation tissue formation in diabetic wound (Karri et al. 2016). Chitosan nanoparticles loaded with adenosine diphosphate (ADP) and fibrinogen also showed accelerated wound healing (Chung et al. 2014). In another study, chitosan–sodium tripolyphosphate nanoparticles encapsulated with *Arrabidaea chica* extract showed cell proliferation during in vivo studies (Servat-Medina et al. 2015). The in vivo studies in male albino rats with chitosan–fibrin nanoparticles showed accelerated wound healing with antimicrobial activity (Vedakumari et al. 2015).

8.4.7   Peptide-Based Nanoparticles (Growth Factors-GFs)

Peptide-based nanoparticles is an emerging method for various biomedical applications. The biologically active polypeptides (growth factors) play an important role in cell growth, proliferation, and metabolism. Almost all wound healing stages such as granulating tissue formation, modulation of inflammatory response, promotion of angiogenesis, matrix formation, remodeling, and re-epithelialization are associated with numerous growth factors and cytokines. These include the family of epidermal growth factor (EGF), platelet-derived growth factor (PDGF), basic fibroblast growth factor (bFGF), transforming growth factor beta (TGF-β), insulin-like growth factor (IGF), and vascular endothelial growth factor (VEGF). The decreased level of GFs in DFUs can be delivered at the wound site through nanoparticles-based delivery. In a study, PLGA incorporated with rhEGF has resulted in the closure of diabetic wounds (Chu et al. 2010). Fibrin-based scaffold incorporated with VEGF- and bFGF-loaded nanoparticles resulted in the complete re-epithelialization, enhanced granulation tissue formation, and collagen deposition in diabetic mice (Losi et al. 2013).

8.4.8   Antibiotics-Based Nanoparticles

The emergence of multidrug-resistant pathogens paved the way for advanced therapeutic targeting by nanobiotics. This makes use of antibiotic linked to nanoparticles which provide enhanced activity than conventional antibiotics in chronic infections. Using nanoantibiotics, the concentration of antibiotics can be reduced and also hence can restrict the emergence of antibiotic-resistant strains.

8.4.9   Antioxidant-Based Nanoparticles (NO-NPs)

Inappropriate inflammation is the major reason for reduced wound healing in patients with diabetes. The use of nitric oxide in treating chronic ulcers has emerged recently with the advantage of antibacterial activity against broad range of biofilm-forming pathogens. They can induce re-epithelialization, angiogenesis, collagen, and fibroblast synthesis and can also elevate the level of inflammatory cells and growth factors. In DFU patients, the generation capacity of nitric oxide is reduced, so the exogenous application of nitric acid at the wound site is a promising therapy. The controlled release of nitric acid at the site of wound by nanoparticles was investigated by several researches. The topical application of NO-NPs in diabetic mice was found to accelerate the closure of wound with elevated blood vessels, fibroblasts, and collagen content and reduced inflammatory cells (Blecher et al. 2012). An in vivo study with diabetic mice also showed the potency of NO-NPs in accelerating the closure of wound and increased anti-inflammatory cytokines along with growth factors especially transforming growth factor beta (TGF-β). The in vivo studies in mice with NO-NPs also showed its potential in mediating proliferation and migration of fibroblasts with increased collagen expression (Han et al. 2012). AuNPs in combination with antioxidant epigallocatechin gallate also showed accelerated wound healing in diabetic mice by enhanced angiogenesis and reduced inflammation (Leu et al. 2012).

8.4.10 Lipid-Based Nanoparticles

Lipid nanotechnology is an emerging field which makes use of lipid nanoparticles. Liposomes are the first nanoparticles used for various medical purposes due to their tolerability. Due to the limitations associated with liposomes, solid lipid nanoparticles and nanostructured lipid carriers were developed. Lipid nanoparticles are capable of protecting the drug, enhancing the in drug stability, and also it provide sustainable release of compounds. The use of solid lipid nanoparticles and nanostructured lipid carriers for the delivery of recombinant human epidermal growth factor (rhEGF) showed reduced wound area, increased epithelial coverage, and enhanced neovascularization and re-epithelialization in diabetic rats compared to controls (Gainza et al. 2014). The same when studied in porcine showed improved wound healing (Gainza et al. 2015). Lipidoid nanoparticles loaded with siTNF-α were reported to down regulate the expression of TNF-α and MCP-1 and accelerated the closure of DFUs (Kasiewicz and Whitehead 2016). Olive oil-based nanostructured lipid carriers loaded with eucalyptus oil showed better cytocompatibility, bioadhesion, physico-chemical properties, and enhancement in proliferation of fibroblast during in vivo studies. The in vitro studies of same further confirmed the enhancement in wound healing process (Saporito et al. 2018). Phenytoin-loaded lipid nanostructured carrier was found to enhance the healing of neuropathic diabetic foot ulcer (Motawea et al. 2019).

8.4.11 siRNA Incorporated Nanoparticles

RNA interference therapy permits the silencing of gene expression by targeting selective molecules in chronic wounds. Nanoparticle-based technology emerged as a strategy to protect the delivery of siRNA from degradation by intracellular RNases.

8.4.12 Stem Cell-Based Nanoparticles

The incorporation of stem cells promotes angiogenesis and re-epithelialization in chronic wounds. Bone marrow-derived mononuclear cells, bone marrow-derived mesenchymal stem cells, placenta-derived stem cells, bone marrow-derived endothelial progenitor cells, and adipose-derived stem cells have been shown for their therapeutic potential in chronic wounds (Blumberg et al. 2012; Gadelkarim et al. 2018). Nanotechnological approaches can provide dynamic microenvironment which targets multiple cell types, and many such studies are under investigation.

8.5 Conclusion

The chronicity and complications associated with wounds have led to the emergence of nanoparticles-based treatments. The biocompatibility, biodegradability, and reduced toxic nature of nanoparticles make them suitable as nanomedicines. Approved nanoparticles for diabetic foot ulcer treatments are limited, and many of them are currently under investigation. Due to the chronic inflammatory stage in DFUs, targeting matrix metalloproteinases (MMPs) through nanotechnological approach can have great promises to cure chronic DFUs.

8.6 Future Perspectives

Nowadays, an increasing number of innovative nanotherapies have emerged in the area of diabetic wound healing. Nanotherapies offer various strategies for treating the chronic diabetic wounds. But there are many questions regarding nanoparticle-mediated diabetic wound healing, and the major signaling pathways involved in it. Further studies are needed to understand the exact mechanisms regarding the healing of diabetic foot ulcer by nanoparticles-mediated approach. The influence of 3D printing, stem cell research, and molecular studies along with computational medicine can revolutionize the future of nanotherapeutics.

References

Alexiadou K, Doupis J (2012) Management of diabetic foot ulcers. Diabetes Ther 3(1).4. https://doi.org/10.1007/s13300-012-0004-9

Basu S, Yudkin JS, Kehlenbrink S, Davies JI, Wild SH, Lipska KJ (2019) Estimation of global insulin use for type 2 diabetes, 2018–30: a microsimulation analysis. Lancet Diabetes Endocrinol 7(1):25–33. https://doi.org/10.1016/s2213-8587(18)30303-6

Behl T, Grover M, Shah K, Makkar R, Kaur L, Sharma S (2019) Role of omega-3-fatty acids in the management of diabetes and associated complications, pp 185–192. https://doi.org/10.1016/b978-0-12-813822-9.00012-6

Blecher K, Martinez LR, Tuckman-Vernon C, Nacharaju P, Schairer D, Chouake J, Friedman JM, Alfieri A, Guha C, Nosanchuk JD, Friedman AJ (2012) Nitric oxide-releasing nanoparticles accelerate wound healing in NOD-SCID mice. Nanomed Nanotechnol 8(8):1364–1371. https://doi.org/10.1016/j.nano.2012.02.014

Blumberg SN, Berger A, Hwang L, Pastar I, Warren SM, Chen W (2012) The role of stem cells in the treatment of diabetic foot ulcers. Diabetes Res Clin Pract 96(1):1–9. https://doi.org/10.1016/j.diabres.2011.10.032

Chen YW, Drury JL, Chung WO, Hobbs DT, Wataha JC (2015) Titanates and Titanate-metal compounds in biological contexts. Int J Med Nano Res 2(1):009

Chereddy KK, Coco R, Memvanga PB, Ucakar B, des Rieux A, Vandermeulen G, Preat V (2013) Combined effect of PLGA and curcumin on wound healing activity. J Control Release 171(2):208–215. https://doi.org/10.1016/j.jconrel.2013.07.015

Chereddy KK, Her CH, Comune M, Moia C, Lopes A, Porporato PE, Vanacker J, Lam MC, Steinstraesser L, Sonveaux P, Zhu H, Ferreira LS, Vandermeulen G, Preat V (2014) PLGA nanoparticles loaded with host defense peptide LL37 promote wound healing. J Control Release 194:138–147. https://doi.org/10.1016/j.jconrel.2014.08.016

Chereddy KK, Lopes A, Koussoroplis S, Payen V, Moia C, Zhu H, Préat V (2015) Combined effects of PLGA and vascular endothelial growth factor promote the healing of non-diabetic and diabetic wounds. Nanomed Nanotechnol 11(8):1975–1984

Chu Y, Yu D, Wang P, Xu J, Li D, Ding M (2010) Nanotechnology promotes the full-thickness diabetic wound healing effect of recombinant human epidermal growth factor in diabetic rats. Wound Repair Regen 18(5):499–505. https://doi.org/10.1111/j.1524-475X.2010.00612.x

Chung TW, Lin PY, Wang SS, Chen YF (2014) Adenosine diphosphate-decorated chitosan nanoparticles shorten blood clotting times, influencing the structures and varying the mechanical properties of the clots. Int J Nanomedicine 9:1655–1664. https://doi.org/10.2147/IJN.S57855

Everett E, Mathioudakis N (2018) Update on management of diabetic foot ulcers. Ann N Y Acad Sci 1411(1):153–165. https://doi.org/10.1111/nyas.13569

Gadelkarim M, Abushouk AI, Ghanem E, Hamaad AM, Saad AM, Abdel-Daim MM (2018) Adipose-derived stem cells: effectiveness and advances in delivery in diabetic wound healing. Biomed Pharmacother 107:625–633. https://doi.org/10.1016/j.biopha.2018.08.013

Gainza G, Pastor M, Aguirre JJ, Villullas S, Pedraz JL, Hernandez RM, Igartua M (2014) A novel strategy for the treatment of chronic wounds based on the topical administration of rhEGF-loaded lipid nanoparticles: in vitro bioactivity and in vivo effectiveness in healing-impaired db/db mice. J Control Release 185:51–61. https://doi.org/10.1016/j.jconrel.2014.04.032

Gainza G, Bonafonte DC, Moreno B, Aguirre JJ, Gutierrez FB, Villullas S, Pedraz JL, Igartua M, Hernandez RM (2015) The topical administration of rhEGF-loaded nanostructured lipid carriers (rhEGF-NLC) improves healing in a porcine full-thickness excisional wound model. J Control Release 197:41–47. https://doi.org/10.1016/j.jconrel.2014.10.033

Gu H, Ho PL, Tong E, Wang L, Xu B (2003) Presenting vancomycin on nanoparticles to enhance antimicrobial activities. Nano Lett 3(9):1261–1263. https://doi.org/10.1021/nl034396z

Han G, Nguyen LN, Macherla C, Chi Y, Friedman JM, Nosanchuk JD, Martinez LR (2012) Nitric oxide-releasing nanoparticles accelerate wound healing by promoting fibroblast migration and collagen deposition. Am J Pathol 180(4):1465–1473. https://doi.org/10.1016/j.ajpath.2011.12.013

Hernández Martínez SP, Rivera González TI, Franco Molina MA, Bollain Y Goytia JJ, Martínez Sanmiguel JJ, Zárate Triviño DG (2019) A novel gold calreticulin nanocomposite based on chitosan for wound healing in a diabetic mice model. Nanomaterials 9(1):75. https://doi.org/10.3390/nano9010075

Huber PDM, Barbosa RM, Duran N, Annichino-Bizzacchi JM (2012) In vivo toxicity of enoxaparin encapsulated in mucoadhesive nanoparticles: topical application in a wound healing model.

Presented at: Nanosafe 2012: international conferences on safe production and use of nanomaterials, Grenoble, France, 13–15 November 2012

Karri VV, Kuppusamy G, Talluri SV, Mannemala SS, Kollipara R, Wadhwani AD, Mulukutla S, Raju KR, Malayandi R (2016) Curcumin loaded chitosan nanoparticles impregnated into collagen-alginate scaffolds for diabetic wound healing. Int J Biol Macromol 93(Pt B):1519–1529. https://doi.org/10.1016/j.ijbiomac.2016.05.038

Kasiewicz LN, Whitehead KA (2016) Silencing TNFalpha with lipidoid nanoparticles downregulates both TNFalpha and MCP-1 in an in vitro co-culture model of diabetic foot ulcers. Acta Biomater 32:120–128. https://doi.org/10.1016/j.actbio.2015.12.023

Kaur P, Sharma AK, Nag D, Das A, Datta S, Ganguli A, Goel V, Rajput S, Chakrabarti G, Basu B, Choudhury D (2018) Novel nano-insulin formulation modulates cytokine secretion and remodeling to accelerate diabetic wound healing. Nanomed Nanotechnol 15(1):47–57. https://doi.org/10.1016/j.nano.2018.08.013

Kobyliak N, Abenavoli L, Kononenko L, Kyriienko D, Spivak M (2018) Neuropathic diabetic foot ulcers treated with cerium dioxide nanoparticles: a case report. Diabetes Metab Syndr: Clinical Research & Reviews. 13. https://doi.org/10.1016/j.dsx.2018.08.027

Kobyliak N, Abenavoli L, Kononenko L, Kyriienko D, Spivak M (2019) Neuropathic diabetic foot ulcers treated with cerium dioxide nanoparticles: a case report. Diabetes Metab Syndr 13(1):228–234. https://doi.org/10.1016/j.dsx.2018.08.027

Kumar PT, Lakshmanan VK, Anilkumar TV, Ramya C, Reshmi P, Unnikrishnan AG, Nair SV, Jayakumar R (2012) Flexible and microporous chitosan hydrogel/nanoZnO composite bandages for wound dressing: in vitro and in vivo evaluation. ACS Appl Mater Interfaces 4:2618–2629

Leu JG, Chen SA, Chen HM, Wu WM, Hung CF, Yao YD, Tu CS, Liang YJ (2012) The effects of gold nanoparticles in wound healing with antioxidant epigallocatechin gallate and alpha-lipoic acid. Nanomed Nanotechnol 8(5):767–775. https://doi.org/10.1016/j.nano.2011.08.013

Losi P, Briganti E, Errico C, Lisella A, Sanguinetti E, Chiellini F, Soldani G (2013) Fibrin-based scaffold incorporating VEGF- and bFGF-loaded nanoparticles stimulates wound healing in diabetic mice. Acta Biomater 9(8):7814–7821. https://doi.org/10.1016/j.actbio.2013.04.019

Mavrogenis AF, Megaloikonomos PD, Antoniadou T, Igoumenou VG, Panagopoulos GN, Dimopoulos L, Moulakakis KG, Sfyroeras GS, Lazaris A (2018) Current concepts for the evaluation and management of diabetic foot ulcers. EFORT Open Rev 3(9):513–525. https://doi.org/10.1302/2058-5241.3.180010

Motawea A, Abd El-Gawad AE-GH, Borg T, Motawea M, Tarshoby M (2019) The impact of topical phenytoin loaded nanostructured lipid carriers in diabetic foot ulceration. Foot 40:14–21. https://doi.org/10.1016/j.foot.2019.03.007

Naraginti S, Kumari PL, Das RK, Sivakumar A, Patil SH, Andhalkar VV (2016) Amelioration of excision wounds by topical application of green synthesized, formulated silver and gold nanoparticles in albino Wistar rats. Mater Sci Eng C Mater Biol Appl 62:293–300. https://doi.org/10.1016/j.msec.2016.01.069

Pereira SG, Moura J, Carvalho E, Empadinhas N (2017) Microbiota of chronic diabetic wounds: ecology, impact, and potential for innovative treatment strategies. Front Microbiol 8:1791. https://doi.org/10.3389/fmicb.2017.01791

Ploderer B, Brown R, Seng LSD, Lazzarini PA, van Netten JJ (2018) Promoting self-care of diabetic foot ulcers through a mobile phone app: user-centered design and evaluation. JMIR Diabetes 3(4):e10105. https://doi.org/10.2196/10105

Rigo C, Ferroni L, Tocco I, Roman M, Munivrana I, Gardin C, Cairns WR, Vindigni V, Azzena B, Barbante C, Zavan B (2013) Active silver nanoparticles for wound healing. Int J Mol Sci 14(3):4817–4840. https://doi.org/10.3390/ijms14034817

Saporito F, Sandri G, Bonferoni MC, Rossi S, Boselli C, Icaro Cornaglia A, Mannucci B, Grisoli P, Vigani B, Ferrari F (2018) Essential oil-loaded lipid nanoparticles for wound healing. Int J Mol Sci 13:175–186. https://doi.org/10.2147/IJN.S152529

Servat-Medina L, Gonzalez-Gomez A, Reyes-Ortega F, Sousa IM, Queiroz Nde C, Zago PM, Jorge MP, Monteiro KM, de Carvalho JE, San Roman J, Foglio MA (2015) Chitosan-tripolyphosphate nanoparticles as Arrabidaea chica standardized extract carrier: synthesis, characterization, biocompatibility, and antiulcerogenic activity. Int J Nanomedicine 10:3897–3909. https://doi.org/10.2147/IJN.S83705

Sherwani MA, Tufail S, Khan AA, Owais M (2015) Gold nanoparticle-photosensitizer conjugate based photodynamic inactivation of biofilm producing cells: potential for treatment of C. albicans infection in BALB/c mice. PLoS One 10(7):e0131684. https://doi.org/10.1371/journal.pone.0131684

Singla R, Soni S, Patial V, Kulurkar PM, Kumari A, S M, Padwad YS, Yadav SK (2017) In vivo diabetic wound healing potential of nanobiocomposites containing bamboo cellulose nanocrystals impregnated with silver nanoparticles. Int J Biol Macromol 105(Pt 1):45–55. https://doi.org/10.1016/j.ijbiomac.2017.06.109

Steffy K, Shanthi G, Maroky AS, Selvakumar S (2018) Enhanced antibacterial effects of green synthesized ZnO NPs using *Aristolochia indica* against multi-drug resistant bacterial pathogens from diabetic foot ulcer. J Infect Public Health 11(4):463–471. https://doi.org/10.1016/j.jiph.2017.10.006

Thomas R, Nair AP, Kr S, Mathew J, Ek R (2014) Antibacterial activity and synergistic effect of biosynthesized AgNPs with antibiotics against multidrug-resistant biofilm-forming coagulase-negative staphylococci isolated from clinical samples. Appl Biochem Biotechnol 173(2):449–460. https://doi.org/10.1007/s12010-014-0852-z

Thomas R, Soumya KR, Mathew J, Radhakrishnan EK (2015) Electrospun polycaprolactone membrane incorporated with biosynthesized silver nanoparticles as effective wound dressing material. Appl Biochem Biotechnol 176(8):2213–2224. https://doi.org/10.1007/s12010-015-1709-9

Vedakumari WS, Prabu P, Sastry TP (2015) Chitosan-Fibrin nanocomposites as drug delivering and wound healing materials. J Biomed Nanotechnol 11(4):657–667

Xiao J, Zhu Y, Huddleston S, Li P, Xiao B, Farha OK, Ameer GA (2018) Copper metal-organic framework nanoparticles stabilized with folic acid improve wound healing in diabetes. ACS Nano 12(2):1023–1032. https://doi.org/10.1021/acsnano.7b01850

Zgheib C, Hilton SA, Dewberry LC, Hodges MM, Ghatak S, Xu J, Singh S, Roy S, Sen CK, Seal S, Liechty KW (2018) Use of cerium oxide nanoparticles conjugated with MicroRNA-146a to correct the diabetic wound healing impairment. J Am Coll Surg 228(1):107–115. https://doi.org/10.1016/j.jamcollsurg.2018.09.017

Chapter 9
Silver Nanoparticles in Wound Infections: Present Status and Future Prospects

Hanna Dahm

Abstract The wounds are infected by one or more bacteria or other microbes. The occurrence of the bacterial infections in wounds is mainly responsible in delayed healing and enhancement of wound. These bacteria include Gram-positive bacteria such as *Streptococcus pyogenes, Enterococcus faecalis, Staphylococcus aureus,* and Gram-negative bacteria including *Pseudomonas aeruginosa, Escherichia coli, Klebsiella* species, and fungi like *Candida* and *Aspergillus.* The use of silver has been known since nineteenth century and after the discovery of penicillin, its use was reduced. However, the occurrence of multidrug-resistant bacteria has led to the search of new antibiotics and alternatives to solve the problem of multidrug-resistance. In this context, scientists have shown much interest on the use of silver and silver nanoparticles as they are very effective against bacterial infections.

This chapter is aimed to discuss the role of silver and silver nanoparticles in wound infections. In addition, the resistance of microbes to silver and silver nanoparticles and the toxicity issues have also been addressed.

Keywords Wounds · Silver · Silver nanoparticles · Bacteria · Fungi · Resistance · Toxicity

9.1 Introduction

Wound is an injury to the body that typically involves laceration or breaking of membrane (such as skin) and usually cause damage to underlying tissues. Microorganisms found on the skin are usually regarded as harmless symbiotic organisms (commensals), pathogens, or probable pathogens. In recent years, the understanding of the host–microorganisms interaction together with the mechanisms of bacterial virulence has been tremendously increased. Studies have shown that chronic wounds are colonized by multiple bacterial species, many of which

H. Dahm (✉)
Department of Microbiology, Nicolaus Copernicus University, Torun, Poland
e-mail: dahm@umk.pl

© Springer Nature Switzerland AG 2020
M. Rai (ed.), *Nanotechnology in Skin, Soft Tissue, and Bone Infections,*
https://doi.org/10.1007/978-3-030-35147-2_9

persist in the wound. The presence of bacteria such as *Pseudomonas aeruginosa* can induce wound enlargement and/or delayed healing.

The occurrence of a wound infection depends on several factors such as: if the integrity or the protective function of the skin is disintegrated or if large amount of different microbial cells enter the wound it initiates an inflammatory response which is characterized by classic signs of pain, redness, swelling, high fever, etc. (Calvin 1998).

Since 1985 the most commonly used terms have included wound contamination, wound colonization, wound infection, and critical colonization (Ayton 1985; Falanga et al. 1994; Kingsley 2001).

- Wound contamination—presence of bacterial cells within wound, without causing any host reaction.
- Wound colonization—the presence of bacteria within the wound which do multiply or initiate a host reaction.
- Critical colonization—bacterial infection resulting in delayed wound healing usually associated with an exacerbation of pain.
- Wound infection—deposition and multiplication of bacteria resulting in associated host reaction in the tissues.

Examples of potential wound pathogens:

Gram-positive cocci Beta haemolytic streptococci (*Streptococcus pyogenes),* Enterococci (*Enterococcus faecalis),* Staphylococci *(Staphylococcus aureus/*MRSA).
Gram-negative aerobic rods *Pseudomonas aeruginosa.*
Gram-negative facultative rods *Enterobacter* species, *Escherichia coli, Klebsiella* species, *Proteus* species.
Anaerobes *Bacteroides, Clostridium.*
Fungi *Candida, Aspergillus.*

Different microbes co-exist in polymicrobial communities and same is the case within the margins of a wound (Bowler et al. 2001; Collier 2004). The presence of microorganisms in the wound does not predict wound infection (Bowler 1998). Protective colonization, in which some bacteria synthesize highly specific proteins and inhibit other bacterial species that are closely related or certain bacteria develop a number of metabolites and end products which inhibits the growth of other microorganisms (Collier 2004).

Once a diagnosis of wound infection is confirmed and antibiotic sensitivities identified, appropriate management regimens should be considered, with a high priority given to reducing the risk of cross infection.

Resistance to antibiotics has become a serious problem in recent years particularly with the rise of epidemic strains of MRSA (Karkman et al. 2019; Wu et al. 2019). The excessive use of antibiotics can only worsen the situation. Henceforth, the use of antibiotics should be according to their known sensitivity. Along with antibiotic therapy, the other two wound management products are compounds containing silver or iodine (Collier 2004).

The main goal of this chapter is to discuss the role of silver nanoparticles in wound infections, their toxicity, and future prospects in use as a new generation of antimicrobial agents.

9.2 Silver-Based Antimicrobials in Wound Infection

The medicinal use of silver is not a new idea. The medicinal potential of silver has been known since 2000 years, and the use of silver and silver-based compounds for antimicrobial applications has been done since the nineteenth century. Silver ions have also been used and an antimicrobial agent ever since the discovery of microbes or the germ theory of diseases.

Since the growth of pathogenic microorganisms and their penetration into the body remained the main problem, a search was made for an antiseptic agent to prevent invasive infection.

The antimicrobial activity of the silver ions was first identified in the nineteenth century, and colloidal silver was accepted by the US Food and Drug Administration (FDA) as being effective for wound management in the 1920s.

However, after the introduction of penicillin in 1940, antibiotics became the standard treatment for bacterial infections and the use of silver diminished. The true renaissance of silver in medicine occurred in the 1960s when silver compounds revolutionized burn wound care. This time it is in the form of 0.5% $AgNO_3$ solution. $AgNO_3$ was combined with a sulphonamide antibiotic in 1968 to produce silver sulphadiazine cream which created a broad-spectrum silver-based antibacterials for the management of burns. More recently, clinicians have turned to wound dressing that incorporate varying levels of silver ion because the emergence and increase of antibiotic-resistant bacteria have resulted in limitations for the antibiotic therapy (Wu et al. 2019).

Infection management include the stimulation of healing in indolent wounds, prophylactic use for patients at risk contracting a wound infection, and the management of critically colonized wounds (Chopra 2007).

Silver has a long history in the treatment of human diseases including epilepsy, neonatal eye disease, venereal disease, cholera, dysentery, and skin infections. Silver nitrate still has a place in burns unit wound clinics today and is frequently a life-saving therapy in cases of *Pseudomonas aeruginosa* infections (Lansdown 2010).

At the time, early evidence was emerging that metallic ions (Ag^+) were effective antibacterial agents at concentration as low as one part per million (ppm).

Silver ions have strong inhibitory and bactericidal effects as well as a broad spectrum of antimicrobial activities. Several proposals have been developed to explain the inhibitory effects of Ag^+ ions on bacteria. It is generally believed that heavy metals react with proteins by combining the -SH groups, which leads to the inactivation of the proteins. Interaction of Ag^+ with thiol group played an essential role in antibacterial activity; however, exact mechanism of these effects is still not fully understood (Liau et al. 1997). Feng et al. (2000) observed significant morphological changes in *E. coli* cells after addition of Ag⁺. A big gap exists between the cytoplasmic membrane and the cell wall, cell walls were damaged, and tightly condensed substances were visible in the centre of cells. X-ray microanalysis of the granules showed a significant amount of silver and sulphur.

After Ag⁺ treatment, similar morphological changes occur in *Staphylococcus aureus*. In *S. aureus* cells, a large amount of phosphorus was detected in the condensed region; probably, it was condensed form of DNA molecules. Authors of these experiments stated that besides the similar morphological changes between these two types of bacteria, minor differences were observed after Ag⁺ treatment.

S. aureus remained integral, the amounts of the granules inside the cells were smaller than that of *E. coli*. It was suggested that *S. aureus* may have a stronger defence system against silver ions.

A variety of animal models of partial and full-thickness burns, infected burns wounds, excised burn wounds, donor sites, and skin flaps evaluated the utility of silver—nylon with and without direct current on wound healing, microcirculation, and wound oedema. Plasma protein extravasation and wound closure (Chu et al. 1988, 1991, 1996; Barillo and Marx 2014).

Already in 1965, Moyer concluded on the basis of in vitro and in vivo studies that a 0.5% solution of silver nitrate represented the lowest concentration at which antibacterial action of *Staphylococcus aureus*, haemolytic streptococci, *Pseudomonas aeruginosa*, and *E. coli* was obtained and had no toxic effect on growing epidermal cells. However, *Aerobacter* species and a number of saprophytes of the human skin were insensitive (Moyer et al. 1965; Klasen 2000).

Different combinations of sulpha drugs (sulphadiazine, sulphamylon acetate) with silver were tested in vitro, but silver sulphadiazine appeared to be the most effective (Stanford et al. 1969; Klasen 2000).

A possible explanation of this phenomenon could be the relatively strong binding of silver sulphadiazine to DNA. The binding differs from that of silver nitrate or other silver salts (Fox and Stanford 1971).

Sulphadiazine does not have antibacterial activity but shows a specific synergetic effect in combination with inhibitory concentration of silver. The effectiveness of silver sulphadiazine would appears to depend on the slow continuous reaction with serum and other Na-Cl-containing body fluids, leading to slow release of silver ions in the wound.

Silver sulphadiazine is a broad-spectrum bactericidal particularly for the treatment of burn wounds. Its mode of action is membrane damaging by binding to cell components including DNA and transcription inhibition by binding to the base pairs in DNA helix (Atiyeh et al. 2007; Rai et al. 2012).

Radioactive silver sulphadiazine was used to investigate whether the silver was resorbed in experimental animals. The presence of silver was only demonstrated in the skin, and not in the blood or other organs. Electron microscopic study of biopsies from burns and epithelized regions round the burns in patients who had been treated with silver sulphadiazine for 21 days showed a silver deposit in the cytoplasm of epidermis cells. The application of the silver sulphadiazine ointment to the burn wounds was found not to be painful (Fox 1968).

Gamelli et al. (1993) concluded that silver sulphadiazine have cytotoxic effect on bone marrow cells. Silver sulphadiazine gave rise to changes in the myeloid cell compartment and observed temporary leucopenia in burns patients treated with silver sulphadiazine might be a results of this.

Fakhry et al. (1995) reported that many attempts to find a better remedy for the treatment of burns than silver sulphadiazine have so far been without success, and silver sulphadiazine is still the most widely used. In fact, in wound treatment, silver quantities should be sufficient to provide sustained bactericidal action (Dunn and Edwards-Jones 2004). The nanosuspensions and nanogels of sulphadiazine were also found to enhance activity against *Staphylococcus aureus*, *Escherichia coli*, and *Pseudomonas aeruginosa causing wounds* (Venkataraman and Nagarsenker 2013).

Antimicrobial activity of silver ion is well defined. Silver has a broad antimicrobial spectrum against bacteria and yeast mold and other pathogenic fungi. Elemental silver requires ionization for antimicrobial efficacy. Silver ion is a highly reactive, readily binding capacity to negatively charged proteins, RNA, DNA, chloride ions, and other (Atiyeh et al. 2007). Bactericidal effect of silver is attributed mainly to the binding of the silver ion to free sulphydryl groups in the bacterium or on its surface leading to inactivation of the enzymes.

Metal silver is relatively inert and is poorly absorbed by mammalian cells. However, in the presence of wound fluids it readily ionizes and becomes highly reactive in binding to proteins and cell membranes (Mooney 2006; Atiyeh et al. 2007). It is important that substances in the wound that chelate free silver ion or precipitate it as an insoluble salt inhibit bacteriostasis. Sodium chloride in wound exudates inhibits the antibacterial action of silver nitrate by precipitating the silver as insoluble silver chloride.

Silver, particularly in the nanocrystalline form, appears to be an effective means of prophylaxis given its rapid and broad-spectrum efficacy. Nanocrystalline silver dressings have demonstrated as effective and antibacterial agent even for antibiotic-resistant bacteria (Wright et al. 1999; Yin et al. 1999; Atiyeh et al. 2007).

Silver ion is the most commonly used topical antimicrobial agents in burn wound care.

9.3 Silver, Wound Infection, and Healing

Bacterial infections are the major obstacles for proper wound healing as it possesses a danger of causing long-term negative effects. The bacterial infection of wounds is one of the major concerns in wound treatment. Keeping the wound free from any bacterial infection is crucial in the proper and timely repair of wounds. Silver due to its bactericidal properties has been used efficiently to treat wounds (Nam et al. 2015).

Early clinical observations indicated that silver nitrate complexes with proteins in skin wounds forms "resistant precipitates" and that the local antibacterial action can be easily controlled. This antiseptic action extends deeply into wounds with silver forming soluble double salts of silver albuminates and silver chloride in the tissues (Lansdown 2006). Silver nitrate is an excellent antibacterial agent and at 0.5% is effective in inhibiting bacteria particularly *Pseudomonas aeruginosa, Streptococcus pyogenes*, and *Staphylococcus aureus* which can prove to be fatal in burn wounds.

The introduction of silver sulphadiazine marked a renaissance in the use of silver in wound care. Silver sulphadiazine represents a second generation of silver antibiotics. Although silver sulphadiazine is sparingly soluble in water, it ionizes readily in body fluids to release silver ions. Silver sulphadiazine is claimed to be effective against up to 95% of bacteria commonly found in skin wounds (Lansdown 2006). Silver sulphadiazine and silver nitrate have been highly successful in controlling infections for many years even though the emergence of sulphonamide-resistant bacteria.

Improved technology permits to enhance the delivery of silver ions to wounds to provide a safer and more efficacious antibacterial action, including methicillin-resistant *Staphylococcus aureus* and vancomycin-resistant enterococci. The variety of silver release dressings differ greatly in composition, mechanism of presumed action, and rates of silver release. Experience gained in the use of silver in wound care has led to the development of silver antibiotics in other medical devices (Lansdown 2006).

The silver ions are the most commonly used topical antimicrobial agents in burn wound care.

The wound repair process involves steps: inflammation around the site of injury, angiogenesis, granulation tissue, repair of the connective tissue and epithelium, and remodelling that leads to a healed wound. Different events and conditions have an influence on the healing of wounds. One factor that impedes wound healing is colonization of the wound by microorganisms (Poon and Burd 2004).

Presence of microorganisms and their products such as toxins and proteases in a wound lead to a prolonged inflammatory response. Many studies support the concept of eradicating infection to help wound healing. Silver-based wound dressings are often used for healing and may have a positive effect on wound healing and therefore can be used to maintain a microorganisms-free, aseptic environment (Warriner and Burrell 2005; Atiyeh et al. 2007). Besides antimicrobial activity, silver may reduce local matrix metalloproteinase levels and enhanced cellular apoptosis (Wright et al. 2002).

9.4   The Effect of Silver Nanoparticles on Wounds

Among the different applications of silver nanoparticles, the biomedical applications are highly taken into consideration due to its antibacterial properties. Due to antibiotic resistance, wound infections have become a big challenge and take longer time to heal.

Silver has been used as antibacterial agent for years and nowadays, taking an advantage of nano size materials, silver nanoparticles are being utilized in wound dressings. However, apart from the use of silver nanoparticles in many applications its action on microorganisms is not completely known. There have been several mechanisms suggested on cell lysis and growth inhibition. Also, the problem with the physical and chemical synthesis methods is that they are costly and involve the use of toxic chemicals which are harmful to the environment (Prabhu and Poulose 2012). The need to develop environmentally friendly and economically feasible technologies for material synthesis led to the search for biomimetic methods of synthesis. There are three major sources of synthesizing silver nanoparticles: bacteria, fungi, and plant extracts (Bawskar et al. 2015; Singh et al. 2018)

Nanoparticles due to their higher surface area to volume ratio provide more surface area for the particles hence increasing its effect. Also, it increases the penetration potential of particles helping in better utilization of its properties.

The antimicrobial nature of silver nanoparticles is the most exploited in the medical field though the anti-inflammatory nature is also considered immensely useful especially in wound infections.

Reports have suggested that presence of silver nanoparticles accelerate wound healing by reducing local matrix metalloproteinase activity and increasing neutrophil apoptosis within the wound. It is proposed that metalloproteins induce inflammation and hence non-healing of wounds (Kirsner et al. 2001; Prabhu and Poulose 2012). A reduction in the levels of pro-inflammatory cytokines was also observed on introduction of silver nanoparticles. It was also reported that silver nanoparticles inhibit the activities of interferon gamma and tumour necrosis factor. The anti-inflammatory effects depicted by silver nanoparticles make it an excellent anti-inflammatory agent. Nanosilver is efficient due to its bactericidal properties on bacteria infecting the wounds and other body fluids.

The most prominent players in silver-based wound healing are Acticoat, Silvercel, and Actisorb, containing silver nanoparticles (AgNPs) (average size of nanoparticles is 15 nm).

Tredget et al. 1998 carried out a comparative study on Acticoat vs silver nitrate solution for burn wounds and demonstrated that the incidence of sepsis was low in Acticoat group and also low pain was observed compared to silver nitrate solution. Fong et al. (2005) also studied the effectiveness of Acticoat in treatment of burn wound compared to Silvazine (Silver sulphadazine and chlorhexidine digluconate). Acticoat reduced the incidence of burn wound cellulitis, also comparing Silvazine, reduced the overall cost of antibiotic usage.

Nanomedicine is a developing field expanding rapidly because of the development of new nanomaterial into a range of products and technologies. Silver nanoparticles (AgNPs) show both unique physicochemical properties (high ratio of surface area to mass) and ample antibacterial activities, which confer them as a major advantage for the development of alternative products against, for example, multidrug-resistant microorganisms (Ahmadi and Adibhesami 2017).

The development of nano chemistry has facilitated the production of micro fine silver particles with greatly increased solubility and release of silver ions (70–100 ppm). Ionization of silver metal is proportional to the surface area of the particles exposed.

Nanosilver not only possesses a broad antimicrobial activity but also has an anti-inflammatory effect and accelerates wound healing (Tian et al. 2007; Nadworny et al. 2010; Kedi et al. 2018).

The antibacterial activity of metals depends on their contact surface. The larger surface of the nanoparticles allows a larger extent of interactions with other organic and inorganic molecules (Ahmadi and Adibhesami 2017). Nanoparticles are defined as particulate dispersion or solid particles with a size in the range of 1–100 nm. The alteration from microparticles to nanoparticles includes an increased surface area among other changes in properties.

Silver nanoparticles smaller in size release more Ag^+ ions, leading to an increase in its antibacterial property.

The higher antimicrobial properties and lower toxicity of AgNPs, compared to those of Ag compounds such as $AgNO_3$ and silver sulphadiazine they could be used for the treatment of wounds' pathogens with greater benefits (Nam et al. 2015).

The truncated triangular nanoparticles exhibited greater silver reactivity due to their high-atom density facets than spherical and rod-shaped nanoparticles. It can be inferred that the high-atom density of the truncated triangular silver nanoparticles enhance its antimicrobial activity. Moreover, lattice plane of triangular nanoparticles allows better contact with the bacteria cell wall and thus able to cause more damage (Nam et al. 2015).

The introduction of silver in the form of nanoparticles has allowed scientific community to enhance its antibacterial properties. The high surface area of nanoparticles increases the rate of interaction between the bacteria and silver ions. Hence, the increase in the bactericidal efficacy lowers minimum inhibitory concentration required for wound healing.

Nanomedicine is a developing field expanding rapidly. Silver nanoparticles show both unique physiochemical properties (high ratio of surface area to mass) and antimicrobial activities. Silver nanoparticles (AgNPs) are attractive because they are non-toxic to human body at low concentration and have broad-spectrum antibacterial action (Jiang et al. 2012).

In recent years, there has been great progress in the application of nanoparticles in biomedical applications. Nanomaterials, which either show antimicrobial activity or elevate the effectiveness and safety of antibiotics administration are called "nanoantibiotics" and their capability of controlling infections in vitro and in vivo has been explored and demonstrated (Ahmadi and Adibhesami 2017).

Silver nanoparticles (AgNPs) have been extensively investigated as an antimicrobial agent in vitro. AgNPs show both unique physiochemical properties and remarkable antimicrobial activities which confer to them a major advantage for the development of alternative factor against microorganisms including multidrug-resistant bacteria, and hence silver nanoparticles are supposed to be the new generation of antimicrobials (Rai et al. 2009; Franci et al. 2015; Alavi and Rai 2019).

Several proposals have been developed to explain the inhibitory effects of Ag^+ ions on bacteria. It is generally believed that heavy metals react with proteins by combining the -SH groups which leads to the inactivation of the proteins. Experiments employing interaction of thiol group with Ag^{+1} played a crucial role in inactivation of bacteria (Liau et al. 1997; Feng et al. 2000). Mechanisms of Ag $^+$ action also include production of reactive oxygen species (ROS) that damage cellular component (Pal et al. 2007), compromising the bacterial cell wall membrane, interruption of energy transduction, inhibition of enzyme activity, and DNA synthesis. It has been found that silver nanoparticles can modulate the signal transduction in bacteria. Phosphorylation of proteins in bacteria influences bacterial signal transduction.

Shrivastava et al. (2007) proposed that silver nanoparticles influence the phosphotyrosine profile of putative bacterial peptides that can affect cellular signalling, which leads to growth inhibition in bacteria. It was also found that silver ions bind to the 30S ribosomal subunit, deactivate the ribosome complex, and prevent protein translation. Klueh et al. (2000) hypothesized that bactericidal activity of the silver nanoparticles is attributable to the Ag^+ ions, which enter the cell and intercalate between the purine and pyrimidine base of DNA. These base pairs showed disturbing effect on the hydrogen bonding between the two antiparallel strands, leading to denaturation of DNA molecule (Klueh et al. 2000; Rai et al. 2012).

The rapid growth in research about antimicrobial activities in vitro strengthens the need for closer evaluation of their potential activities in vivo.

Bacteria are thought to play a critical role in delayed healing by altering host cell function. Strategies to control the risk of infection and the level of bacterial activity are generally directed toward number of bacteria, strength of their virulence, and the immune status of the host (Robson 1997). The studies showed that AgNPs beside high antimicrobial activities had the potential to promote wound healing through facilitated anti-inflammatory action (Tian et al. 2007; Liu et al. 2010; Kedi et al. 2018). Then AgNPs not only had a beneficial effect on acceleration of the wound-healing process but also improved the tensile properties of the repaired skin (Fig. 9.1).

Silver nanoparticles are mostly included in wound treatment systems to obtain clinically desired results with fast and effective healing. In vitro experiments have depicted that silver in its nanoparticles form reduced mitochondrial activity without causing skin cell lysis or disrupting the nuclear integrity of skin cells. The reduction in the mitochondrial activity implies decrease in the presence of bacteria hence proving the antibacterial potential of silver nanoparticles (Nam et al. 2015).

The ability of silver nanoparticles to cause reduction in the growth of bacteria without causing any damage to skin cells sets the basis for clinical safety and antimicrobial activity. Tian et al. (2007) and Liu et al. (2010) studied in vivo wound-healing potential of topically delivered silver nanoparticles and reported fast healing and enhanced scarring appearance in dose-dependent pattern. For the study, thermal injury mouse model was used and it was observed that the average healing time of mouse inoculated with silver nanoparticles was much less than those of the negative control group. Also, the appearance of the healed areas with silver nanoparticles was similar to normal skin whereas silver sulphadizine-treated groups depicted hypertrophic scarring. Therefore, the wound dressing coated with nanosilver was significantly more efficient in hindering bacterial growth at the wound site than the silver sulphadiazine solution (Figs. 9.2 and 9.3).

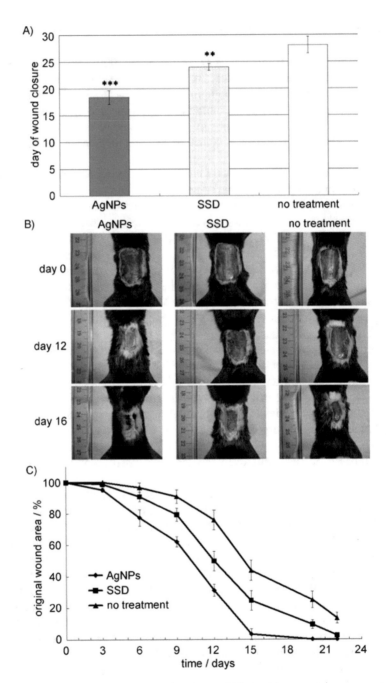

Fig. 9.1 The effects of AgNPs on wound healing: excisional skin wounds were created on the dorsa of mice, and they were divided into three groups for treatment with AgNPS, silver sulphadiazine (SSD), no treatment (control). (**a**) Time to complete wound closure in each group (**p« 0.01, ***p « 0.001). (**b**) Wound appearance from the three groups at various time points. (**c**) Rate of wound closure at various time points after wounding. *X. Liu X, Lee PY, Ho CM, Lui VC, Chen Y, Che CM, Tam PK, Wong KK (2010) Silver nanoparticles mediate differential responses in keratinocytes and fibroblasts during skin wound healing. ChemMedChem 5:468–475. Copyright Wiley-VCH Verlag GmbH & Co. KGaA. Reproduced with permission*

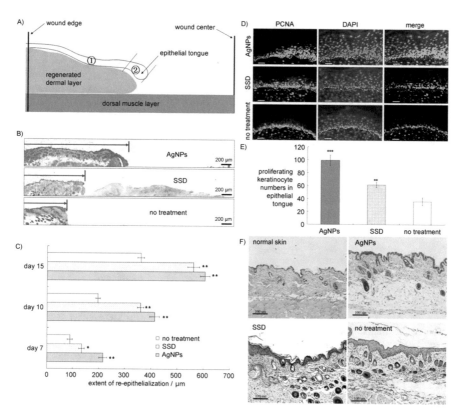

Fig. 9.2 Re-epithelialization and proliferation of keratinocytes by AgNPs during healing. (**a**) Schematic side view of a wound indicating the location of proliferating cells after examination. Region 1 represents the re-epithelialization area, and region 2 represents the epithelial tongue. (**b**) Wounds were excised and stained with HE on day 7 after wounding and the degree of wound closure was examined histologically. Proliferating cells arising from the wound edge at the left migrate toward the wound center at right; the blue bar indicates the leading edge of the epithelium. (**c**) The extent of re-epithelization on days 7, 10, and 15 after wounding was measured histologically in the three experimental groups ($^{*}p \ll 0.005$, $^{**}p \ll 0.01$). (**d**) IHC staining of proliferating cells in the epithelial tongue area on day 15 after wounding. The dashed line in each image indicates the division between the epithelial layer and the dermal layer; scale bars: 20 μm. (**e**) Average numbers of proliferating cells in the epithelial tongue area on day 15 after wounding ($^{**}p \ll 0.01$, $^{***}p \ll 0.001$). (**f**) Histological morphology of healed wounds in animals from the three experimental groups relative to normal skin. *Liu X, Lee PY, Ho CM, Lui VC, Chen Y, Che CM, Tam PK, Wong KK (2010) Silver nanoparticles mediate differential responses in keratinocytes and fibroblasts during skin wound healing. ChemMedChem 5:468–475. Copyright Wiley-VCH Verlag GmbH & Co. KGaA. Reproduced with permission*

Although silver has been used in commercially available products, such advancements in wound care would lead to positive health implications. The use of nanoparticles and their modification at the molecular and nano level increases the efficacy of wound healing. These developments also notably reduce the time required for the wound to reach its normal homeostatic equilibrium and reduce the risk of unnecessary complications (Nam et al. 2015).

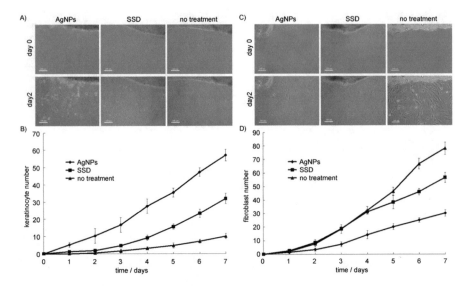

Fig. 9.3 The effect of AgNPs or SSD on keratinocytes and fibroblast obtained from the dorsal skin mice and cultured in appropriate media with either AgNPs or SSD. (**a**) The number of keratinocytes in the three experimental groups after 2 days of culture. (**b**) Keratinocyte numbers in the outgrowth area counted and averaged over the course of 7 days. (**c**) The number of fibroblast grown from the dermal margin after 2 days of culture. (**d**) Fibroblast numbers in the outgrowth area counted and averaged over the course of 7 days. *Liu X, Lee PY, Ho CM, Lui VC, Chen Y, Che CM, Tam PK, Wong KK (2010) Silver nanoparticles mediate differential responses in keratinocytes and fibroblasts during skin wound healing. ChemMedChem 5:468–475. Copyright Wiley-VCH Verlag GmbH & Co. KGaA. Reproduced with permission*

In the processing of skin tissue repair, the moisture provided by the dressing promoted ulcers healing and reduced pain of patients. An attractive novel wound-dressing material is silver nanoparticles/bacterial cellulose composites (Wu et al. 2014). The aggregation tendency of silver nanoparticles can undermine their unique properties at nanoscale. One strategy to prevent aggregation is controlled deposition of metal particles through hybridization by using a nanoporous material as template to ensure a well-defined spatial distribution. The electrostatic interactions between silver ions, dipole moments of cellulose molecules, and the nanospace in the cellulose fibres serve as nanoreactor. The in vitro experimental results demonstrated that AgNPs-bacterial cellulose had low cytotoxicity because of the slow releasing of silver ions and little leakage of Ag nanoparticles, which is an essential characteristic for biomaterials as wound dressing (Wu et al. 2014).

To date, there are a less number of reports on a synergistic effect of AgNPs in combination with antibiotics against bacteria. Ahmadi and Adibhesami (2017) studied the effect of AgNPs alone and in combination with tetracycline on inoculated wounds with Pseudomonas aeruginosa in mice. Wound infection assessed using total count of bacterial load and also wound healing monitored. In all groups, treatments applied topically in the wound bed: AgNPs, tetracycline, AgNPs along with tetracycline, and normal saline in control group. The tetracycline along with AgNPs achieved 100% wound closure on day 12. In the AgNPs group, the percentage of wound contraction has close figures compared to tetracycline and normal saline as 98, 99, and 79%, respectively. By day 12, all of the treated groups with AgNPs, tetracycline, and AgNPs along with tetracycline showed decreases in surface bacterial concentration compared with control group. Also significant decrease in deep skin bacterial counts in the AgNPs, tetracycline, and AgNPs along with tetracycline compared with control group at any time point was observed. Application of AgNPs along with tetracycline was more effective than AgNPs and tetracycline alone to reduce the bacterial load whilst wound macroscopic contraction increased.

Wypij et al. (2018) demonstrated remarkable enhancement of antimicrobial activity and reduced dosage against bacteria and yeast by combining silver nanoparticles with antibiotics. The reduction in the dosage of antimicrobial agent also reduced its toxicity to mammalian cell lines. Thus, silver nanoparticles in combination with antibiotics possess the ability to kill drug-resistant bacteria. Birla et al. (2009) found that antibacterial activity of silver nanoparticles in combination with antibiotics against *E. coli, Staphylococcus aureus*, and *Pseudomonas aeruginosa* and found that silver nanoparticles in combination with antibiotics showed strong antibacterial activity against the bacteria exhibiting resistance to various antibiotics. Gajbhiye et al. (2009) studied the fungicidal activity of nanoparticles alone and in combination with commercially available antifungal agent fluconazole. They found that not only silver nanoparticles can inhibit the fungal growth, but also there was an increase in the antifungal activity of fluconazole in combination with silver nanoparticles. Bonde et al. (2012) reported bactericidal potential of phytonanoparticles alone and in combination with commercially available antibiotics: gentamycin, ampicillin, tetracycline, streptomycin against pathogenic bacteria *E. coli, Staphylococcus aureus, Pseudomonas aeruginosa*. They observed that silver nanoparticles in combination with gentamycin showed the maximum activity against *E. coli*, whilst tetracycline in combination with nanoparticles showed maximum activity against *Staphylococcus aureus*. They concluded that activity of standard antibiotics was significantly increased in the presence of silver nanoparticles and that can be used against antibiotic-resistant pathogens effectively.

9.5 Mechanisms of Silver Resistance

The lack of standardized methods to determine bacterial susceptibility to silver complicates interpretation of silver susceptibility and resistance data.

There are a few reports of silver resistance in bacteria and few include data that help clarify resistance mechanisms (Chopra 2007). McHugh et al. (1975) described the first instance when a silver-resistant strain of *Salmonella typhimurium* emerged in a hospital burns unit. It was reported that a silver-resistant determinant occurred on a conjugally transferable plasmid, which also encoded resistance to mercuric chloride, ampicillin, chloramphenicol, tetracycline, streptomycin, and sulphonamides. The silver-resistant determinant contains seven genes and two open-reading frames of unknown function. Bridges et al. (1979) isolated silver-resistant *Pseudomonas aeruginosa* from burn patients. A loss of resistance on subculture suggests that resistance may have been plasmid mediated. Li et al. (1997) concluded that activation of an endogenous silver efflux system together with porin mutation provides the basis for silver resistance. The mechanism of silver resistance may have involved intracellular detoxification of silver ions by plasmid.

Silver resistance in bacteria has a molecular, morphological, and genetic basis. A silver-resistant strain of E. coli isolated from a burn wound containing two large plasmids failed to absorb or retain silver, whereas in a sensitive strain silver accumulation was five-fold higher. Electron microscopy and molecular techniques have shown that silver resistance encodes in a pericytoplasmic protein—SilE and that this is expressed in the presence of metallothionein (a silver-induced, cysteine-rich metal-binding protein). Cytoplasmic changes in a sensitive strain of Staphylococcus aureus have been identified as electron-light regions in the cytoplasm associated with denatured DNA.

The lack of standardized methods to determine bacterial susceptibility to silver complicates interpretation of silver susceptibility and resistance data.

Silver-based dressing release different amounts of silver ions in different ways via different materials. Some of the higher silver release formulations produce ionic silver concentrations that reach 70–100 ppm (measured in ionic water) and kill relevant bacteria within 30 min (Burrell 2003).

Dressings that release low levels of silver ions are likely to be more dangerous in terms of selection for resistance, especially if the silver ion concentration is sublethal. Faster acting dressings will inevitably present less risk because organisms are more likely to be killed, thereby eliminating possibilities for enrichment of the resistant populations through growth and division, especially in the context of mutational development of resistance (Chopra 2007).

There is no direct evidence that silver-resistant mechanisms confer cross-resistance to antibiotics. However, silver-resistant genes and antibiotic-resistant genes have been reported in the context of plasmid-mediated silver resistance.

Some silver-based dressings appear to provide an effective alternative to antibiotics in the management of wound infection. However, dressings that release low levels of silver ions are likely to be more problematic in terms of selection for resistance, especially if the silver concentration is sublethal. In order to minimize the risk of silver-resistant clinicians should choose dressings that release high levels of silver ions and that demonstrate rapid bactericidal activity (Chopra 2007).

9.6   Toxicity of Silver Nanoparticles

Toxicity of silver is reported in the form of argyria, where there is large deposition of silver ions on the open wound. However, there are no usual reports of allergy to silver (Rai et al. 2009). Silver nanoparticles in most studies are suggested to be non-toxic.

AgNPs promote wound healing through their powerful antibacterial properties, as well as their ability to decrease inflammation (Liu et al. 2010). The question remains as to whether silver nanoparticles can elicit effects on the various skin cell types present. This is important in the wound-healing process, as re-epithelialization and wound contraction are two components that are mediated by two different respective cell types: keratinocytes and fibroblasts.

Burd et al. (2007) studied cytotoxicity of silver nanoparticles impregnated commercially dressings. It was found that three out of five silver dressing depicted cytotoxicity effects in keratinocytes and fibroblast cultures. The question as to whether silver nanoparticles can affect skin cell types—keratinocytes and fibroblasts—during the wound-healing process still remains. Silver nanoparticles can increase the rate of wound closure. This was achieved through the promotion of proliferation and migration of keratinocytes. Silver nanoparticles can drive the differentiation of fibroblasts into myofibroblasts, thereby promoting wound contraction. Braydich-Stolle et al. (2005) studied the toxicity of silver nanoparticles on C18-4 cell, a cell line with spermatogonial stem cells. The results of the above study depicted that the cytotoxicity of silver nanoparticles to the mitochondrial activity increases with an increase in the concentration of silver nanoparticles.

Due to substantial experiences with adverse silver reactions and side effects, it is appropriate to keep the possibility of a toxic silver effect in burn patients treated with slow sustained release silver-coated wound dressings. The agent and system of delivery should maximize the lethal effect for bacteria and minimize the damage to human cells. Ultimately, no matter how sophisticated the delivery system the agent, silver, cannot be expected to make a selective kill even though it has been reported that its toxicity toward bacteria was greater than the human cells. The ultimate aim remains the choice of a product with a superior profile of antimicrobial activity over cellular toxicity (Atiyeh et al. 2007).

9.7 Conclusion

To sum up, the wounds are mainly caused by bacteria and fungi which are usually treated with different antibiotics. Unfortunately due to the emergence of antibiotic resistance, some strains of bacteria have become resistant to almost all the available antibiotics, for example, *Staphylococcus aureus*, *Pseudomonas aeruginosa*, and *Acinetobacter baumannii*. There is a revival of interest among the researchers and clinicians for the use of silver, and more recently, silver nanoparticles are supposed to be the ray of hope as a new generation of antimicrobials owing to their use singly and in combination which has been proved to be beneficial to treat multidrug-resistant microbes as a broad-spectrum antimicrobial agent. However, the toxicity issue is the main problem, and there is a need to carry out thorough studies for the evaluation of toxicity of nanoparticles to the environment and human beings.

References

Ahmadi M, Adibhesami M (2017) The effect of silver nanoparticles on wounds contaminated with *Pseudomonas aeruginosa* in mice: an experimental study. Iran J Pharm Res 16(2):661–669

Alavi M, Rai M (2019) Recent advances in antibacterial applications of metal nanoparticles (MNPs) and metal nanocomposites (MNCs) against multidrug-resistant (MDR) bacteria. Expert Rev Anti-Infect Ther 17(6):419–428. https://doi.org/10.1080/14787210.2019.1614914

Atiyeh BS, Costagliola M, Hayek SN, Dibo SA (2007) Effect of silver on burn wound infection control and healing: review of literature. Burns 33:139–148

Ayton M (1985) Wound care: wounds that won't heal. Nurs Times 81(46):16–19

Barillo DJ, Marx DE (2014) Silver in medicine: a brief history BC 335 to present. Burns 40:3–8

Bawskar MS, Deshmukh SD, Bansod S, Gade AK, Rai MK (2015) Comparative analysis of bio-synthesised and chemosynthesised silver nanoparticles with special reference to their antibacterial activity against pathogens. IET Nanobiotechnol 9(3):107–113

Birla SS, Tiwari VV, Gade AK, Ingle AP, Yadav AP, Rai MK (2009) Fabrication of silver nanoparticles by *Phoma glomerata* and its combined effect against *Escherichia coli, Pseudomonas aeruginosa* and *Staphylococcus aureus*. Lett Appl Microbiol 48(2):173–179

Bonde SR, Rathod DP, Ingle AP, Ade RB, Gade AK, Rai MK (2012) *Murraya koenigii*-mediated synthesis of silver nanoparticles and its activity against three human pathogenic bacteria. Nanosci Methods 1:25–36

Bowler PG (1998) The anaerobic and aerobic microbiology of wounds: A review. Wounds 10(6):170–178

Bowler P, Duerden B, Armstrong D (2001) Wound microbiology and associated approaches to wound management. Clin Microbiol Rev 14(2):244–269

Braydich-Stolle L, Hussain S, Schlager JJ, Hofmann MC (2005) In vitro cytotoxicity of nanoparticles in mammalian gemline stem cells. Toxicol Sci 88(2):412–419

Bridges K, Kidson A, Lowbury EJ et al (1979) Gentamicin—and silver—resistant *Pseudomonas* in a burns unit. Br Med J 1:446–449

Burd A, Kwok CH, Hung SC, Chan HS, Gu H, Lam WK, Huang L (2007) A comparative study of the cytotoxicity of silver-based dressings in monolayer cell, tissue explant, and animal models. Wound Repair Regen 15:94–104

Burrell RE (2003) A scientific perspective on the use of topical silver preparations. Ostomy Wound Manage 49(Suppl. 5A):19–24

Calvin M (1998) Cutaneous wound repair. Wounds 10(1):12–32

Chopra I (2007) The increasing use of silver-based products as antimicrobial agents: a useful development or a cause for concern? J Antimicrob Chemother 59:587–590

Chu CS, McManus AT, Pruitt BA Jr, Mason AD Jr (1988) Therapeutic effects of silver nylon dressings with weak current on *Pseudomonas aeruginosa*—infected burn wounds. J Trauma 28:1488–1492

Chu CS, McManus AT, Okerberg CV, Mason AD Jr, Pruitt BA Jr (1991) Weak direct current accelerates split-thickness graft healing on tangentially excised second degree burns. J Burn Care Rehabil 12:285–293

Chu CS, Matylevich NP, McManus AT, Masson AD Jr, Pruitt BA Jr (1996) Direct current reduces wound edema after full thickness burn injury in rats. J Trauma 40(5):738–742

Collier M (2004) Recognition and management of wound infection. J World Wide Wounds

Dunn K, Edwards-Jones V (2004) The role of Acticoat with nanocrystalline silver in the management of burns. Burns 30:1–9

Fakhry SM, Alexander J, Smith D, Meyer AA, Petterson HD (1995) Regional and institutional variation in burn care. J Burn Care Rehabil 16:86–90

Falanga V, Grinnell F, Gilchrest B, Maddox YT, Moshell A (1994) Workshop on the pathogenesis of chronic wounds. J Invest Dermatol 102(1):125–127

Feng QL, Wu J, Chen GQ, Cui FZ, Kim TN, Kim JO (2000) A mechanistic study of the antibacterial effect of silver ions on *Escherichia coli* and *Staphylococcus aureus*. J Biomed Mater Res 52(4):662–668

Fong J, Wood F, Fowler BA (2005) A silver coated dressing reduces the incidence of early burn wound cellulitis and associated costs of inpatient treatment: comparative patient care audits. Burns 31(5):562–567

Fox CL (1968) Silver sulfadiazine—a new topical agent. Arch Surg 96:184–188

Fox CL, Stanford JW (1971) Anti-bacterial action of silver sulphadiazine and DNA binding. In: Matter P, Barcaly TL, Konikova Z (eds) Research in burns. Huber, Bern, pp 133–138

Franci G, Falanga A, Galdiero S, Palomba L, Rai M, Morelli G, Galdiero M (2015) Silver nanoparticles as potential antibacterial agents. Molecules 20:8856–8874. https://doi.org/10.3390/molecules20058856

Gajbhiye M, Kesharwani J, Ingle A, Gade A, Rai M (2009) Fungal-mediated synthesis of silver nanoparticles and their activity against pathogenic fungi in combination with fluconazole. Nanomedicine 5(4):382–386

Gamelli RL, Paxton TP, O'Reilly M (1993) Bone marrow toxicity by silver sulphadiazine. Surg Gynec Obstet 177:115–120

Jiang B, Larson JC, Drapala PW, Perez-Luna VH, Kang-Mieler JJ, Brey EM (2012) Investigation of lysine acrylate containing poly(N-isopropylacrylamide) hydrogels as wound dressings in normal and infected wounds. J Biomed Mater Res 100:668–676

Karkman A, Katariina P, Joakim Larsson DG (2019) Fecal pollution can explain antibiotic resistance gene abundances in anthropogenically impacted environments. Nat Commun 0:80. https://doi.org/10.1038/s41467-018-07992-3

Kedi PBE, Meva FE, Kotsedi L, Nguemfo EL, Zangueu CB, Ntoumba AA, Mohamed HEA, Dongmo AB, Maaza M (2018) Eco-friendly synthesis, characterization, in vitro and in vivo anti-inflammatory activity of silvernanoparticle-mediated *Selaginella myosurus* aqueous extract. Int J Nanomedicine 12(13):8537–8548. https://doi.org/10.2147/IJN.S174530.

Kingsley A (2001) A proactive approach to wound infection. Nurs Stand 15(30):50–54, 56, 58

Kirsner R, Orsted H, Wright B (2001) Matrix metalloproteinases in normal and impaired wound healing: a potential role of nanocrystaline silver. Wounds 13:5–10

Klasen HJ (2000) A historical review of the use of silver in the treatment of burns. Part I early uses. Burns 30:1–9

Klueh U, Wagner V, Kelly S, Johnson A, Bryers JD (2000) Efficacy of silver coated fabric to prevent bacterial colonization and subsequent device-based biofilm formation. J Biomed Mater Res 53:621–631

Lansdown ABG (2006) Silver in health care: antimicrobial effects and safety in use. Cuur Probl Dermatol 33:17–34. In: Biofunctional Textiles and the Skin, Hipler U.C., Elsner P. (eds)

Lansdown ABG (2010) Silver in health and disease. Its antimicrobial efficacy and safety in use. Royal Society of Chemistry, London

Li XZ, Nikaido H, Williams KE (1997) Silver-resistant mutants of *Escherichia coli* display active efflux of Ag$^+$ and are deficient in porins. J Bacteriol 179:6127–6132

Liau SY, Read DC, Pugh WJ, Furr JR, Russel AD (1997) Interaction of silver-nitrate with readily identiflabe groups-relationship to the antibacterial action of silver ions. Lett Appl Microbiol 25:279–283

Liu X, Lee P, Ch H, Lui V, Chen Y, Ch C, Tam P, Wong KY (2010) Silver nanoparticles mediate differential responses in keratinocytes and fibroblasts during skin wound healing. ChemMedChem 5(3):468–475

McHugh GL, Moellering RC, Hopkins CC et al (1975) *Salmonella typhimurium* resistant to silver nitrate, chloramphenicol and ampicillin. Lancet 1:235–240

Mooney EK (2006) Silver dressings (safety and efficacy reports). Plast Reconstr Surg 117(2):666–669

Moyer CA, Brentano L, Gravens DL, Margraf HW, Monafo WW (1965) Treatment of large human burns with 0.5% silver nitrate solution. Arch Surg 90:812–867

Nadworny PL, Wang JF, Tredget EE, Burrell RE (2010) Anti-inflammatory activity of nanocrystal-line silver-derived solutions in porcine contact dermatitis. J Inflam 7:20

Nam G, Rangasamy S, Purushothaman B, Song JM (2015) The application of bactericidal silver nanoparticles in wound treatment. Nanomater Nanotechnol 5:23

Pal S, Tak YK, Song JM (2007) Does the antibacterial activity of silver nanoparticles depend on the shape of the nanoparticle? A study of the gram-negative bacterium *Escherichia coli*. Appl Environ Microbiol 73(6):1712–1720

Poon VKM, Burd A (2004) In vitro cytotoxity of silver: implication for clinical wound care. Burns 30:140–147

Prabhu S, Poulose EK (2012) Silver nanoparticles: mechanism of antimicrobial action, synthesis, medical application, and toxicity effects. Int Nano Lett 2:32–42

Rai MK, Yadav AP, Gade AK (2009) Silver nanoparticles as a new generation of antimicrobials. Biotechnol Adv 27(1):76–83

Rai MK, Deshmukh SD, Ingle AP, Gade AK (2012) Silver nanoparticles: powerful nanoweapon against multidrug-resistant bacteria. Appl Microbiol 112:841–852

Robson MC (1997) Wound infection. A failure of wound healing caused by an imbalance of bacteria. Surg Clin N Am 77:637–650

Shrivastava S, Bera T, Poy A, Singh G, Ramachandrarao P, Dash D (2007) Characterisation of enhanced antibacterial effects of novel silver nanoparticles. Nanotechnology 18:1–9

Singh J, Dutta T, Kim K, Rawat M, Samddar P, Kumar P (2018) Green' synthesis of metals and their oxide nanoparticles: applications for environmental remediation. J Nanobiotechnol 16:84. https://doi.org/10.1186/s12951-018-0408-4

Stanford W, Rappole BW, Fox Jr CL (1969) Clinical experience with silver sulfadiazine, a new topical agent for control of pseudomonas infection in burn patients. *J Trauma* 9(5):377–388

Tian J, Wong KK, Ho CM, Lok CN, Yu WY, Che CM et al (2007) Topical delivery of silver nanoparticles promotes wound healing. ChemMedChem 2:129–136

Tredget EE, Shankowsky HA, Groeneveld A, Burrell R (1998) A matched – pair, randomized study evaluating the efficacy and safety of Acticoat silver – coated dressing for the treatment of burn wounds. *J Burn Care Rehabil* 19:531–537

Venkataraman M, Nagarsenker M (2013) Silver sulfadiazine nanosystems for burn therapy. AAPS PharmSciTech 14(1):254–264. https://doi.org/10.1208/s12249-012-9914-0

Warriner R, Burrell R (2005) Infection and the chronic wound: a focus on silver. Adv Skin Wound Care 18(8):2–12

Wright JB, Lam K, Hansen D, Burrell RE (1999) Efficacy of topical silver against fungal burn wound pathogens. *Am J Inf Control* 27(4):344–350

Wright J, Lam K, Buret A, Olson M, Burrell R (2002) Early healing events in a porcine model of contaminated wounds: effects of nanocrystalline silver on matrix matalloproteinases, cell apoptosis, and healing. *Wound Repair Regeneration*, 10:141

Wu J, Zheng Y, Song W, Luan J, Wen X, Wu Z, Chen X, Wang Q, Guo S (2014) *In situ* synthesis of silver-nanoparticles/bacterial cellulose composites for slow-released antimicrobial wound dressing. Carbohydr Polym 102:762–771

Wu S, Huang J, Zhang F, Qingping W, Zhang J, Pang R, Zeng H, Yang X, Chen M, Wang J, Dai J, Xue L, Lei T, Wei X (2019) Prevalence and characterization of food-related methicillin resistant *Staphylococcus aureus* (MRSA) in China. Front Microbiol 10:304. https://doi.org/10.3389/fmicb.2019.00304

Wypij M, Świecimska M, Czarnecka J, Dahm H, Rai M, Golińska P (2018) Antimicrobial and cytotoxic activity of silver nanoparticles synthesized from two haloalkaliphilic actinobacterial strains alone and in combination with antibiotics. Appl Microbiol 124:1411–1424

Yin HQ, Langford R, Burrell RE (1999) Comparative evaluation of the antimicrobial activity of ACTICOAT antimicrobial barrier dressing. J Burn Care Rehabil 20:195–200

Chapter 10
Applications of Chitosan and Nanochitosan in Formulation of Novel Antibacterial and Wound Healing Agents

Mehran Alavi

Abstract Applications of chitosan and nanochitosan biomaterials in biomedical field are based on important advantages of this biopolymer including biocompatibility, biodegradability, hemostatic, antimicrobial activities, acceleration in wound healing process, nearly controlled release of antimicrobial agents and growth factors. However, low solubility of chitosan in physiological pH condition is important disadvantage which can be resulted in fast metabolism of this biopolymer by enzymes of gastrointestinal tract. Other striking drawbacks in chitosan application are low degree of stability, mechanical resistance, and porosity which can have negative effects on wound healing. Hence, it can be used as biocomposites/nanobiocomposites forms via interaction with natural and synthetic polymers or other materials. Considering these facts, recent advancements related to wound healing and antibacterial agents based on combination of chitosan with major natural polymers involving cellulose, collagen, alginic acid, hyaluronic acid, starch, and chondroitin sulfate are presented in this chapter.

Keywords Chitosan · Nanochitosan · Wound healing · Antibacterial agents · Natural polymer · Bio-nanocomposites

Nomenclature

AND	Andrographolide
ChNF	Chitosan nanofibril
ChNC	Chitosan nanocrystal
CN	Chitosan nanoparticle
CNC	Cellulose nanocrystal
CNF	Cellulose nanofibril
CNW	Cellulose nanowhiskers

M. Alavi (✉)
Laboratory of Nanobiotechnology, Department of Biology, Faculty of Science,
Razi University, Kermanshah, Iran

© Springer Nature Switzerland AG 2020
M. Rai (ed.), *Nanotechnology in Skin, Soft Tissue, and Bone Infections*,
https://doi.org/10.1007/978-3-030-35147-2_10

CPP   Cell-penetrating peptide
DA   Deacetylation
ECM   Extracellular matrix
EDTAD   Ethylenediaminetetraacetic acid dianhydride
IαI   Inter-α-inhibitor
KGM   Konjac glucomannan
MRSA   Methicillin resistant *Staphylococcus aureus*
MSSA   Me   thicillin sensitive *Staphylococcus aureus*
MTGase   Microbial transglutaminase
NC   Nanocellulose
NLC   Nanostructured lipid carrier
PVA   Polyvinyl alcohol
PVP   Polyvinyl pyrrolidone
S   Stearic acid
SLN   Solid lipid nanoparticle
TSG-6   TNF-stimulated gene 6
VEGF   Vascular endothelial growth factor

10.1   Introduction

The first abundant nitrogen-containing organic material and second frequent natural polymer in earth is chitin. This polymer is polysaccharide of N-acetyl-D-glucosamine with β-(1 → 4) linkage. Natural form of chitin is crystalline microfibrils which exist in several living organisms specifically shells of shrimp and crab. Exoskeleton of crustaceans and cell wall of fungi are the main source of this biopolymer (Arrouze et al. 2019). In the case of industrial facet, chitin can be obtained as waste product of krill, shellfish, oysters, fungi, clams, and squid. For production of purified polymer from these organisms, dissolution of $CaCO_3$ and elimination of related proteins are required. The main derivative of chitin is chitosan which can be generated by deacetylation (DA) treatment (about ≥50%) in the alkaline condition such as sodium hydroxide at higher temperature (120 °C). Removal of proteins, mineral materials, pigments, and acetyl groups are four steps in chitosan production. Solubility capacity of this polymer in acidic aqueous solution is related to protonation of amine group on the position of carbon-2 of the repeated unit of D-glucosamine. Amount of solubility is dependent on percentage of DA. As, DA of chitin with more and less than 60% (about 50%) are respectively insoluble in acidic and soluble in neutral media (Chen et al. 2018). There are two functional groups for chitosan including hydroxyl and amine groups which contribute in chemical and biological reactions (Fig. 10.2a). Higher reactivity of chitosan than cellulose is resulted from functional group of NH_2. Interactions of this polymer with metal cations are the basis of removal of toxic metals from wastewater. For example, modification of C-4 of chitosan   in   two   steps   of   reduction   and   esterification   by   respectively

2-pyridinecarboxaldehyde and ethylenediaminetetraacetic acid dianhydride (EDTAD) was useful in removal of Cu^{2+} and Cr^{6+} ions from aqueous solution (Moreira et al. 2018). This polymer can chelate transition metals and immobilize enzymes. In this way, composite of bio-based activated carbon with chitosan illustrated absorption values of 2.38 and 3.44 mmol g^{-1} for Cd^{2+} and Cu^{2+} cations, respectively, at 24.85 °C and pH 6 conditions (Elwakeel et al. 2018). For the case of enzyme immobilization, synthesis of galacto-oligosaccharide by β-galactosidase immobilized on chitosan showed 4.7 times the cumulative productivity than soluble enzyme. Modification of chitosan by aldehyde group is important for improvement of covalent bonding and stabilization of enzyme (Urrutia et al. 2018). Nanoderivatives of chitosan can be in different forms such as chitosan nanofibril (ChNF), chitosan nanocrystal (ChNC), chitosan nanocapsule, and chitosan film. Sodium sulfate and tripolyphosphate can be used for cross-linking of chitosan nanoparticles (CNs) (Garrido-Maestu et al. 2018).

Interactions of chitosan or nanochitosan with natural polymers are considerable issues in biomedical field specifically antibacterial and wound healing applications which are objectives of this chapter. Here, collagen, alginic acid, hyaluronic acid, starch, and chondroitin sulfate as biopolymers have been described as contents of chitosan biocomposites/nano-biocomposites.

10.2 Antibacterial Activities of Chitosan

Gram positive and Gram negative bacteria have different cell wall structure specifically in the case of peptidoglycan. Gram negative bacteria have thin peptidoglycan than Gram positive. Chitosan with NH_3^+ group in its structure can adsorb on cell wall by electrostatic interaction (Alavi and Rai 2019b). In this way, lipopolysaccharide and teichoic acid are important anionic parts of cell wall for Gram negative and Gram positive bacteria, respectively. Binding of chitosan with these parts can be resulted in damaging cell wall integrity and leakage of macromolecules from bacteria (Ma et al. 2017). Interaction of CNs with OmpA protein in outer membrane of Gram negative bacteria with chitosan may contribute in enhancing antibacterial activities (Garrido-Maestu et al. 2018).

10.3 Wound Healing Activities of Chitosan

Epidermis, dermis, and subcutaneous fat layer are three major parts of skin. These parts can be disrupted as superficial (epidermis), partial (epidermis and dermis), and full (epidermis, dermis, and subcutaneous layer) wounds (Fig. 10.1). Healing process in both chronic and acute forms of skin wounds has four stages including inflammation, migration, proliferation, and maturation or remodeling. Three weeks and 3 months are healing period for acute and chronic wounds, respectively (Patrulea

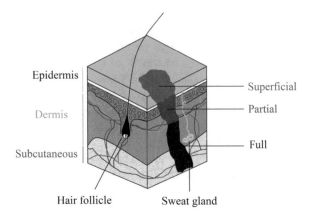

Fig. 10.1 Three layers of skin organ and three types of wounds based on thickness wound

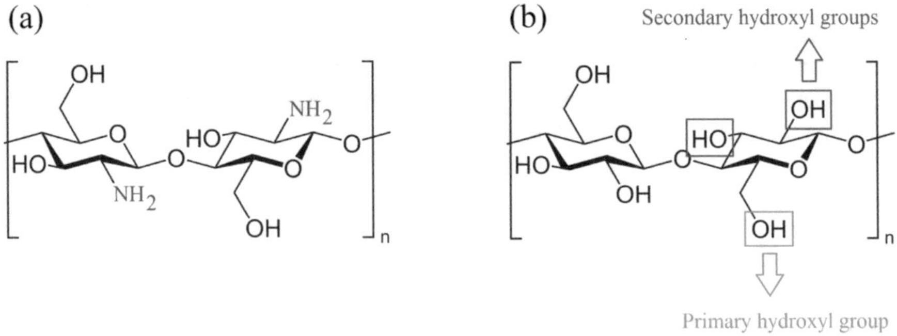

Epidermis — Superficial

Dermis — Partial

Subcutaneous — Full

Hair follicle   Sweat gland

(a)

(b)

Secondary hydroxyl groups

Primary hydroxyl group

Fig. 10.2 Structural formula of chitosan (**a**) and primary and secondary hydroxyl groups of cellulose polymer for modification (**b**)

et al. 2015). Several factors are needed for accelerating wound healing that involves wound cleansing, moist environment with exchange of gases, thermal insulation, low wound adherence and low dressing replacement, removal of bacteria, blood, and excess exudate (Boateng et al. 2008). Other problem related to wound healing is desiccation of wounds which can cause trauma after removal of wound dressings (Michalska-Sionkowska et al. 2018). There are three wound dressings including artificial, biological, and traditional dressings. In biological dressing type, application of biopolymer such as chitosan, alginate, collagen, cellulose, elastin, and hyaluronic acid is common. Among the biopolymer, biocompatibility and biodegradability of chitosan are two major advantages for using this polymer in wound dressing.

10.4 Chitosan/Cellulose

Cellulose is first abundant natural polymer in our planet. This polysaccharide is linear polysaccharide with β-(1 → 4) linkage of D-glucose unites as formula of $(C_6H_{10}O_5)_n$. Important functional groups of cellulose for modification are two secondary hydroxyl groups and one primary hydroxyl group on the surface of D-glucose (Fig. 10.2b). Major natural source of this polymer is cell walls of plant species. Also, bacteria specifically *Acetobacter xylinum* can produce extracellular cellulose with advantage and disadvantage of higher crystalline structure and porosity, respectively, than herbal cellulose. In this regard, spaces between cellulose microfibrils are filled by lignin and hemicellulose. Nanocellulose (NC) with unique properties of nanomaterials such as large surface area and higher reactivity than cellulose has been applied in several industrial and medicinal fields. There are two forms of NC including cellulose nanofibril (CNF) and cellulose nanocrystal (CNC) (Alavi 2019). Chitosan nanofibril/CNF with weight ratio of 1:1 and concentration of 100 µg/disc demonstrated antibacterial activities against *Stenotrophomonas maltophilia* pathogens (Zarayneh et al. 2018). In another study, nanocomposites of chitosan-xylan/cellulose nanowhiskers (CNW) with 12% weight ratio of CNW to chitosan showed significant antibacterial effects against *S. aureus* followed by *E. coli* after 24 h incubation (Bao et al. 2018). Considerable antibacterial activities against *S. aureus*, *E. coli*, *Pseudomonas aeruginosa,* and *Bacillus subtilis* and improved mechanical properties including young's modulus and strength tensile were observed for nanocomposite film of CNC-styrylquinoxalin-grafted-chitosan (Fardioui et al. 2018).

10.5 Chitosan/Alginic Acid

Linear copolymer of β-D-mannuronic (M) and α-L-guluronic acid (G) with β-$(1 \rightarrow 4)$ linkage is alginic acid. This natural polymer can be isolated from cell walls of seaweeds such as brown algae specifically *Laminaria hyperborea* and biofilm of *Pseudomonas aeruginosa* bacteria. Number and length of M and G blocks are dependent on extraction source. For example, approximately 60% amount of G block is determined for *L. hyperborean* compared to other alginate sources with 14–30% (Lee and Mooney 2012). Biocompatibility of alginate can be effected by impurities resulted from extraction methods. Content of M and G blocks also is important in this property. As, higher amount of M block compared to G block can lead to reduction of biocompatibility. Other property of alginate, viscosity, is related to molecular weight. Alginate with higher molecular weight has higher viscosity as well as better mechanical trait than lower one. However, one disadvantage of higher molecular weight is difficulty of gel formation of this polymer in solution (Park et al. 2017). There are three major salts of alginic acid including sodium alginate ($NaC_6H_7O_6$), calcium alginate ($C_{12}H_{14}CaO_{12}$), and potassium alginate ($KC_6H_7O_6$). Sodium alginate is natural polymer with anionic, biocompatibility, and biodegradability properties (Fig. 10.3). Also, amphiphilic and cell adhesive derivatives of alginates can be obtained by application of hydrophobic materials and particular peptides.

There are several studies related to polyelectrolyte complex of chitosan with alginate. In the case of antibacterial activities, significant effects on *E. coli* and *S. aureus* were observed for hydrogels of lysozyme-loaded chitosan/alginate (Wu

Fig. 10.3 Structural
formula of sodium alginate

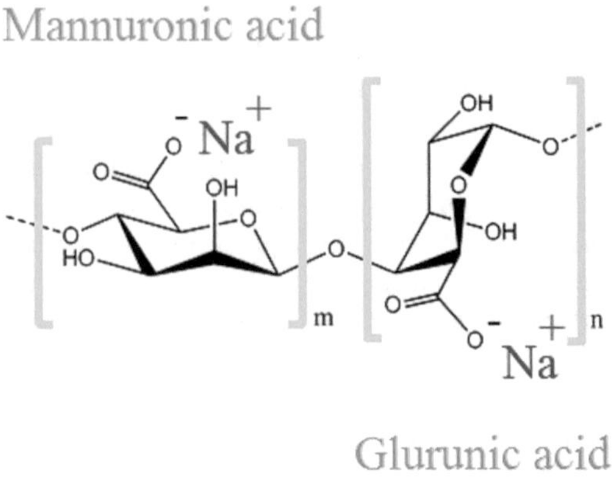

Mannuronic acid

Glurunic acid

et al. 2018). In another study, immersion method was used to blend chitosan, alginate, *Aloe vera* gel, and silver NPs as nanocomposites in different weight ratio with
antibacterial abilities. Antibacterial activities of these nanocomposites compared to
gentamicin antibiotic showed significant results for chitosan-*Aloe vera*-AgNPs and
alginate-*Aloe vera*-Ag NPs (Gómez Chabala et al. 2017). Improved antibacterial
efficiency of these nanocomposites may be resulted from unique antibacterial
capacities of silver NPs (Alavi and Karimi 2018a, b, 2019; Alavi and Rai 2019a;
Taran et al. 2016). In case of wound dressing, wet spin method was used for preparation of chitosan-coated alginate fiber with antibacterial effects on *E. coli*,
Staphylococcus epidermidis, methicillin resistant and sensitive *Staphylococcus
aureus* (MRSA and MSSA). Results of this study illustrated more bacterial reduction rate (100%) for longer fibers with 100 cm than fibers with 50 cm (98%)
(Dumont et al. 2018). Prepared microspheres of chitosan/alginate with Ca^{2+} ions
cross-linking process showed significant reduction in biofilm formation of *E. faecalis*, *P. aeruginosa*, *P. vulgaris*, and *S. aureus* at 40 μg concentration (Thaya et al.
2018). Composite of chitosan/alginate was coated by AgNPs for improving of antibacterial activities against *E. coli* and *S. aureus*. This study showed lower cytotoxicity of these modified biocomposites at 25 μM and higher antibacterial effect at
100 μM with 7.7 and 7 mm of IZD respectively for *E. coli* and *S. aureus* (Zhang
et al. 2018).

10.6   Chitosan/Collagen

The major structural protein in extracellular matrix (ECM), connective tissue, and
skin organ (3/4 of skin dry weight in human) of vertebrates is collagen. This protein
is composed of triple helix (two identical chains of α1 plus one chain of α2) of
amino acids sequence specifically glycine, proline, alanine, and hydroxyproline.
Fibroblast cells in skin are responsible for collagen synthesis. In human, there are
five most common collagen types involving types I, II, III, IV, and V. Among these

types, more percentage (90%) is associated to collagen type I (Shoulders and Raines 2009). In order to improve degradability rate and hemostatic effect of collagen, the solution of collagen-chitosan was applied with w/v of 2% in 0.01 mol/L acetic acid as volume ratio of 2:3 of collagen and chitosan, respectively. In this study, organo-montmorillonite and extract of *Callicarpa nudiflora* plant were used, respectively, to increase porous and antibacterial properties in membrane structure of collagen/alginate. In incubation period of 12, 24, and 36 h, this composite membrane showed antibacterial activity of 27.03 ± 0.20, 49.77 ± 0.33, and 68.60 ± 0.10, respectively (Yu et al. 2018). In another investigation, oligoarginine (R8) with function of cell-penetrating peptide (CPP) was used for modification of collagen/chitosan gel. Disc diffusion assay for collagen/chitosan and collagen/chitosan/CPP showed IZDs of 11.43 ± 0.88 and 17.7 ± 0.98 mm, respectively. Wound healing activity as wound closure rate after 14 days for control, collagen/chitosan, and collagen/chitosan/CPP gel were 89 ± 4.53, 93 ± 4.71, and 96 ± 4.47%, respectively (Li et al. 2018). In order to improve antibacterial activities of biological wound dressing, gentamicin sulfate antibiotic was coated on chitosan/collagen/hyaluronic acid film. Hyaluronic acid with weight ratio of 1, 2, and 5% w/w illustrated different antibacterial effect on *P. aeruginosa* as 27.5 ± 0.5, 23.0 ± 1.0, and 25.0 ± 2.0 mm of IZDs (Michalska-Sionkowska et al. 2018). Microbial transglutaminase (MTGase) as biocatalyst can be used for grafting of collagen on chitosan. Fan and coworkers (2014) used Konjac glucomannan (KGM) polysaccharide for increasing biocompatibility and biodegradability of chitosan-collagen peptide composite hydrogel (Fan et al. 2014). In this study, grafting of collagen peptide on chitosan and linking of KGM to composite were performed by MTGase and Schiff-base reaction, respectively. Cytotoxicity assay results of this hydrogel demonstrated more than 90% viability of NIH-3T3 cells after 5 days incubation (Liu et al. 2018).

10.7 Hyaluronic Acid

Glycosaminoglycans are divided into two groups of sulfated and non-sulfated polysaccharides with negative charge which contribute to structural stability of most tissues. Hyaluronic acid or hyaluronan is a non-sulfated glycosaminoglycan which is one of the important components of the ECM with functions in cell migration and proliferation (Belvedere et al. 2018). This anionic polymer may have high molecular weight and can be found in extracellular capsule of group A streptococcus bacteria as virulence factors (Henningham et al. 2018). Promotion and moderation of inflammation response in wound healing process are two major functions of hyaluronic acid (Hussain et al. 2017). Granulation stability in tissue matrix can be moderated by this polymer. Hyaluronic acid by binding with TSG-6 (TNF-stimulated gene 6) and serum proteinase inhibitor IαI (inter-α-inhibitor) can moderate inflammation process (Tighe and Garantziotis 2018). Anionic property of this glycosaminoglycan contributes to free-radical scavenging abilities (Vecchies et al. 2018). Based on these abilities, composites and nanocomposites formulation of this polymer with chitosan have been used for healing of wounds. For example, for increasing physiological activities of chitosan, L-glutamic acid was applied as chitosan-L-glutamic acid compound in 0.5% of acetic acid solution. This compound was used for reduction of $AgNO_3$ (AgNPs formation) followed by loading on hyaluronic acid for spongy dressing material with higher antibacterial effects on *E. coli* and *S. aureus* (Lu et al. 2017). There are applications of diterpenes as antimicrobial and anti-inflammation agents in wound healing formulations of chitosan-hyaluronic acid. For instance, andrographolide (AND) diterpene was firstly encapsulated in solid lipid nanoparticle (SLN) and nanostructured lipid carrier (NLC) to increase permeability in stratum corneum of skin. Then, these nanoparticles were loaded in chitosan-hyaluronic acid sponge. In this study, antioxidant and wound healing results were evaluated. In this way, complete wound closure was observed after 21 days for chitosan-hyaluronic acid/NLC (with composition of Geleol: Brij 58: 40% Labrafac) compared to control and chitosan-hyaluronan composite with respectively 85.3% and 95.3% rates (Sanad and Abdel-Bar 2017). Growth factors such as vascular endothelial growth factor (VEGF) have major effect on wound tissue regeneration by angiogenesis and therefore providing nutrient environment to accelerate wound healing process (Wang et al. 2018). Two steps strategy with antibacterial and angiogenesis properties in short-term and long-term activities was performed by vancomycin-loaded carboxymethyl chitosan/aldehyde hyaluronic acid hydrogels and VEGF-encapsulated poly (lactic-co-glycolic acid) microspheres, respectively, having various pore sizes. In this context, more antibacterial effect was observed in the case of *S. aureus* pathogen. In addition, histological studies showed wound healing acceleration in animal models after 14 days (Huang et al. 2018). Mechanical stability in wound dressings is an important property which chitosan-hyaluronic acid composites do not have. In electrospinning method, polycaprolactone was used for improvement of mechanical stability of these composites. In this study, nanofibrous scaffold (chitosan/polycaprolactone-hyaluronic acid) with diameter of 362.2 nm (similar to collagen diameter) illustrated reduction in *E. coli* adhesion on this bilayer scaffold. In addition, vero cell showed significant proliferation, growth, and migration on the scaffold (Chanda et al. 2018). In another study, layer by layer assembly method was used for production of non-woven cotton-chitosan-hyaluronic acid wound dressing. Silver nanoparticles (≤ 13 nm) also were coated on this dressing in order to enhance antibacterial activities. In this way, higher concentration of hyaluronic acid (1%) and significant swelling percent were obtained (Fahmy et al. 2018).

10.8   Starch

Two components of starch are linear amylose (20–30%) and amylopectin (70–80%) with linear and linear-branched forms, respectively. Unites of both forms are α-D-glucose by glycosidic bonds of $\alpha(1 \rightarrow 4)$ and $\alpha(1 \rightarrow 6)$ in amylose and amylopectin, respectively. This biopolymer can make gelation under heat condition by retrogradation process (Torres et al. 2013). Biodegradability, biocompatibility, stimulus roles in adhesion, proliferation, differentiation and regeneration of cells in wound healing region are important effects of this biopolymer (Waghmare et al. 2018). In addition, this biopolymer is utilized as filler material in bio-nanocomposites. Striking disadvantages of starch are weak mechanical and high hydrophilic properties which have caused less application of this biopolymer as hydrogel in wound dressing aspect. To solve these drawbacks, other materials and biomaterials such as polyvinyl alcohol (PVA) and chitosan in composite form were used. For improvement of antibacterial activities against *P. aeruginosa, S. aureus,* and *E. coli* bacteria, ZnO NPs were incorporated in hydrogel membrane of PVA/starch/chitosan. In this case, several parameters involving mechanical, antibacterial, and cytotoxicity properties were evaluated as in vitro and in vivo studies. Histopathology results of this investigation demonstrated positive effects on all stages of wound healing process after 14 days of experiment compared to control groups (Baghaie et al. 2017). In another study, PVA and glutaraldehyde were used to increase mechanical stability of starch nanofibers for preparation of wound dressing in electrospinning method. The starch nanofibers with diameter of 162.1 ± 27.02 nm had higher mechanical strength as value as 16.58 kPa (Waghmare et al. 2018). Also, mechanical properties of nanostarch with approximately size diameter of 30 nm were improved by chitosan-polyvinyl pyrrolidone (PVP) through solution casting method. With respect to antibacterial survey, two bacteria involving *S. aureus* MTCC 1688 and *P. aeruginosa* MTCC 3615 were evaluated by disc diffusion assay. In this work, three percentages of nanostarch with 1%, 3%, and 5% were used for measurement of concentration effect of these nanocrystals. Results showed more IZDs of 11.6 ± 0.7 and 12.3 ± 0.2 mm for *S. aureus* and *P. aeruginosa* pathogens respectively in higher concentration of nanostarch (Poonguzhali et al. 2018a). In similar study, 1% and 3% nanostarch was coated on chitosan-PVP membrane via NaCl leaching method. Stearic acid (S) was used in symmetric and asymmetric wound dressings to compare hydrophilic and hydrophobic effects of membrane. *S. aureus* MTCC 1688, *Bacillus subtilis* MTCC 2414, *E. coli* MTCC 443, and *P. aeruginosa* MTCC 3615 were selected to assess antibacterial activities of this bio-nanocomposite. In this way, higher sensitivities were observed for *S. aureus* and *B. subtilis* than Gram negative bacteria. Moreover, histological analysis demonstrated higher value of granulation tissue and hair follicle formation after 14 and 21 days, respectively, for nanostarch (1%) in asymmetric wound dressing of chitosan-PVP-S (Poonguzhali et al. 2018b).

10.9   Chondroitin Sulfate

N-acetylgalactosamine and glucuronic acid are sugar units of chondroitin sulfate with sulfating at C-4 and C-6 position of *N*-acetylgalactosamine as glycosaminoglycan polymer (Stephenson and Yong 2018). In connective tissue such as cartilage, this polymer is important proteoglycan structure. This polymer can also be found in skin and cornea. Combination of chitosan with chondroitin sulfate produces scaffolds and sponges biomaterials with antimicrobial and anti-inflammatory properties. In this regard, incorporation of chondroitin 4-sulfate in film with chitosan-gelatin-ZnO particles demonstrated higher wound contraction percentage as value of 86.5 ± 1.6% compared to control group (with only chitosan) by 79.0 ± 4.2% (Cahú et al. 2017). Moreover, application of chitosan-chondroitin sulfate aerogel for 14 days period of in vitro and in vivo experiments illustrated significant activity for re-epidermization and leukocyte infiltration (Concha et al. 2018). It is worth noting that this polymer has less application in wound healing than to other medical fields such as cartilage engineering.

10.10 Conclusion and Future Perspectives

In this chapter, several ways for combination of chitosan and nanochitosan with natural polymers including cellulose, collagen, alginic acid, hyaluronic acid, starch, and chondroitin sulfate are presented in order to remove drawbacks of chitosan applications in wound healing. Each of these biopolymers can be used for improvement of antibacterial and wound healing process. In this way, selection of suitable biopolymer is important task which is related to types and stages of wounds. In addition, combination of these polymers can be influenced by various derivatives of each part. On the whole, there is need for new approaches such as use of organic and inorganic nanoparticles in order to obtain new wound healing agents with minimum drawbacks.

References

Alavi M, Karimi N (2018a) Antiplanktonic, antibiofilm, antiswarming motility and antiquorum sensing activities of green synthesized Ag–TiO2, TiO2–Ag, Ag–Cu and Cu–Ag nanocomposites against multi-drug-resistant bacteria. Artif Cells Nanomed Biotechnol 46:S399–S413

Alavi M, Karimi N (2018b) Characterization, antibacterial, total antioxidant, scavenging, reducing power and ion chelating activities of green synthesized silver, copper and titanium dioxide nanoparticles using Artemisia haussknechtii leaf extract. Artif Cells Nanomed Biotechnol 46:2066–2081

Alavi M (2019) Modifications of microcrystalline cellulose (MCC), nanofibrillated cellulose (NFC), and nanocrystalline cellulose (NCC) for antimicrobial and wound healing applications. E-Polymers 19:103–119

Alavi M, Karimi N (2019) Biosynthesis of Ag and Cu NPs by secondary metabolites of usnic acid and thymol with biological macromolecules aggregation and antibacterial activities against multi drug resistant (MDR) bacteria. Int J Biol Macromol 128:893–901

Alavi M, Rai M (2019a) Recent advances in antibacterial applications of metal nanoparticles (MNPs) and metal nanocomposites (MNCs) against multidrug-resistant (MDR) bacteria. Expert Rev Anti-Infect Ther 17:419–428. https://doi.org/10.1080/14787210.2019.1614914

Alavi M, Rai M (2019b) Recent progress in nanoformulations of silver nanoparticles with cellulose, chitosan, and alginic acid biopolymers for antibacterial applications. Appl Microbiol Biotechnol 103: 8669–8676. https://doi.org/10.1007/s00253-019-10126-4

Arrouze F, Desbrieres J, Rhazi M, Essahli M, Tolaimate A (2019) Valorization of chitins extracted from North Morocco shrimps: comparison of chitin reactivity and characteristics. J Appl Polym Sci 136:47804

Baghaie S, Khorasani MT, Zarrabi A, Moshtaghian J (2017) Wound healing properties of PVA/starch/chitosan hydrogel membranes with nano zinc oxide as antibacterial wound dressing material. J Biomater Sci Polym Ed 28:2220–2241. https://doi.org/10.1080/09205063.2017.1390383

Bao Y, Zhang H, Luan Q, Zheng M, Tang H, Huang F (2018) Fabrication of cellulose nanowhiskers reinforced chitosan-xylan nanocomposite films with antibacterial and antioxidant activities. Carbohydr Polym 184:66–73. https://doi.org/10.1016/j.carbpol.2017.12.051

Belvedere R, Bizzarro V, Parente L, Petrella F, Petrella A (2018) Effects of Prisma® skin dermal regeneration device containing glycosaminoglycans on human keratinocytes and fibroblasts. Cell Adhes Migr 12:168–183. https://doi.org/10.1080/19336918.2017.1340137

Boateng JS, Matthews KH, Stevens HNE, Eccleston GM (2008) Wound healing dressings and drug delivery systems: a review. J Pharm Sci 97:2892–2923

Cahú TB, Silva RA, Silva RPF, Silva MM, Arruda IRS, Silva JF, Costa RMPB, Santos SD, Nader HB, Bezerra RS (2017) Evaluation of chitosan-based films containing gelatin, chondroitin 4-sulfate and ZnO for wound healing. Appl Biochem Biotechnol 183:765–777

Chanda A, Adhikari J, Ghosh A, Chowdhury SR, Thomas S, Datta P, Saha P (2018) Electrospun chitosan/polycaprolactone-hyaluronic acid bilayered scaffold for potential wound healing applications. Int J Biol Macromol 116:774–785. https://doi.org/10.1016/j.ijbiomac.2018.05.099

Chen G-W, Lin Y-H, Lin C-H, Jen H-C (2018) Antibacterial activity of emulsified pomelo (Citrus grandis Osbeck) peel oil and water-soluble chitosan on Staphylococcus aureus and Escherichia coli. Molecules (Basel, Switzerland) 23:840

Concha MS, Vidal A, Giacaman A, Ojeda J, Pavicic F, Oyarzun-Ampuero FA, Torres C, Cabrera MP, Moreno-Villoslada I, Orellana SL (2018) Aerogels made of chitosan and chondroitin sulfate at high degree of neutralization: biological properties toward wound healing. J Biomed Mater Res B Appl Biomater 106:2464–2471. https://doi.org/10.1002/jbm.b.34038

Dumont M, Villet R, Guirand M, Montembault A, Delair T, Lack S, Barikosky M, Crepet A, Alcouffe P, Laurent F, David L (2018) Processing and antibacterial properties of chitosan-coated alginate fibers. Carbohydr Polym 190:31–42. https://doi.org/10.1016/j.carbpol.2017.11.088

Elwakeel KZ, Aly MH, El-Howety MA, El-Fadaly E, Al-Said A (2018) Synthesis of chitosan@ activated carbon beads with abundant amino groups for capture of cu (II) and cd (II) from aqueous solutions. J Polym Environ 26(9):3590–3602

Fahmy HM, Aly AA, Abou-Okeil A (2018) A non-woven fabric wound dressing containing layer—by—layer deposited hyaluronic acid and chitosan. Int J Biol Macromol 114:929–934. https://doi.org/10.1016/j.ijbiomac.2018.03.149

Fan L, Wu H, Zhou X, Peng M, Tong J, Xie W, Liu S (2014) Transglutaminase-catalyzed grafting collagen on chitosan and its characterization. Carbohydr Polym 105:253–259. https://doi.org/10.1016/j.carbpol.2014.01.065

Fardioui M, Meftah Kadmiri I, Aek Q, Bouhfid R (2018) Bio-active nanocomposite films based on nanocrystalline cellulose reinforced styrylquinoxalin-grafted-chitosan: antibacterial and mechanical properties. Int J Biol Macromol 114:733–740. https://doi.org/10.1016/j.ijbiomac.2018.03.114

Garrido-Maestu A, Ma Z, Paik S-Y-R, Chen N, Ko S, Tong Z, Jeong KC (2018) Engineering of chitosan-derived nanoparticles to enhance antimicrobial activity against foodborne pathogen Escherichia coli O157:H7. Carbohydr Polym 197:623–630. https://doi.org/10.1016/j.carbpol.2018.06.046

Gómez Chabala LF, Cuartas CEE, López MEL (2017) Release behavior and antibacterial activity of chitosan/alginate blends with aloe vera and silver nanoparticles. Mar Drugs 15:328

Henningham A, Davies MR, Uchiyama S, Sorge NM, Lund S, Chen KT, Walker MJ, Cole JN, Nizet V (2018) Virulence role of the GlcNAc side chain of the Lancefield Cell Wall carbohydrate antigen in non-M1-serotype group a Streptococcus. MBio 9:e02294–e02217

Huang J, Ren J, Chen G, Li Z, Liu Y, Wang G, Wu X (2018) Tunable sequential drug delivery system based on chitosan/hyaluronic acid hydrogels and PLGA microspheres for management of non-healing infected wounds. Mater Sci Eng C 89:213–222. https://doi.org/10.1016/j.msec.2018.04.009

Hussain Z, Thu HE, Katas H, Bukhari SNA (2017) Hyaluronic acid-based biomaterials: a versatile and smart approach to tissue regeneration and treating traumatic, surgical, and chronic wounds. Polym Rev 57:594–630

Lee KY, Mooney DJ (2012) Alginate: properties and biomedical applications. Prog Polym Sci 37:106–126

Li M, Han M, Sun Y, Hua Y, Chen G, Zhang L (2019) Oligoarginine mediated collagen/chitosan gel composite for cutaneous wound healing. Int J Biol Macromol 122:1120–1127. https://doi.org/10.1016/j.ijbiomac.2018.09.061

Liu L, Wen H, Rao Z, Zhu C, Liu M, Min L, Fan L, Tao S (2018) Preparation and characterization of chitosan—collagen peptide/oxidized konjac glucomannan hydrogel. Int J Biol Macromol 108:376–382. https://doi.org/10.1016/j.ijbiomac.2017.11.128

Lu B, Lu F, Zou Y, Liu J, Rong B, Li Z, Dai F, Wu D, Lan-less G (2017) In situ reduction of silver nanoparticles by chitosan-l-glutamic acid/hyaluronic acid: enhancing antimicrobial and wound-healing activity. Carbohydr Polym 173:556–565. https://doi.org/10.1016/j.carbpol.2017.06.035

Ma Z, Garrido-Maestu A, Jeong KC (2017) Application, mode of action, and in vivo activity of chitosan and its micro-and nanoparticles as antimicrobial agents: a review. Carbohydr Polym 176:257–265

Michalska-Sionkowska M, Kaczmarek B, Walczak M, Sionkowska A (2018) Antimicrobial activity of new materials based on the blends of collagen/chitosan/hyaluronic acid with gentamicin sulfate addition. Mater Sci Eng C 86:103–108. https://doi.org/10.1016/j.msec.2018.01.005

Moreira ALDSL, de Souza Pereira A, Speziali MG, Novack KM, Gurgel LVA, Gil LF (2018) Bifunctionalized chitosan: a versatile adsorbent for removal of Cu (II) and Cr (VI) from aqueous solution. Carbohydr Polym 201:218–227

Park H, Lee HJ, An H, Lee KY (2017) Alginate hydrogels modified with low molecular weight hyaluronate for cartilage regeneration. Carbohydr Polym 162:100–107

Patrulea V, Ostafe V, Borchard G, Jordan O (2015) Chitosan as a starting material for wound healing applications. Eur J Pharm Biopharm 97:417–426

Poonguzhali R, Basha SK, Kumari VS (2018a) Nanostarch reinforced with chitosan/poly (vinyl pyrrolidone) blend for in vitro wound healing application. Polym-Plast Technol Eng 57:1400–1410. https://doi.org/10.1080/03602559.2017.1381255

Poonguzhali R, Khaleel Basha S, Sugantha Kumari V (2018b) Fabrication of asymmetric nanostarch reinforced chitosan/PVP membrane and its evaluation as an antibacterial patch for in vivo wound healing application. Int J Biol Macromol 114:204–213. https://doi.org/10.1016/j.ijbiomac.2018.03.092

Sanad RA-B, Abdel-Bar HM (2017) Chitosan–hyaluronic acid composite sponge scaffold enriched with Andrographolide-loaded lipid nanoparticles for enhanced wound healing. Carbohydr Polym 173:441–450. https://doi.org/10.1016/j.carbpol.2017.05.098

Shoulders MD, Raines RT (2009) Collagen structure and stability. Annu Rev Biochem 78:929–958. https://doi.org/10.1146/annurev.biochem.77.032207.120833

Stephenson EL, Yong VW (2018) Pro-inflammatory roles of chondroitin sulfate proteoglycans in disorders of the central nervous system. Matrix Biol 71-72:432–442. https://doi.org/10.1016/j.matbio.2018.04.010

Taran M, Rad M, Alavi M (2016) Characterization of Ag nanoparticles biosynthesized by Bacillus sp. HAI4 in different conditions and their antibacterial effects. J Appl Pharm Sci 6:094–099

Thaya R, Vaseeharan B, Sivakamavalli J, Iswarya A, Govindarajan M, Alharbi NS, Kadaikunnan S, Al-Anbr MN, Khaled JM, Benelli G (2018) Synthesis of chitosan-alginate microspheres with high antimicrobial and antibiofilm activity against multi-drug resistant microbial pathogens. Microb Pathog 114:17–24. https://doi.org/10.1016/j.micpath.2017.11.011

Tighe RM, Garantziotis S (2018) Hyaluronan interactions with innate immunity in lung biology. Matrix Biol 78-79:84–99. https://doi.org/10.1016/j.matbio.2018.01.027

Torres FG, Commeaux S, Troncoso OP (2013) Starch-based biomaterials for wound-dressing applications. Starch 65:543–551. https://doi.org/10.1002/star.201200259

Urrutia P, Bernal C, Wilson L, Illanes A (2018) Use of chitosan heterofunctionality for enzyme immobilization: β-galactosidase immobilization for galacto-oligosaccharide synthesis. Int J Biol Macromol 116:182–193. https://doi.org/10.1016/j.ijbiomac.2018.04.112

Vecchies F, Sacco P, Decleva E, Menegazzi R, Porrelli D, Donati I, Turco G, Paoletti S, Marsich E (2018) Complex coacervates between a lactose-modified chitosan and hyaluronic acid as radical-scavenging drug carriers. Biomacromolecules 19(10):3936–3944. https://doi.org/10.1021/acs.biomac.8b00863

Waghmare VS, Wadke PR, Dyawanapelly S, Deshpande A, Jain R, Dandekar P (2018) Starch based nanofibrous scaffolds for wound healing applications. Bioactive Mater 3:255–266. https://doi.org/10.1016/j.bioactmat.2017.11.006

Wang CG, Lou YT, Tong MJ, Zhang LL, Zhang ZJ, Feng YZ, Li S, Xu HZ, Mao C (2018) Asperosaponin VI promotes angiogenesis and accelerates wound healing in rats via up-regulating HIF-1α/VEGF signaling. Acta Pharmacol Sin 39:393

Wu T, Huang J, Jiang Y, Hu Y, Ye X, Liu D, Chen J (2018) Formation of hydrogels based on chitosan/alginate for the delivery of lysozyme and their antibacterial activity. Food Chem 240:361–369. https://doi.org/10.1016/j.foodchem.2017.07.052

Yu X, Guo L, Liu M, Cao X, Shang S, Liu Z, Huang D, Cao Y, Cui F, Tian L (2018) Callicarpa nudiflora loaded on chitosan-collagen/organomontmorillonite composite membrane for anti-bacterial activity of wound dressing. Int J Biol Macromol 120(Pt B):2279–2284. https://doi.org/10.1016/j.ijbiomac.2018.08.113

Zarayneh S, Sepahi AA, Jonoobi M, Rasouli H (2018) Comparative antibacterial effects of cellulose nanofiber, chitosan nanofiber, chitosan/cellulose combination and chitosan alone against bacterial contamination of Iranian banknotes. Int J Biol Macromol 118:1045–1054

Zhang H, Peng M, Cheng T, Zhao P, Qiu L, Zhou J, Lu G, Chen J (2018) Silver nanoparticles-doped collagen–alginate antimicrobial biocomposite as potential wound dressing. J Mater Sci 53:14944–14952. https://doi.org/10.1007/s10853-018-2710-9

Chapter 11
Nanobiotechnological Strategies for Treatment of Tegumentary and Visceral Leishmaniasis Including Resistance Strains

Marco Vinicius Chaud, Venâncio Alves Amaral, Fernando Batain, Kessi Marie Moura Crescencio, Carolina Alves dos Santos, Márcia Araújo Rebelo, and Victória Soares Soeiro

Abstract Leishmaniasis is a vector-borne chronic infectious disease caused by a group of protozoan parasites of the genus *Leishmania*. The most severe form of the disease is visceral leishmaniasis, which is fatal if not treated properly. Leishmaniasis is one of the neglected tropical diseases caused by different species of the protozoan parasite *Leishmania*, and leishmaniasis is a major public health problem worldwide. *Leishmania*, in the amastigote development period, lives inside tissue-resident macrophages as well as migrating monocytes in distinct anatomical locations. Their hidden location is responsible for impairing the accession of drug therapy. Drug delivery systems should allow the adverse effects caused by parenteral routes of administration to be avoided as well as enhancing the antileishmanial activity and reducing the toxicity of the medication. Access to essential drugs for the treatment of leishmaniasis is challenging in the developing countries that have the highest burden of cases. In the absence of effective vector control measures, drug treatment of the host associated with the nano-theranostic vaccines is the most promising alternative against leishmaniasis. Development of vaccines against leishmaniasis does not appear to follow any specific pattern. However, it is possible to notice an effort from countries developing vaccines in recent years. Research efforts regarding the development of DNA vaccines, recombinant proteins or peptides, and adjuvants are increasing and seem to be among the best feasible alternatives for a

M. V. Chaud (✉) · V. A. Amaral · F. Batain · K. M. M. Crescencio · V. S. Soeiro
Laboratory of Biomaterials and Nanotechnology, University of Sorocaba,
Sorocaba, São Paulo, Brazil
e-mail: marco.chaud@prof.uniso.br

C. A. dos Santos
College of Pharmacy, University of Sorocaba, Sorocaba, São Paulo, Brazil

M. A. Rebelo
College of Pharmacy, Max Planck University Center, Indaiatuba, São Paulo, Brazil

© Springer Nature Switzerland AG 2020
M. Rai (ed.), *Nanotechnology in Skin, Soft Tissue, and Bone Infections*,
https://doi.org/10.1007/978-3-030-35147-2_11

successful vaccine. Advances in research, development, and innovation in drug delivery systems show that new dosage forms can enhance the efficacy, safety, and amenability of the old drugs including antimonials, amphotericin B, imiquimod, and buparvaquone. However, the strategy of vaccination by the cutaneous route has been an exponential development, allowing immunization against cutaneous, mucocutaneous, and visceral leishmaniasis.

Keywords Leishmaniasis · Vaccine · Nanocarriers · Transdermal drug delivery · Neglected disease · Drug resistance

Nomenclature

AmB	Amphotericin B
Amb-d	Amphotericin B deoxycholate
AmB-UDL	Amphotericin B ultra-deformation liposome
CL	Cutaneous leishmaniasis
DALYs	Disability-adjusted life-years
DNA	Deoxyribonucleic acid
HIV	Human immunodeficiency virus
HSV-2	Herpes simplex virus type 2
IgG	Immunoglobulin G
L-AmB	Liposomal amphotericin B
MA	Meglumine antimoniate
ML	Mucocutaneous leishmaniasis
SEDDS	Self-emulsifying drug delivery systems
SNEDDS	Self-nanoemulsifying drug delivery systems
SDEDDS	Self-double-emulsifying drug delivery systems
UDL	Ultra-deformation liposome
US FDA	Food and Drug Administration
VL	Visceral leishmaniasis
WHO	World Health Organization

11.1 Introduction

Leishmaniasis is a neglected tropical disease caused by protozoan parasites from more than 20 species of *Leishmania*. Both wild and domesticated animals, especially dogs and cats, are intermediate hosts of these parasites. The parasites are transmitted to humans, the definitive host, by the bites of the infected female hematophagous phlebotomine (Old World) or *Lutzomyia* (New World) sand-fly insect vector (Van Griensven and Diro 2012).

In the cycle of *Leishmania*, the parasite invades the local phagocytic host cells; then, the promastigote infective form transforms and multiplies as the amastigote-form inside the phagolysosome by binary fission within tissue-resident macrophages. The macrophage phagolysosomes, positioned in different anatomical zones, present important physiological and structural barriers that antileishmanial drugs must overcome.

The primary forms of leishmaniasis in the skin and soft tissues are cutaneous leishmaniosis (CL), visceral or kala-azar leishmaniosis (VL), and mucocutaneous leishmaniosis (ML).

Cutaneous leishmaniasis lesions typically present as papules that progress to nodules or open ulcers without lymphangitis or adenopathy. In visceral leishmaniases in patients who develop symptoms, the presentation is insidious, with the development of splenomegaly, recurrent fevers, anemia, pancytopenia, weight loss, and weakness occurring progressively for weeks or even months (Van Griensven and Diro 2012).

Almost all clinically symptomatic (nonimmune) patients die within months if not treated. In mucocutaneous leishmaniasis, the lesions can damage the mucous membranes and surrounding tissues. This disabling form of leishmaniasis can lead to the sufferer being rejected by the community because of disability-adjusted life-years (DALYs). Bailey et al. performed a multi-language systematic review of the psychological impact and inactive cutaneous leishmaniasis, and calculated that the DALY burden was seven times greater than the latest study estimates. They conclude that there was need to include the leading social impacts, particularly major depressive disorder (Bailey et al. 2019). This study placed highlights on the neglected diseases, especially all leishmaniases.

Visceral leishmaniasis, also known as kala-azar, is the most serious form of the disease; the cutaneous form is the most common; and the mucocutaneous form occurs less frequently than the cutaneous form. The involvement of the nasal and/or oral mucosa is more severe, which may lead to sequelae and death.

Moreover, the psychosocial stigma arising from this disease is something that has not yet been measured and is directly related to DALYs (Lessa et al. 2007; Diniz et al. 2011).

Currently, the leishmaniases have reached urban centers, particularly the most densely populated areas. With the decrease of green areas around the cities, the main reservoir of hosts became pets. According to this possibility, the leishmaniases can affect people of all age groups.

The epidemiology of cutaneous and mucocutaneous leishmaniasis in the region of the Americas is complex, with intraspecific and interspecific variation in transmission cycles, reservoir hosts, sand-fly vectors, clinical manifestations, and multiple circulating *Leishmania* species in the same geographic area.

Anthroponotic CL is predominantly urban and peri-urban, and shows patterns of spatial clustering similar to those of anthroponotic VL in Southeast Asia. Estimates show that the annual global incidence is 1.0 million cases of CL and 0.3 million cases of VL (Alvar et al. 2012). In 2017, 20.8 of 22.1 (94%) new cases reported to WHO occurred in seven countries: Brazil, Ethiopia, India, Kenya, Somalia, South Sudan, and Sudan. Almost 90% of mucocutaneous leishmaniasis cases have been reported in the Plurinational State of Bolivia, Brazil, and Peru (WHO/PAHO Department of Neglected Infectious Diseases 2019). However, the estimates that best reflect how much leishmaniasis is a neglected illness is expressed as DALYs lost, provided it is considered the major depressive disorder.

To date, *Leishmania* and human immunodeficiency virus (HIV) coinfection has been reported in more than 35 countries. Since 2001, the incidence of this coinfection has decreased in response to the administration of antiretroviral treatment of HIV (Van Griensven et al. 2018).

Access to essential drugs for the treatment of leishmaniasis is challenging in the developing countries that have the highest burden of cases. Few antibiotics are available that have antileishmanial activity, such as amphotericin B, pentamidine, and miltefosine (an alkyl phospholipid). However, decreases in efficacy, resistance, and toxicity have been noted against these drugs (Sundar et al. 2014).

The dry antileishmanial pipeline further indicates the slow pace of drug discovery in this field where resistance is a major barrier (Okwor et al. 2016). Alternatives to current treatment (Fig. 11.1) options for skin (LC) and soft tissue (LV) infections

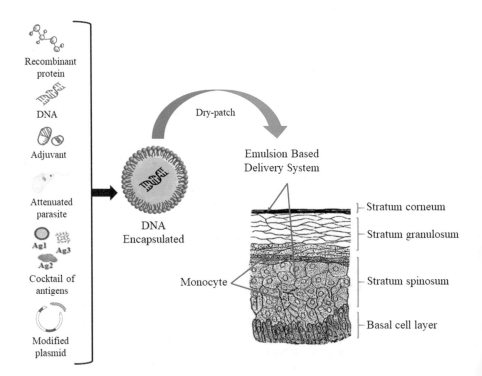

Fig. 11.1 Nanobiotechnological perspectives for treatment of leishmaniasis

are needed for more effective treatment of leishmaniasis disease now and in the future.

This review article aims to survey and summarize previous studies in the treatment of cutaneous and visceral leishmaniasis and to show the advances in nanobiotechnological knowledge in the field of vaccine prevention that may reduce the damage and social impact caused by these diseases.

11.2   Current Treatment and Unresponsive Drugs

Systemic treatment approaches with pentavalent antimonials, liposomal amphotericin B, fluconazole, and miltefosine are increasingly used despite the absence of supportive evidence (Mosimann et al. 2018).

The mainstay treatment for all forms of leishmaniasis is pentavalent antimony in the form of sodium stibogluconate or meglumine antimonate. Pentavalent antimonials have been used for therapy for leishmaniasis in humans since 1911 and are administered by parenteral routes. In the 1980s, the use of 20 mg pentavalent antimonials per kilogram of body weight per day for 20 days (instead of 10 mg/kg/day) of antimony was recommended up to a maximum daily dose of 850 mg (Herwaldt and Berman 1992; Arevalo et al. 2002). The leishmaniasis treatment has evolved; the daily dose of antimony and the duration of therapy have been progressively increased to combat unresponsiveness to treatment. Studies have been performed on *Leishmania infantum* with amphotericin B deoxycholate (AmB-d), and meglumine antimoniate (MA), where AmB was administered at a dose of 0.7 mg/kg/day for 28 days (20 mg/kg total dose): similar initial cure rates (62.6% for AmB) and relapse rates were reported for AmB and antimonials (Laguna et al. 1999; Van Griensven et al. 2014). However, these studies have been merely exploratory or casual tests, without bringing any advance in knowledge.

Until this time no prospective clinical trial has been conducted for the systemic treatment of leishmaniasis. Although published studies of liposomal amphotericin B, a polyene antibiotic, are scarce, because of its safety profile it is recommended by the WHO and other international organizations as the preferred treatment for VL.

Lipid formulations of amphotericin B (L-AmB) have been successfully used in the treatment of leishmaniasis. L-AmB was first introduced in 1996 and was the more widely studied lipid formulation in clinical trials. The lipid formulation is significantly less nephrotoxic than AmB-D and offers a shorter duration of treatment than pentavalent antimonial. L-AmB has been safely and effectively administered in very high doses for a few days or in a single day (Mistro et al. 2017).

L-AmB is a cost-effective alternative as compared to pentavalent antimonial or AmB-D; the degree of the net benefit is related to the extent of reduction in drug acquisition costs. L-AmB is a very safe and highly effective treatment for primary VL in *L. infantum* endemic areas and in the *Leishmania donovani* South Asian focus where it was recently recommended as first-line treatment by the WHO expert committee on the control of leishmaniasis (WHO 2010). Therefore, L-AmB cannot be recommended as first-line treatment for VL in all regions, except for patients at increased risk of death with pentavalent antimonials-based treatments. Additional research is needed to better define the indication of L-AmB for other forms of leishmaniasis and to design optimal and combination regimens for drug delivery for HIV co-infected patients (Balasegaram et al. 2012; Mosimann et al. 2018).

Imiquimod, (1-(2-methyl propyl)-1-imidazo(4,5-c)quinoline-4-amine) that has been approved by the US FDA for topical use as a 5% cream is an immunomodulator thought to act through stimulation of production of local interferon and other cytokines (Kulakov and Cooper 2011). This drug exhibits antiviral activities in some in vitro and animal models. Imiquimod treatment of primary genital herpes simplex virus infection in guinea pigs reduced the level of genital disease by 90%. The authors further investigated its utility as suppressive therapy of recurrent disease in animals that had recently recovered from primary genital HSV-2 disease (Harrison et al. 1994).

Among the significant challenges of leishmaniasis treatment are the clinical manifestations that may appear similar to a wide variety of other conditions. The clinical differentiation that mimics the cutaneous lesions of leishmaniasis requires specific professional evaluation. However, the major challenges of leishmaniasis treatment are developing an effective optimal drug, that is, responsive, prophylactic, toxicologically secure, efficacious with combined therapies, and an efficient drug delivery system. A delay in diagnosis, especially in visceral leishmaniasis, has potential to prove leishmaniasis fatal in immunosuppressed patients, such as those with leukemia or HIV; these are aggressive and refractory to treatment (Handler et al. 2015).

Because of the limited medicines and techniques available of antileishmanial drugs, it is of vital importance that effective monitoring of antileishmanial drug use be done to prevent the emergence of resistance (Sundar et al. 2014). The main challenge in the management of antileishmanial drug unresponsive, is the expectation shortly of new technologies for specific target drug release.

In North Bihar, India, the cure rate has dropped to 64% and even lower in subsequent studies. The reasons for the emergence of resistance were the extensive abuse of the primary drug. Sodium stibogluconate was prescribed in inappropriate doses and duration by both qualified medical practitioners and 'witch doctors,' which led to overuse and misuse of this drug (Jha et al. 1992; Rai and Bandyopadhyay 2001). This negligence and carelessness resulted in its subtherapeutic blood levels and increased the resistance of parasites to sodium stibogluconate.

Unresponsive antimonials is a fundamental determinant of treatment failure in anthroponotic cutaneous leishmaniasis. The increase of pentavalent antimony compound-resistant parasites in causative agents of anthroponotic induced by *L. tropica* may be the result of lowered susceptibility to pentavalent antimony, including meglumine antimonite, insufficient treatment duration, low dosage uptake, and the nature of the anthroponotic transmission cycle, which is the only measure to control the disease (den Boer et al. 2018).

Grogl et al. (1992) reported that in vitro sensitivity to pentavalent antimony of 35 *Leishmania* isolates as determined by the semi-automated microdilution technique showed an 89% and 86% correlation with clinical outcome after pentostam and glucantime treatment, respectively. Strains from pentavalent antimony-treated patients with American cutaneous and mucocutaneous disease who fail at least one complete course of pentostam are as highly unresponsive to this drug as laboratory-proven drug-resistant *Leishmania* strains. Furthermore, the results indicate that drug resistance is a problem and that at least in some instances, failure to respond to treatment is caused by the parasite as well as patient factors. The degree of resistance of a strain to antimony in association with host-specific factors will determine whether the clinical response to treatment with this drug is a total cure or a partial response followed by relapse(s), and possibly secondary unresponsiveness, resulting in total resistance to antimony.

Clinical resistance to amphotericin B is uncommon, although with the increasing use of amphotericin B in auto-assembled lipid formulations [(liposomes, niosomes, nanoparticles, liquid crystal, self-emulsifying drug delivery system (SEDDS)], which have a longer half-life, there could be possibilities of resistance associated with this drug (Bhattacharyya and Bajpai 2013; Zaioncz et al. 2017; Jain et al. 2018). The alkyl phospholipid (miltefosine), as the lipid formulation administered by the oral route, has a long half-life (6–10 days), which renders it vulnerable to resistance. In this case, patients tend to discontinue the drug prematurely because of gastrointestinal side effects if not counselled beforehand.

Patients with incomplete treatment, with the drug long half-life, will lead to persistence of subtherapeutic levels of the drug along with the parasites, leading to tolerance and drug resistance; this will cause an exponential rise in these refractory parasites (Bryceson 2001; Sundar et al. 2014).

Sitamaquine (8-aminoquinoline) has a short half-life (24–30 h), preventing emergence of rapid resistance. The selection of a sitamaquine-resistant clone of *Leishmania donovani* in the laboratory and the phase II clinical trials pointing out some adverse effects such as methemoglobinemia and nephrotoxicity are considered for a further development decision (Loiseau et al. 2011).

To discriminate resistant and susceptible strains, a clear definition of drug resistance, with the establishment of resistance 'breakpoints' and associated molecular markers, should be studied at a more significant extent for proper input to drug policy makers. As markers of validated genomic resistance are not yet available, monitoring resistance depends on a standard parasite susceptibility test in vitro. The control of *Leishmania* infection relies initially on drug therapy. Knowledge about the mechanism of action of the drugs and the mechanisms involved in the resistance is needed for designing effective drug-specific dosage forms and new treatment regimen against leishmaniases or identifying new aims (Sundar et al. 2014; Loiseau and Bories 2006). Many groups of researchers have focused on the development of an appropriate *Leishmania* vaccine. DNA vaccines have induced an appropriate immune response against *Leishmania infantum* (Moafi et al. 2019).

Considering the life cycle of *Leishmania* spp. in a susceptible mammal during feeding, the parasite continues to infect phagocytic cells either at the site of cutaneous infection or in secondary lymphoid organs, with eventual parasitemia. The sand-fly becomes infected through feeding on a host either with an active skin lesion in cutaneous leishmaniasis or with parasitemia in visceral leishmaniasis. Parasites convert to promastigotes within the sand-fly midgut lumen, and the promastigotes migrate from the midgut lumen and transform into highly infectious metacyclic promastigotes (Esch and Petersen 2013).

11.3   Drug Delivery System Against Leishmaniasis

The conventional treatment is poorly selective. Thus, alternatives by the parenteral route are a smart drug delivery system to surpass the anatomical and physiological barriers and control pharmacokinetic properties, improve efficacy, and reduce drug toxicity. Smart drug delivery systems using micro- or nanostructure and system lipid-based formulations can result in higher concentrations and slower release of drugs in several mammalian body organs, including the spleen, liver, and kidneys.

Nano-enabled auto-assembled lipid-based drug delivery systems make up a technological platform to overcome challenges encountered with current failed leads in the treatment of leishmaniasis.

11.3.1   Transdermal Drug Delivery Nanocarrier as Strategy for Leishmanicidal Activity

Side effects, toxicity, resistance, cost-effectiveness, and other therapeutic issues promote an urgent need to identify and develop new strategies and alternative targets with known effective drugs for the treatment of leishmaniasis.

By the transdermal route, the targets can be macrophages and other types of mononuclear phagocytic cells able to phagocytize specific nanostructure loading with leishmanicidal drugs. The nanostructure must be carefully designed to be phagocytosed by macrophages, as a "Trojan horse" upon reaching the deeper parts of the skin will be phagocytosed and may combat the promastigotes forms that infect phagocytic cells. However, the use of the transdermal route is the major challenge. The cutaneous tissue has the physiological function of a drainage organ and the skin is a barrier especially against xenobiotics.

Thus, the search for strategies to provide and increase the cutaneous permeation of the drugs used in the treatment of leishmaniasis is extremely important. Among those strategies are the use of emulsion-based systems such as liposomes, self-emulsifying drug delivery systems (SEDDS), lyotropic liquid crystals, microemulsions, nanoemulsions, solid lipid nanoparticles, and Pickering emulsions.

In the study conducted by Van Bocxlaer et al. (2016), the skin barrier of BALB/C mice contaminated with cutaneous leishmaniasis was characterized as to its physiology and integrity, as well as the identification of the influence of these factors on the cutaneous permeation of drugs. The drugs tested were caffeine, ibuprofen, and drugs used in the treatment of leishmaniasis, amphotericin B, buparvaquone, and paromomycin sulfate. Skin infected with *Leishmania major* showed changes in the structure of the epidermis and dermis caused by the presence of inflammatory cells, besides presenting the increase of the loss of trans-epidermal water and the increased skin permeation of caffeine, ibuprofen, buparvaquone, and paromomycin sulfate, compared to uninfected skin. Both infected and uninfected skin were impermeable to AmB. This finding demonstrates that the alteration of the skin barriers provided the increase in the permeability of the drugs to healthy skin (Van Bocxlaer et al. 2016).

11.3.2 Liposome-Based Formulation

Conventional liposomes were not able to permeate the deeper layers of the skin, because they are retained in the stratum corneum. Thus, to provide increased permeability of these systems, various modifications have been performed such as transfersomes, niossomes, and ethosomes (Tanriverdi 2018).

For the past 50 years, liposomes have been utilized in the treatment of leishmaniasis, and treatment has evolved together with advances in knowledge on relationships between liposome structure, administration route, pharmacokinetics, and biodistribution of leishmanicidal drugs. Understanding the strategic utility of the intravenous administration of liposomal pentavalent antimony and liposome-entrapped pentosan for selective delivery to the liver and spleen macrophages infected with visceral leishmaniasis took place in the early past 80 years (Alving et al. 1978; New et al. 1981).

In the first decade of the twenty-first century, the molecular structure of potassium tartrate and of the organic antimonials (III), and their metabolism and mechanism of action, were still being investigated. Later, the clinical use of this compound was interrupted because of severe side effects. Studies suggested that pentavalent antimony, less toxic, acts as a prodrug that is converted to active and more toxic trivalent antimony. New data suggest that thiols (glutathione, cysteine, cysteinyl-glycine) and ribonucleotides may mediate the action of these drugs as a reducing agent (Frézard et al. 2001, 2009).

In the specific case of pentavalent antimonial drugs, the advances included the development of liposomes, complex antimony-quercetin and cyclodextrin-based formulations for improved drug bioavailability. The earlier insights into their chemistry and mechanism of action did result in novel strategies for improved treatment of leishmaniasis (Ruiz et al. 2014; Souza et al. 2019).

The use of liposomes has been so far one of the most efficient means for improving antimonial effectiveness against visceral leishmaniasis. At least four different properties make liposomes the most appropriate carrier system for antimonials: their ability to encapsulate and retain large amounts of water-soluble compounds (Akbarzadeh et al. 2013); their natural tendency to be captured by the macrophages of the reticuloendothelial system, which are the same cells that harbor *Leishmania* parasites; their relative safety; and their high versatility with respect to lipid composition, volume, and composition of internal compartment, vesicle size, and lamellarity (Frézard et al. 2009). The spectacular effect of liposome encapsulation was attributed to the marked targeting of antimony pentavalent to infection sites. On the basis of parasite suppression in the liver or spleen, liposome-encapsulated meglumine antimoniate and sodium stibogluconate administered intravenously were more than 700 times more active compared to either of the free drugs (Collins et al. 1993).

It is often considered that the relatively high cost of phospholipids used to prepare liposomes represents a major obstacle in the development of liposomal formulations. In a liposome-based treatment, a much lower amount of antimony would be used and the cost would be determined mainly by lipids, assuming that the cost of lipids is about US$ $10/g^{-1}$ and that a 5 mL vial of glucantime is about US$1–2.

Based on the high levels of efficacy and safety of the AmB liposome, the World Health Organization (WHO) has recommended the use of this formulation for the treatment of leishmaniasis (WHO 2010). In general, AmB-liposomes are less nephrotoxic than free AmB, as they are taken up selectively by macrophages. The mild urticarial rash and renal impairment resolved after therapy.

11.3.3 Cyclodextrin-Based Formulation

The cyclodextrin carrier system is a feasible strategy to improve the absorption of oral drugs, and the oral bioavailability of water-insoluble drugs, owing to the enhanced drug solubility and dissolution rate (Gidwani and Vyas 2015). Preparation of a meglumine antimoniate/β-cyclodextrin through heating of an equimolar mixture in water, followed by freeze-drying, enhanced the absorption of Sb by the oral route and rendered the antimonial drug orally active in a murine model of cutaneous leishmaniasis (Demicheli et al. 2004). The results found in this study allow concluding that the slow release property of meglumine antimoniate/β-cyclodextrin nanoassemblies induced the migration of complex along the gastrointestinal tract, which would permeate the intestinal epithelium by simple diffusion.

AmB-γ-cyclodextrin in gel dosage form exhibited high in vitro leishmanicidal efficacy with the wider therapeutic index when compared with AmB deoxycholate, depending on *Leishmania* spp., and also in vivo activity in an experimental model of cutaneous leishmaniasis (Ruiz et al. 2014).

11.3.4 Self-Emulsifying Drug Delivery System

The self-emulsifying drug delivery systems (SEDDS) present some subdivisions, among which are the self-nanoemulsifying drug delivery system (SNEDDS) and the self-double-emulsifying drug delivery systems (SDEDDS). SNEDDS provide increased drug permeation in the stratum corneum (Pratiwi et al. 2017) and SDEDDS provide increased permeation in the stratum corneum and epidermis (Wang et al. 2016), in skin permeation studies of antileishmanial drugs. SNEDDS is a drug carrier with promissory potential for the treatment of cutaneous and mucocutaneous leishmaniasis. However, when curcumin was used as a model drug in the treatment of leishmaniasis, the analysis of the results was better for SEDDS than SNEDDS (Khan et al. 2018, 2019).

A study was performed by Khan et al. with SEDDS for the hydrophobic polyphenol pigment curcumin to enable its potential use in cutaneous and mucocutaneous leishmaniasis. The result analysis demonstrated that the SEDDS formulations of curcumin can be used as a promising tool in the treatment of cutaneous and mucocutaneous leishmaniasis (Khan et al. 2018).

Buparvaquone (BCS Class II drug) is a hydroxynaphthoquinone that has in vitro activity in the nanomolar range. Nevertheless, it failed to translate clinically as a viable treatment for visceral leishmaniasis because of poor aqueous solubility. A self-nanoemulsifying system (SNEDDS) with high loading and thermal stability with the ability to enhance the solubility equilibrium of buparvaquone in gastrointestinal media has shown enhanced oral bioavailability compared to aqueous buparvaquone dispersions, resulting in an increased plasma AUC0–24 by 55% that is fourfold higher. Buparvaquone-SNEDDS demonstrated potent in vitro efficacy in the nanomolar range (<37 nM) and was able to inhibit parasite replication in the spleen almost completely (Smith et al. 2018).

11.3.5 Transfersomes

In the topical route, the transfersomes remain intact after contact with the skin. Permeation of the transferosomes can occur through two mechanisms: (1) acting as a permeation enhancer, causing an opening in the layer of the intercellular lipids of the stratum corneum, thus allowing the drug molecules to permeate through the stratum corneum; and (2) when the ultra-deformation of the liposome (UDL) occurs, this deformation modifies the behavior of the vesicle and presses the intracellular lipid layer of the tight junction, promoting permeation in the stratum corneum. This mechanism has the advantage of increasing the capacity to absorb and maintain water, avoiding dehydration; a process similar to osmosis occurs, although the transfersomes can also induce hydration, causing a dilation in the pores of the skin (Agrawal et al. 2018; Bhasin et al. 2018; Kumar 2018).

In a study accomplished by Perez et al., AmB-loaded transferosomes were formulated to improve the topical release of this drug, and its permeation through the skin, and antifungal and antileishmanial activity in vitro, were analyzed. The transferosomes had a diameter of 107 ± 8 nm and an encapsulation efficiency of 75%, with a total accumulation of the AmB in the skin 40 times greater when compared to AmBisome. In relationship to the antileishmanial activity, the system presented 100% and 75% of anti-promastigote and anti-amastigote activity, respectively, for *Leishmania braziliensis*. The ultra-deformable liposomes containing amphotericin

B (AmB-UDL) showed comparable antifungal and antileishmanial activities with AmBisome, only AmB-UDL provided a considerable increased AmB skin deposition. Therefore, the AmB-UDL formulation would be advantageous over other liposomal AmB formulations for topical leishmanicidal treatment that require a targeted delivery of AmB to the viable epidermis and dermis (Perez et al. 2016).

Topical administration of drugs for the treatment of leishmaniasis was evaluated to sodium stibogluconate-loaded transferosomes have been formulated for the treatment of cutaneous leishmaniasis. The transferosomes obtained had a diameter of 195.1 nm and encapsulation efficiency of 35.26% of the model drug. The ex vivo skin permeation assay showed a retention of the drug for the deeper layers of the skin 10 times greater than the control. In the antileishmanial activity in the intramacrophage amastigote model of *Leishmania tropica*, an IC_{50} value was shown 4 times lower in comparison to the pure drug solution, besides the increase in the index of selectivity. In the in vivo study, greater antileishmanial activity was observed through wound healing and parasite load reduction (Dar et al. 2018).

11.3.6 Ethosomes

The ethosomal system, which is composed of phospholipid ethanol and water, differs from the elemental composition of a conventional liposome. Ethosomes are much more efficient for the delivery of drugs to the skin in terms of quantity and depth (Touitou et al. 2000; Dongare et al. 2015).

The mechanisms of permeation of the ethosomes to the topical route are still not well understood. However, some studies indicate that skin diffusion possibly occurs in two ways: (1) the presence of ethanol in the formulations of the ethosomes acts as an enhancer of the skin permeation, the fluidity of the membrane, and reducing the packaging density of the lipid multilayers of the stratum corneum, and (2) the synergistic effect of the phospholipids occurs with the increase of the fluidity of the lipid membrane from the action of the ethanol present in the composition of the ethosomes. Thus, this system can easily permeate the skin, melting the cutaneous lipids and releasing the drug (Varsha and Arum Kumar 2018).

While screening the literature, we did not find studies using ethosomes as a system for drug release in the treatment of leishmaniasis. However, because of the structural characteristics of this vesicle, as well as mechanisms of topical action and efficiency of encapsulation of hydrophilic and lipophilic drugs, we understand that ethosomes and trans-ethosomes have potential for enhancing the transdermal delivery for use in the topical administration of leishmanial medicines and that this vesicular carrier may be used for drug delivery targeting macrophages.

11.3.7 Niosomes

Niosomes or nonionic surfactant vesicles appear to be similar in terms of their physical properties to liposomes and have been shown to modify the tissue distribution of the entrapped niosomal drug (Ge et al. 2019). The niosomes have the ability to modify tissue distribution and efficacy of antileishmanial drugs, with efficacy against protozoan infection of the reticuloendothelial system (Baillie et al. 1986).

Niosomes loaded with sodium stibogluconate were shown to be more active than free drug against experimental murine visceral leishmaniasis, an effect apparently dependent on maintaining high drug levels in the infected reticuloendothelial system (Aflatoonian et al. 2016).

The niosomes can come into contact with the skin and reach the stratum corneum; when they come in contact with the stratum corneum, niosomes interact with the cell surface by the process of fusion, aggregation, and adhesion. The presence of the cholesterol molecules interferes in the fluidity, resulting in a greater thermodynamic activity of the drug on the surface of the stratum corneum, modifying its structure, promoting relaxation of the multilayer lipid packaging, and acting as a driving force for drug permeation (Lohani and Verma 2017).

In a study carried out by Khazaeli et al. (2014), niosomes were formulated with itraconazole, and the antileishmanial effect was evaluated by in vitro susceptibility of *Leishmania tropica*. The niosomes developed by the research group had a diameter of 9.5 ± 0.35 µm, with 20.9% being the higher encapsulation efficiency among the formulations. In the in vitro study, the growth rate of promastigotes treated with niosome-treated itraconazole was significantly lower when compared to the pure drug, with IC_{50} equal to 0.24 µg/mL and IC_{50} equal to 0.43 µg/mL, respectively. The multiplication rate and the mean number of amastigotes in the macrophages were evaluated, and the results showed a significantly lower value in the macrophages treated with niosomes (34.9 and 3.0), and the pure drug presented a relatively higher result (62.0 and 3.8) (Khazaeli et al. 2014). However, in this study, no specific route of administration was suggested.

Aflatoonian et al. (2016) accomplished a study to verify the efficacy of the combination of the niosome topical dapsone gel and intralesional injection of meglumine antimoniate compared to intralesional meglumine antimoniate and cryotherapy in the treatment of cutaneous leishmaniasis. This study followed a randomized clinical trial of 73 participants divided into two groups. At the end of the study it was verified that 82.9% of the participants in the group treated with the niosomes presented complete response of the lesion. The researchers concluded with the study that the ds-anapsid gel can be used as an alternative drug or adjuvant, with low cost and approximately without any adverse effect in the treatment of cutaneous leishmaniasis. However, they recommend additional studies to evaluate the efficacy and adverse effects of this niosomal system in comparison with other types of topical treatment.

Conventional treatments for leishmaniasis contain drugs with high toxicity rates and are related to parasitic resistance, and the use of such liposome-based drug delivery systems and their variations as transferosomes, ethosomes and niosomes have an important role in reducing toxicity by encapsulation of the drug, besides acting in the protection against enzymatic degradation, immunological inactivation, and reducing the exposure of the drug in healthy tissues (Wang and Chao 2017).

11.3.8 Microemulsion, Nanoemulsion, and Pickering Emulsion

Skin permeation tests are performed in healthy skin, but the formulation will be administered in tissues affected by the disease. The intact stratum corneum becomes a limiting factor to verify the efficiency of the developed system, requiring further studies and tests taking into account the damaged skin (Sousa et al. 2016).

Microemulsified and nanoemulsified vehicles are adaptable for various types of drug, with a mucocutaneous bioadhesion, low cost, and easy fabrication. Nanoemulsions also have a selective toxicity that does not affect the skin and mucous membranes, allowing activity in several concentrations, and the application for topical use (Caldeira et al. 2015). Among the treatments of topical use for leishmaniasis, these systems present several advantages over common pharmaceutical formulas (gels, creams, ointments), with an effective action against the disease and with lower toxicity in use (Oliveira et al. 2015).

Through nanobiotechnology in emulsions, a controlled and targeted release of the drugs can be performed. This property is possible because of the small size of the drop, which performs the permeation of lipophilic compounds through the skin, potentializing the topical effect of the drug and reaching specific tissues and cells, besides increasing the permeation of drugs in the parasites (Sousa et al. 2016; Cardoso et al. 2018).

In cutaneous leishmaniasis disease, it is important that the formulation presents a penetration of the drug into the skin until the dermis, acting on the parasites internalized in macrophages. In some specific cases, it is necessary that the system has a high retention rate and a low permeation, acting on local lesions and combating bacterial and fungal infections (Bastos de Mattos et al. 2015). Hydrophilic compounds have difficulty permeating through biological membranes of the pathogens. As a solution, nanoemulsified systems can act as a vehicle for the drug, increasing the bioavailability and applicability of it (Cardoso et al. 2018). Then, nanoemulsion systems are more promising than microemulsion because these can fuse with the pathogen membrane.

The interaction of the cationic load of the system with the anionic load of the parasite promotes a destabilization of the cell membrane, resulting in cell lysis and death of the promastigote and amastigote leishmania forms. The antileishmanial properties are linked to the small size of drops of the oily phase, which possess a high superficial tension. This property causes the cell membranes to be damaged, causing a synergistic effect with the formulation of the system. Consequently, there is a reduction in side effects (Rodrigues et al. 2018).

The vegetable oils have an important role in nanobiotechnology as nanoemulsions are very useful for the treatment of leishmaniasis because of their lower toxicity and their biodegradability, and also are renewable resources, being employed as new drugs or pharmaceutical adjuvants for topical systems (Bastos de Mattos et al. 2015). One of the main motivations of exploring nanobiotechnology in emulsions associated with natural products is the search for increased antileishmanial activity already known that can be combined with drugs for the elimination of the parasite more efficiently (Tabatabaie et al. 2018).

One of the examples of the application of nanoemulsions for the treatment of leishmaniasis is an association of the system with photodynamic therapy, which uses photosensitizing agents to create reactive oxygen species capable of eliminating the parasite. By combining the two strategies, there is an increase in inhibitory activity against the promastigote and amastigote stages of *L. amazonensis* and promastigote *L. infantum*, significantly reducing the amastigote form within the macrophages. These properties represent an improvement of the nanoemulsion technique and performance, making it an alternative for the eradication of the leishmania (Siqueira et al. 2017).

One of the disadvantages found in micro- and nanoemulsified systems is the irritating potential of the formulation caused by the use of surfactants. To solve this problem, nanoparticles (of synthetic or natural origin) are used to stabilize the emulsion rather than the surfactants. This methodology is given the name of Pickering emulsion.

Pickering emulsions have advantages such as better stability, low toxicity, and less pollution to the environment because of the absence of surfactant. In the pharmaceutical area, it is described that this type of emulsion can increase the pharmacological bioavailability and perform the controlled release of drugs. Concerning leishmaniasis, Pickering emulsions can encapsulate up to 47% of amphotericin B (more effective than commercial products). However, there are few studies on the technology applied to leishmaniasis, especially about activity in vitro, and testing of release and toxicity, which can prove the efficacy of the system in parasites (Richter et al. 2018). For many reasons, the Pickering emulsion is system emulsion based with great potential to combat the human and animal forms of *Leishmania* spp. The Pickering emulsion has a high permeation rate by the transdermal route; the cost of its production is less than that of liposomes, niosomes, and transferosomes. This system for drug delivery can be performed by a cutaneous, oral, or parenteral route.

11.4   Vaccines and New Perspectives

Immunization is one of the most efficient means for the prevention of illness. The skin is an attractive target for topical vaccine delivery.

Efforts to find a vaccine for the prevention of leishmaniasis are supported by the fact that patients once cured of leishmaniasis, when exposed again to the parasite, present an immune response and generally do not return to contract the disease. This finding justifies the development of vaccines to immunize people who are at risk of infection. The design of new vaccine drug delivery for leishmaniasis implies that the development of noninvasive or needle-free delivery is a global priority together with adjuvants and antigens delivered for the cutaneous and subcutaneous route that can result in immune response.

There is an increasing recognition of the skin as an organ of the immune system. Langerhans cells are found in close proximity to the stratum corneum and represent a network of immune cells that underlie and cover 25% of the area of total surface area (Gupta et al. 2005). The concept and principal aim of transcutaneous immunization is to produce an efficacious and safe product. Transcutaneous immunization is an important strategy for dose sparing in pandemic and enhanced immunity in elderly people (Glenn et al. 2007).

As already mentioned, under normal circumstances, the stratum corneum is an effective barrier. Thus, significant delivery of the active drug compound through the skin requires some disruption of the stratum corneum. There are different ways of breaking the barrier of the stratum corneum. The simplest is by hydrating the cutaneous tissue using an occlusive system, and the most efficient and safe is the dry-patch delivery system. This formulation provides a unique opportunity to formulate a dry, excipient-stabilized vaccine for noninvasive immunization against leishmaniasis, more acceptable and more suitable for mass use. The dry-patch delivery system can be designed to carry antigen encapsulated. Among the various approaches for topical immunization, the vesicular lipid-based system has gained much attention (Motlekar and Youan 2006). The recent development in vesicular system design for transdermal vaccine is the use of an elastic vesicle, for example, ultra-deformable liposomes, niosomes, transfersomes, and ethosomes. However, nanoemulsion, Pickering nanoemulsion, and γ-cyclodextrin are systems with great potential.

Gupta et al. (2005) compared the respective immune responses for transfersomes, niosomes, and liposomes by measuring serum IgG antibody titer. The results of the analyses showed that in comparison to transfersomes, niosomes and liposomes elicited a weaker immune response. Thus, transfersomes hold promise for effective noninvasive topical delivery of antigens (Gupta et al. 2005).

Several types of vaccines against *Leishmania* were studied. The main classes comprise vaccines using live cells, dead cells, recombinant protein; and the DNA of the parasite. Vaccines comprising recombinant proteins consist of genetically engineered cells with genes encoding antigenic proteins. These vaccines can be obtained by administration of parasite proteins expressed as heterologous proteins in other organisms, or different nonpathological bacteria or virus are genetically modified to contain genes encoding *Leishmania* antigenic molecules and used in vaccination to take advantage of the immunostimulant characteristics of these organisms to induce immune responses against leishmanial proteins.

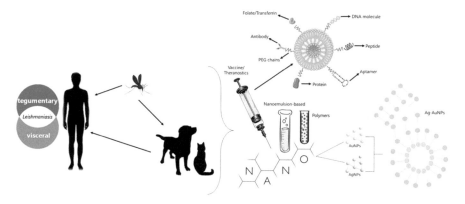

Fig. 11.2 Graphical representation of *Leishmania* cycle: recent updates and perspectives for prevention and treatment

The types of vaccines protected by patent applications worldwide for leishmaniasis before 2019 are distributed in recombinant protein (100), DNA vaccine (23), adjuvant (20), attenuated parasite (15), and others (<20) (Thomaz-Soccol et al. 2017).

Development of vaccines against leishmaniasis does not appear to follow any specific pattern. However, it is possible to notice an effort from countries developing its evolution in recent years.

Research efforts regarding development of DNA vaccines, recombinant proteins or peptides, and adjuvants are growing and seems to be among the best feasible alternatives for a successful vaccine (Fig. 11.2).

11.5   Conclusion

The advances in research, development, and innovation in drug delivery systems show that new dosage forms can enhance efficacy and secure compliance of the old drugs, including antimonials, amphotericin B, imiquimod, and buparvaquone. On the other hand, the strategy of vaccination by the cutaneous route has an exponential development, and can be used for immunization against cutaneous, mucocutaneous, and visceral leishmaniasis.

New drug delivery systems, whether emulsion based or polymers based, may prove to be a promising alternative to innovative carriers from synthetic, vegetal, or biotechnological material pharmacologically effective to attract the attention of the pharmaceutical field.

Leishmaniases and other neglected diseases as well as chronic diseases can be curable or delayed if these can be diagnosed at the earliest stage. Advanced theranostic platforms were designed for diagnosis, accurate targeting, and controlled delivery with an advantageous and simultaneous combination of immunological, therapeutic, and diagnostic properties.

The ultimate tool to eliminate tegumentary and visceral leishmaniasis, including resistance strains, will likely focus on biomimetically inspired self-assembly systems. Then, key tools in the frontier of immune theranostics will have emerged from nanoscale science and with creative (immune) engineering from nanoscale lipid vesicles such as the liposomes, niosomes, ethosomes, transfersomes, and dendrimers, cyclodextrin bio-optimized to prevent inflammation activation, and treating of the immune system to recognize and eliminate pathogens prophylactically (vaccines).

References

Aflatoonian M, Fekri A, Rahnam Z, Khalili M, Pardakhti A, Khazaeli P, Bahadini K (2016) The efficacy of combined topical niosomal dapsone gel and intralesional injection of meglumine antimoniate in comparison with intralesional meglumine antimoniate and cryotherapy in the treatment of cutaneous leishmaniasis. J Pak Assoc Dermatol 26(4):353–360. https://doi.org/10.1088/1361-6528/28/6/065101

Agrawal HG, Raval AG, Patel YK, Prajapati K (2018) Transfersome: a recent and novel approaches in transdermal drug delivery system. WJPPS 7(10):1621–1643. https://doi.org/10.20959/wjpps201810-12541

Akbarzadeh A, Rezaei-Sadabady R, Davaran S, Joo SW, Zarghami N, Hanifehpour Y, Nejati-Koshki K (2013) Liposome: classification, preparation, and applications. Nanoscale Res Lett 8(1):102. https://doi.org/10.1186/1556-276X-8-102

Alvar J, Vélez ID, Bern C, Herrero M, Desjeux P, Cano J, de Boer M (2012) Leishmaniasis worldwide and global estimates of its incidence. PLoS One 7(5):e35671. https://doi.org/10.1371/journal.pone.0035671

Alving CR, Steck EA, Chapman WL, Waits VB, Hendricks LD, Swartz GM, Hanson WL (1978) Therapy of leishmaniasis: superior efficacies of liposome-encapsulated drugs. Proc Natl Acad Sci U S A 75:2959–2963. https://doi.org/10.1073/pnas.75.6.2959

Arevalo I, Ward B, Miller R, Meng T, Najar E, Alvarez E, Llanos-Cuentas A (2002) Successful treatment of drug-resistant cutaneous leishmaniasis in humans by use of imiquimod, an immunomodulator. Clin Infect Dis 33:1847–1851. https://doi.org/10.1086/324161

Bailey F, Mondragon-Shem K, Haines LR, Olabi A, Alorfi A, Ruiz-Postigo JA, Alvar J, Hotez P, Adams ER, Vélez ID, Al-Salem W, Eaton J, Acosta-Serrano A, Molyneux DH (2019) Cutaneous leishmaniasis and co-morbid major depressive disorder: a systematic review with burden estimates. PLoS Negl Trop Dis 13(2):e0007092. https://doi.org/10.1371/journal.pntd.0007092

Baillie AJ, Coombs GH, Dolan TF, Laurie J (1986) Non-ionic surfactant vesicles, niosomes, as a delivery system for the anti-leishmanial drug, sodium stibogluconate. J Pharm Pharmacol 38(7):502–505. https://doi.org/10.1111/j.2042-7158.1986.tb04623.x

Balasegaram M, Ritmeijer K, Lima MA, Burza S, Ortiz Genovese G, Milani B, Chappuis F (2012) Liposomal amphotericin B as a treatment for human leishmaniasis. Expert Opin Emerg Drugs 17(4):493–510

Bastos de Mattos C, Fretes Argenta D, de lima Melchiades G, Norberto Sechini Cordeiro M, Luis Tonini M, hoehr Moraes M, Scherer Koester L (2015) Nanoemulsions containing a synthetic chalcone as an alternative for treating cutaneous leshmaniasis: optimization using a full factorial design. Int J Nanomedicine 10:5529–5542. https://doi.org/10.2147/IJN.S83929

Bhasin B, Patel SP, Road VLM (2018) An overview of transfersomal drug delivery. Int J Pharm Sci Res 9(6):2175–2184. https://doi.org/10.13040/IJPSR.0975-8232.9(6).2175-84

Bhattacharyya A, Bajpai M (2013) Oral bioavailability and stability study of a self-emulsifying drug delivery system (SEDDS) of amphotericin B. Curr Drug Deliv 10(5):542–547. https://doi. org/10.2174/15672018113109990001

Bryceson AA (2001) A policy for leishmaniasis with respect to the prevention and control of drug resistance. Tropical Med Int Health 6(11):928–934. https://doi. org/10.1046/j.1365-3156.2001.00795.x

Caldeira LR, Fernandes FR, Costa DF, Frézard F, Afonso LCC, Ferreira LAM (2015) Nanoemulsions loaded with amphotericin B: a new approach for the treatment of leishmaniasis. Eur J Pharm Sci 70:125–131. https://doi.org/10.1016/j.ejps.2015.01.015

Cardoso VS, Vermelho A, Ricci E Jr, Rodrigues IA, Mazzotto AM, Supuran CT (2018) Antileishmanial activity of sulphonamide nanoemulsions targeting the β-carbonic anhydrase from *Leishmania* species. J Enzyme Inhib Med Chem 33(1):850–857. https://doi.org/10.1080/14756366.2018.1463221

Collins M, Carter K, Baillie A, O'Grady J (1993) The distribution of free and non-ionic vesicular sodium stibogluconate in the dog. J Drug Target 1(2):133–142. https://doi. org/10.3109/10611869308996069

Dar MJ, Din FU, Khan GM (2018) Sodium stibogluconate loaded nano-deformable liposomes for topical treatment of leishmaniasis: macrophage as a target cell. Drug Deliv 25(1):1595–1606. https://doi.org/10.1080/10717544.2018.1494222

Demicheli C, Ochoa R, Da Silva JBB, Falcão CAB, Rossi-Bergmann B, De Melo AL, Frézard F (2004) Oral delivery of meglumine antimoniate-β-cyclodextrin complex for treatment of leishmaniasis. Antimicrob Agents Chemother 48(1):100–103. https://doi.org/10.1080/10717544.2018.1494222

den Boer M, Davidson RN, Oliaee RT, Sharifi I, Afgar A, Kareshk AT, Daneshvar H (2018) Unresponsiveness to meglumine antimoniate in anthroponotic cutaneous leishmaniasis field isolates: analysis of resistance biomarkers by gene expression profiling. Tropical Med Int Health 23(6):e6212. https://doi.org/10.1111/tmi.13062

Diniz JLCP, da Rochas Costa MO, Gonçalves DU (2011) Mucocutaneous leishmaniasis: clinical markers in presumptive diagnosis. Braz J Otorhinolaryngol 77(3):380–384

Dongare S, Raut S, Bonde S, Tayshete S, Gurav S (2015) Ethosomes as novel vesicular carriers for enhanced drug delivery. Int J Pharm Technol 6(3):2981–2997

Esch KJ, Petersen CA (2013) Transmission and epidemiology of zoonotic protozoal diseases of companion animals. Clin Microbiol Rev 26(1):58–85. https://doi.org/10.1128/CMR.00067-12

Frézard F, Demicheli C, Ferreira CS, Costa MAP (2001) Glutathione-induced conversion of pentavalent antimony to trivalent antimony in meglumine antimoniate. Antimicrob Agents Chemother 45(3):913–916. https://doi.org/10.3390/molecules14072317

Frézard F, Demicheli C, Ribeiro RR (2009) Pentavalent antimonials: new perspectives for old drugs. Molecules 14:2317–2336. https://doi.org/10.3390/molecules14072317

Ge X, Wei M, He S, Yuan W (2019) Advances of non-ionic surfactant vesicles (niosomes) and their application in drug delivery. Pharmaceutics 11(55):1–16. https://doi.org/10.3390/pharmaceutics11020055

Gidwani B, Vyas A (2015) A comprehensive review on cyclodextrin-based carriers for delivery of chemotherapeutic cytotoxic anticancer drugs. Biomed Res Int 2015(ID 198268):1–15. https://doi.org/10.3390/molecules14072317

Glenn GM, Flyer DC, Ellingsworth LR, Frech SA, Frerichs DM, Seid RC, Yu J (2007) Transcutaneous immunization with heat-labile enterotoxin: development of a needle-free vaccine patch. Expert Rev Vaccines 6(5):809–819. https://doi.org/10.1586/14760584.6.5.809

Grogl M, Thomason TN, Franke ED (1992) Drug resistance in leishmaniasis: its implication in systemic chemotherapy of cutaneous and mucocutaneous disease. Am J Trop Med Hyg 47(1):117–126

Gupta PN, Mishra V, Rawat A, Dubey P, Mahor S, Jain S, Vyas SP (2005) Non-invasive vaccine delivery in transfersomes, niosomes and liposomes: a comparative study. Int J Pharm 293(1-2):73–82. https://doi.org/10.1016/j.ijpharm.2004.12.022

Handler MZ, Patel PA, Kapila R, Al-Qubati Y, Schwartz RA (2015) Cutaneous and mucocutaneous leishmaniasis: differential diagnosis, diagnosis, histopathology, and management. J Am Acad Dermatol 73(6):911–926. https://doi.org/10.1016/j.jaad.2014.09.014

Harrison CJ, Miller RL, Bernstein DI (1994) Posttherapy suppression of genital herpes simplex virus (HSV) recurrences and enhancement of HSV-specific T-cell memory by imiquimod in Guinea pigs. Antimicrob Agents Chemother 38:2059–2064. https://doi.org/10.1128/AAC.38.9.2059

Herwaldt BL, Berman JD (1992) Recommendations for treating leishmaniasis with sodium stibogluconate (pentostam) and review of pertinent clinical studies. Am J Trop Med Hyg 46(3):296–306. https://doi.org/10.1128/AAC.38.9.2059

Jain S, Yadav P, Swami R, Swarnakar N, Kushwah V, Katiyar S (2018) Lyotropic liquid crystalline nanoparticles of amphotericin B: implication of phytantriol and glyceryl monooleate on bioavailability enhancement. AAPS PharmSciTech 19(4):1699–1711

Jha TK, Singh NK, Jha N (1992) Therapeutic use of sodium stibogluconate in kala-azar from some hyperendemic districts of N. Bihar. J Assoc Physicians India 40:868–888

Khan M, Nadhman A, Sehgal S, Siraj S, Yasinzai M (2018) Formulation and characterization of a self-emulsifying drug delivery system (SEDDS) of curcumin for the topical application in cutaneous and mucocutaneous leishmaniasis. Curr Top Med Chem 18(18):1603–1609. https://doi.org/10.2174/1568026618666181025104818

Khan M, Ali M, Shah W, Shah A, Yasinzai MM (2019) Curcumin-loaded self-emulsifying drug delivery system (cu-SEDDS): a promising approach for the control of primary pathogen and secondary bacterial infections in cutaneous leishmaniasis. Appl Microbiol Biotechnol 103(18):7481–7490. https://doi.org/10.1007/s00253-019-09990-x

Khazaeli P, Sharifi I, Talebian E, Heravi G, Moazeni E, Mostafavi M (2014) Anti-leishmanial effect of itraconazole niosome on in vitro susceptibility of *Leishmania tropica*. Environ Toxicol Pharmacol 38(1):205–211. https://doi.org/10.1016/j.etap.2014.04.003

Kulakov E, Cooper A (2011) Topical imiquimod use in treatment-resistant mycosis fungoides. Br J Dermatol 165(29):e1365. https://doi.org/10.1111/j.1365-2133.2011.10277.x

Kumar A (2018) Transferosome: a recent approach for transdermal drug delivery. J Drug Delivery Ther 8(5s):100–104. https://doi.org/10.22270/jddt.v8i5-s.1981

Laguna F, López-Vélez R, Pulido F, Salas A, Torre-Cisneros J, Torres E, Alvar J (1999) Treatment of visceral leishmaniasis in HIV-infected patients: a randomized trial comparing meglumine antimoniate with amphotericin B. AIDS 13(9):1063–1069. https://doi.org/10.1097/00002030-199906180-00009

Lessa MM, Lessa HA, Castro TWN, Oliveira A, Scherifer A, Machado P, Carvalho EM (2007) Mucosal leishmaniasis: epidemiological and clinical aspects. Braz J Otorhinolaryngol 73(6):843–847

Lohani A, Verma A (2017) Vesicles: potential nano carriers for the delivery of skin cosmetics. J Cosmet Laser Ther 19(8):485–493. https://doi.org/10.1080/14764172.2017.1358451

Loiseau PM, Bories C (2006) Mechanisms of drug action and drug resistance in *Leishmania* as basis for therapeutic target identification and design of antileishmanial modulators. Curr Trop Med Chem 6(5):539–550. https://doi.org/10.2174/156802606776743165

Loiseau PM, Cojean S, Schrével J (2011) Sitamaquine as a putative antileishmanial drug candidate: from the mechanism of action to the risk of drug resistance. Parasite 18(2):115–119. https://doi.org/10.1051/parasite/2011182115

Mistro S, Gomes B, Rosa L, Miranda L, Camargo M, Badaró R (2017) Cost-effectiveness of liposomal amphotericin B in hospitalised patients with mucocutaneous leishmaniasis. Trop Med Int Health 22(12):e-112. https://doi.org/10.1111/tmi.12996

Moafi M, Rezvan H, Sherkat R, Taleban R (2019) Leishmania vaccines entered in clinical trials: a review of literature. Int J Prev Med 10:95. https://doi.org/10.4103/ijpvm.IJPVM_116_18

Mosimann V, Neumayr A, Paris DH, Blum J (2018) Liposomal amphotericin B treatment of Old World cutaneous and mucosal leishmaniasis: a literature review. Acta Trop 182:246–250. https://doi.org/10.1016/j.actatropica.2018.03.016

Motlekar NA, Youan BBC (2006) The quest for non-invasive delivery of bioactive macromolecules: a focus on heparins. J Control Release 113(2):91–101. https://doi.org/10.1016/j.jconrel.2006.04.008

New RRC, Chance ML, Heath S (1981) The treatment of experimental cutaneous leishmaniasis with liposome-entrapped pentostam. Parasitology 37:253–256. https://doi.org/10.1017/S0031182000080501

Okwor I, Uzonna J, Kumar A, Pandey SC, Samant M (2016) Slow pace of antileishmanial drug development. PAO 94(3):e4. https://doi.org/10.1017/pao.2018.1

Oliveira MM, Calixto G, Graminha M, Cerecetto H, Gozález M, Chorilli M (2015) Development, characterization, and in vitro biological performance of fluconazole-loaded microemulsions for the topical treatment of cutaneous leishmaniasis. Biomed Res Int 2015:396894. https://doi.org/10.1155/2015/396894

Perez AP, Altube MJ, Schillreff P, Apezteguia G, Celes FS, Zacchino S, Morilla MJ (2016) Topical amphotericin B in ultradeformable liposomes: formulation, skin penetration study, antifungal and antileishmanial activity in vitro. Colloids Surf B Biointerfaces 139:190–198. https://doi.org/10.1016/j.colsurfb.2015.12.003

Pratiwi L, Fudholi A, Martien R, Pramono S (2017) Self-nanoemulsifying drug delivery system (SNEDDS) for topical delivery of mangosteen peels (*Garcinia mangostana* L.): formulation design and in vitro studies. J Young Pharm 9(3):341–346. https://doi.org/10.5530/jyp.2017.9.68

Rai S, Bandyopadhyay S (2001) Problems in management of Kala Azar: experience from Bihar. Med J Armed Forces India 57:117–119. https://doi.org/10.5530/jyp.2017.9.68

Richter AR, Feitosa JPA, Paula HCB, Goycoolea FM, de Paula RCM (2018) Pickering emulsion stabilized by cashew gum-poly-*L*-lactide copolymer nanoparticles: synthesis, characterization and amphotericin B encapsulation. Colloids Surf B Biointerfaces 164:201–209. https://doi.org/10.1016/j.colsurfb.2018.01.023

Rodrigues IA, Ramos ADS, Falcão DQ, Ferreira JLP, Basso SL, Silva JRDA, Amaral ACF (2018) Development of nanoemulsions to enhance the antileishmanial activity of *Copaifera paupera* oleoresins. Biomed Res Int 2018:9781724. . 9p. https://doi.org/10.1155/2018/9781724

Ruiz HK, Serrano DR, Dea-Ayuela MA, Bilbao-Ramos PE, Bolás-Fernández F, Torrado JJ, Molero G (2014) New amphotericin B-gamma cyclodextrin formulation for topical use with synergistic activity against diverse fungal species and *Leishmania* spp. Int J Pharm 473(1-2):148–157. https://doi.org/10.1016/j.ijpharm.2014.07.004

Siqueira LBO, Cardoso VS, Rodrigues IA, Vazquez-Villa AL, Santos EP, Guimarães CSCC, Vermelho SB, Ricci E Jr (2017) Development and evaluation of zinc phthalocyanine nanoemulsions for use in photodynamic therapy for *Leishmania* spp. Nanotechnology 28(6):65101. https://doi.org/10.1088/1361-6528/28/6/065101.

Smith L, Serrano DR, Mauger M, Bolás-Fernández F, Dea-Ayuela MA, Lalatsa A (2018) Orally bioavailable and effective buparvaquone lipid-based nanomedicines for visceral leishmaniasis. Mol Pharm 15(7):2570–2583. https://doi.org/10.1021/acs.molpharmaceut.8b00097

Sousa GD, Kishishita J, Aquino KAS, Presgrave OAF, Leal LB, Santana DP (2016) Biopharmaceutical assessment and irritation potential of microemulsions and conventional systems containing oil from *Syagrus cearensis* for topical delivery of amphotericin B using alternative methods. AAPS PharmSciTech 18(5):1833–1842. https://doi.org/10.1208/s12249-016-0663-3

Souza JKC, Barbosa VT, Souza JCC, Menezes JB, Grillo LAM, Dornelas CB (2019) Preparation and evaluation of the pentavalent antimony-quercetin complex (SbV-QUE). Braz J Health Rev 2(4):3091–3103. https://doi.org/10.34119/bjhrv2n4-074

Sundar S, Singh A, Singh OP (2014) Strategies to overcome antileishmanial drugs unresponsiveness. J Trop Med 2014:e-646932. https://doi.org/10.1155/2014/646932

Tabatabaie F, Samarghandi N, Zarrati S, Maleki F, Ardestani MS, Elmi T, Mosawi SH (2018) Induction of immune responses by DNA vaccines formulated with dendrimer and poly(methyl methacrylate) (PMMA) nano-adjuvants in BALB/c mice infected with *Leishmania major*. Open Access Macedonian J Med Sci 6(2):229–236. https://doi.org/10.3889/oamjms.2018.061

Tanriverdi ST (2018) Preparation and characterization of caffeine loaded liposome and etho-some formulations for transungual application. Turk J Pharm Sci 15(2):178–183. https://doi.org/10.4274/tjps.22931

Thomaz-Soccol V, Ferreira da Costa ES, Karp SG, Letti LA Jr, Soccol FT, Soccol CR (2017) Recent advances in vaccines against *Leishmania* based on patent applications. Recent Pat Biotechnol 12(1):21–32. https://doi.org/10.2174/1872208311666170510121126

Touitou E, Dayan N, Bergelson L, Godin B, Eliaz M (2000) Ethosomes: novel vesicular carri-ers for enhanced delivery. Characterization and skin penetration properties. J Control Release 65(3):403–418. https://doi.org/10.1016/S0168-3659(99)00222-9

Van Bocxlaer K, Yardley V, Murdan S, Croft SL (2016) Drug permeation and barrier damage in *Leishmania*-infected mouse skin. J Antimicrob Chemother 71(6):1578–1585. https://doi.org/10.1093/jac/dkw012

Van Griensven J, Diro E (2012) Visceral leishmaniasis. Infect Dis Clin N Am 26:309–322

Van Griensven J, Carrillo E, López-Vélez R, Lynen L, Moreno J (2014) Leishmaniasis in immunosuppressed individuals. Clin Microbiol Infect 20(4):286–299. https://doi.org/10.1111/1469-0691.12556

Van Griensven J, Simegn T, Endris M, Diro E (2018) Visceral leishmaniasis and HIV co-infection in Northwest Ethiopia: antiretroviral treatment and burden of disease among patients enrolled in HIV care. Am J Trop Med Hyg 98(2):486–491. https://doi.org/10.4269/ajtmh.17-0142

Varsha K, Arum Kumar KV (2018) Ethosomal gel: a new strategy for gouty arthritis. World J Pharm Med Res 4(8):312–316

Wang Q, Chao Y (2017) Multifunctional quantum dots and liposome complexes in drug delivery. J Biomed Res 32(2):91–106. https://doi.org/10.7555/JBR.31.20160146

Wang Q, Hu C, Zhang H, Zhang Y, Liu T, Qian A, Xia Q (2016) Evaluation of a new solid non-aqueous self-double-emulsifying drug-delivery system for topical application of quercetin. J Microencapsul 33(8):785–794. https://doi.org/10.1080/02652048.2016.1264494

WHO/PAHO Department of Neglected Infectious Diseases (2019) Leishmaniases: epidemio-logical report of the Americas, vol. 7, pp 1–7. https://www.who.int/leishmaniasis/resources/who_paho_era7/en/

World Health Organization (WHO) (2010) Control of the leishmaniasis. World Health Organ Tech Rep Ser 949:22–26

Zaioncz S, Khalil N, Mainardes R (2017) Exploring the role of nanoparticles in amphotericin B delivery. Curr Pharm Des 23(3):509–521. https://doi.org/10.2174/1381612822666161027103640

Chapter 12
Additive Manufacturing and Nanotherapeutics: Present Status and Future Perspectives in Wound Healing

Parneet Kaur Deol, Amoljit Singh Gill, Sushant Prajapati, and Indu Pal Kaur

Abstract In the past decades, additive manufacturing had emerged as a cost-effective and clinically acceptable means for fabrication of diverse and biologically compatible materials of complex geometrical structure. This technology can use an array of materials (mainly biopolymers) as carriers, which can print the incorporated cells, drug, or even nanoparticles in desired shape with high accuracy and precision.

In this chapter, we have highlighted the current status and the future scope of fabricating the tailor-made nanotherapeutics and additive manufacturing techniques for effective wound healing. Current market demand of the tailor-made wound dressings/implants has contributed positively towards the use of additive manufacturing in their fabrication as it can address specific problems associated with various phases (namely hemostasis, inflammation, proliferation, and remodeling) of wound healing phenomenon. Additive manufacturing fabricated materials can either work as carriers for nanostructured therapeutic agents like silver nanoparticles, nanoparticle loaded antibiotics and antioxidants or they can print biomaterials (with or without drug) in complex nanoporous scaffolds.

Keywords Nanotherapeutics · Additive manufacturing · Wound healing · Nanomaterials · 3D scaffolds

P. K. Deol
Department of Pharmaceutics, G.H.G. Khalsa College of Pharmacy, Gurusar Sadhar, Ludhiana, Punjab, India

A. S. Gill
Department of Mechanical Engineering, Punjab Technical University, Kapurthala, Punjab, India

S. Prajapati
Department of Biotechnology and Medical Engineering, NIT, Rourkela, India

I. P. Kaur (✉)
Department of Pharmaceutics, University Institute of Pharmaceutical Sciences, Panjab University, Chandigarh, India

© Springer Nature Switzerland AG 2020
M. Rai (ed.), *Nanotechnology in Skin, Soft Tissue, and Bone Infections*,
https://doi.org/10.1007/978-3-030-35147-2_12

205

12.1 Introduction

Wound healing is a highly coordinated and evolutionary stagnant process carried out by variety of cells following different biochemical pathways to replace or repair the damaged cells or tissues for restoring their original structure and function (Hamdan et al. 2017). Wounds can take days to few years to heal depending upon the type of wound and the person's health (Rani and Ritter 2016). Wound healing is the effective synchronization of cell–cell, cell–proteins and Cell–extra cellular matrix (ECM) interaction leading to complete healing. Different cell types, namely macrophage, fibroblast, endothelial, poly-morphonuclear leucocytes, neutrophils, etc., coordinate the healing process with tight control by numerous growth factors, chemokines, and cytokines. The imbalance in any of the aforementioned interaction or factors could lead to improper healing or chronic wounds, characterized with unsolved inflammation, weakened fibroblast function, reduced angiogenesis, and bacterial infection (Hamdan et al. 2017).

Normal wound healing consists of four overlapping and sequential phases, namely hemostasis, inflammation, proliferation, and remodeling. Hemostasis is the immediate response (seconds to minutes) of the body defense system to the injury. Here, the blood clotting occurs which consists of polymerized matrix of fibrinogen and fibronectin along with platelet aggregation (Mele 2016). The inflammation phase takes hours to days where the creation of the immune barrier occurs upon the initiation of various molecular events. This phase is mainly coordinated by neutrophils, macrophages, and poly-morphonuclear leucocytes, which appear at the wound site at different time interval post injury (Rani and Ritter 2016). They are responsible for effective removal of bacteria, foreign and other contaminants from the body by the process called phagocytosis (Guo and DiPietro 2010). The macrophages here also initiate angiogenesis and fibroplasia within 3–5 days (Rani and Ritter 2016). Then comes the proliferation phase, also known as fibroblastic phase, which lasts as long as 3 weeks. Here, the macrophages release angiogenesis factor which gives rise to capillary buds and neovasculature and also fibroblast stimulating factor which is responsible for the activation of fibroblasts (Guo and DiPietro 2010). The collagen and the proteoglycans produced by the fibroblast along with neovasculature form the granulation tissue, which fills the tissue defects (Rani and Ritter 2016). The granulation tissue replaces the fibrin formed clot and the fibroblasts differentiate into myofibroblasts, which have special contractile properties that bring edges of wound together for better healing (Mele 2016). Then the epithelial cells proliferate and move to the granulation tissue for re-epithelialization, form a barrier for microbes and prevent fluid loss (Das and Baker 2016). The final phase of remodeling lasts for 3 weeks to few years and involves complete functional regeneration of the tissue. The fibroblasts here continue to produce network of collagen along with other ECM proteins in an orderly fashion to provide strength to the wound followed by shrinking of underlying connective tissues in size for bringing the wound edges closer together (Rani and Ritter 2016).

A successful wound healing necessitates the optimization of patient-specific wound condition in addition with the ideal healing niche. In the current scenario, there are many products in the market which effectively act on the wound environment providing a protected and pathogen-free moist area (Murphy and Evans 2012). Generally, there are two major categories of wounds, namely acute and chronic. The acute wounds can be peripheral involving both the epidermis and the papillary region of the dermis or the subcutaneous layer (Dreifke et al. 2015). Chronic wounds are the result of damage of all skin layers comprising epidermis, dermis, and subcutaneous layer, and are generally resulted from other diseases like diabetic foot ulcers, pressure ulcers from spinal cord injury, and some neurodegenerative processes (Dreifke et al. 2015). Acute wounds heal over a short period with no to minimal scarring, whereas chronic wounds heal much slowly often taking months to show progress. According to an evaluation on 5000 patients by the United States Wound Registry, it was observed that a preliminary reason for most of the chronic wounds is generally an underlying condition (Fife and Carter 2012). World Health Organization (2016) reported that four times increase in number of diabetes patients, from 1980 to 2014, has significantly increased the incidence of chronic wounds, thus putting a high cost burden on the healthcare system. In the USA alone, approximately 6.5 million people were affected by non-healing wounds in 2009 with total cost of treatment reaching a whopping 25 billion USD per year (Sen et al. 2009; Han and Ceilley 2017).

The traditional wound healing market has witnessed an influx of novel medical technologies addressing various phases of healing owing to a growing knowledge on wound etiology and pathology. The global market is expected to reach $22 billion by 2022, expanding at a compound annual growth rate of 3.7% from 2016 to 2022 (Han and Ceilley 2017). Presently, many treatment procedures are being employed for the treatment of both the acute and chronic wounds. Skin grafts, biomaterials, stem cells, nanotherapeutics to name a few (Fig. 12.1).

Bioengineered skin grafts, either biosynthetic or cultured, have shown a promising effect in repairing the damaged tissues and are not only biocompatible but also bring minimal risk of immunogenic rejection (Murphy and Evans 2012). Stem cells are also potent means for wound repair because of their capability of differentiating into various specialized cells in the body. In this technique, stem cells isolated from bone marrow, blood and umbilical cord, are applied at the infected area for its reconstruction (Dreifke et al. 2015). Many other approaches are also explored for complete tissue reconstruction like application of growth factors (eicosanoids, cytokines, platelet-derived growth factors (PDGF)), antibiotics, anti-inflammatory drugs, hyperbaric oxygen, and many others (Murphy and Evans 2012).

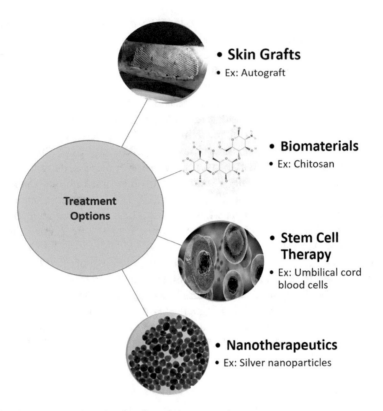

Fig. 12.1 Treatment options for chronic and acute wounds

12.2 Current Status and Scope of Nanotherapeutics in Wound Healing

The global nanotechnology industry reached over $1.5 trillion in 2014, becoming a major economic force (Sahoo et al. 2007; Zhou et al. 2014). Compared to conventional wound care products, nanotechnology-driven therapeutics offer unique opportunities where a specific biochemical process is influenced within the impaired healing process. It employs nanosized (1–100 nm) tools for the purpose of diagnosis, prevention, and ultimately treatment comprising discrete areas of application such as drug delivery, therapies, in vivo and in vitro diagnosis, and active implants (Hafner et al. 2014). The special properties of nanosized particles like electric conductivity, antimicrobial activity, high surface to volume ratio, swelling, and contraction make them a versatile resource which can be explored to improve drug solubility, drug targeting, controlled drug release and also to improve the transportation across various biological barriers (Hafner et al. 2014). The main objective is to achieve improved bioavailability, efficacy, safety, and pharmacokinetics which cannot be possible by the conventional dosages. In wound healing, nanomaterials can either act as intrinsic therapeutic agents or can act as carriers for them.

12.2.1   Nanomaterials as Intrinsic Therapeutic Agents

Metal and metal oxide nanomaterials (like silver, gold, copper, zinc oxide) as well as nonmetallic carbon nanomaterials exhibit excellent properties such as low in vivo toxicity, and bacteriostatic and bactericidal activities.

Silver is a known bactericidal agent and is commonly used to treat burns, wound infection, and a variety of ulcers. Positively charged silver ions bind with a range of negatively charged proteins and disrupt the microbial respiration and their cell membrane, thus adversely affecting the microbial replication mechanism (Lansdown 2002; Graham 2005; Fong and Wood 2006). Further, it has an inherent anti-inflammatory activity, which makes it a suitable candidate for both acute and chronic wounds (Wong et al. 2009). Despite the broad antimicrobial activity of ionic silver products, patient suffers from serious disadvantages such as skin discoloration (silver nitrate), eschar formation (silver sulfadiazine), tissue irritation (due to non-specific binding of silver ions), and high frequency of dressing replacement (due to non-specific inactivation of ionic silver in the wound bed by chloride ions and proteins) (Klasen 2000; Wasiak et al. 2013). These shortcomings of ionic silver products led to the development of slow-releasing nanocrystalline silver products. Due to their large surface area, these products show efficient antimicrobial activity. Further, these nanosized silver particles loaded dressings can release antimicrobial silver ions over 7 days vis-à-vis conventionally used gels and films which can sustain the release of an active ingredient, over a period of 1–2 days. Presently two such products, ActicoatTM (Smith & Nephew plc., UK), and Polymem® silver (Ferris Mfg. Corp., USA), are marketed for wound healing applications. These nanocrystalline silver dressings require much less frequent dressing changes compared to the dressings containing ionic silver and result in a reduced distress to the wound bed and improved patient compliance (Klasen 2000; Murphy and Evans 2012). Apart from silver, other metals and their oxides have also found applications in wound healing. Gold nanoparticles (Leu et al. 2012; Randeria et al. 2015), magnesium fluoride nanoparticles (Jacob et al. 2006), cerium oxide nanoparticles (Chigurupati et al. 2013), copper nanoparticles (Rakhmetova et al. 2010), titanium dioxide nanoparticles (Archana et al. 2013), and iron oxide nanoparticles (Ziv-Polat et al. 2010) alone or in conjugation with other biomolecules have reported beneficial effect in wound healing. Their mechanism of action ranges from antioxidant action (e.g., for cerium oxide nanoparticles) to antibacterial action (e.g., for gold and zinc oxide nanoparticles).

Carbon nanomaterials like graphene, carbon nanotubes, fullerenes and the various forms of diamond have attracted great attention for their potential antibacterial action. The observed antimicrobial properties of carbon nanomaterials are attributed to the combined mechanisms of bacterial membrane perturbation caused by sharp edges and oxidative stress induction. Additionally, an abundance of functionalized hydroxyl, epoxy, and carboxyl groups on the surface enhance their hydrophilicity and biocompatibility and significantly facilitate its surface modification with other molecules or polymers (Liu et al. 2011; Ji et al. 2016; Maas 2016).

12.2.2 Nanomaterials as Carriers for Therapeutic Agents

Polymer and lipid based nanocarriers, gold nanoparticles and nanofibers loaded with antibiotics, antioxidants, nitric oxide, growth factors, and nucleic acid derivatives have been extensively explored for beneficial applications in wound healing.

Turos et al. (2007) developed antibiotic conjugated polyacrylate nanoparticles with significantly increased antimicrobial activity in comparison to the non-conjugated antibiotic formulation. Similarly, poly(butyl acrylate-styrene) nanoparticles conjugated to N-thiolated beta-lactam antibiotic have been prepared with conventional and polymerizable surfactants, which showed higher antimicrobial activity while maintaining low toxicity (Garay-Jimenez et al. 2009). Lipidic nanoparticles like liposomes (Das et al. 2016a, b), solid lipid nanoparticles (Kuchler et al. 2009, 2010a), and exosomes (Rani and Ritter 2016) have shown great promise in successfully delivering the drugs for effective wound healing. They have been tested for delivering bioactive molecules such as opioids like morphine (Kuchler et al. 2010b) and resveratrol (Gokce et al. 2012), antioxidants like curcumin and silver sulfadiazine, and even siRNA for wound healing. The encapsulation of these growth factors in polymeric or lipidic nanoparticles not only resulted in extended release product but also demonstrated the ability to protect proteins from early degradation by various proteolytic enzymes including matrix metalloproteinases (Chu et al. 2010; Lai et al. 2014).

Gold nanoparticles are biocompatible and extensively used in tissue regeneration, targeted drug delivery, and wound healing. These nanoparticles can be easily integrated with other biomolecules like antimicrobials, growth factors, and peptides by attaching at the gold surface, thereby increasing their potency to kill microbes. Vancomycin-conjugated gold nanoparticles were reported to increase vancomycin's activity against vancomycin-resistant enterococci by 50-fold, and showed significant activity against E. coli, a gram-negative bacterium that is usually unaffected by vancomycin (Gu et al. 2003). Chen et al. (2015) functionalized gold nanodots with antimicrobial peptides in order to inhibit the growth of drug-resistant bacteria and promote healing in a rodent wound model (Chen et al. 2015).

In recent times, scientists have focused on developing nanofiber-based dressings that can mimic the native dermal extra cellular matrix (ECM) and have high surface area-to-volume ratio and high porosity. Polymers like chitosan, gelatin, poly(lactic-co-glycolic acid) (PLGA), alginate, polyurethane, and caprolactone are very commonly used to prepare these dressings. In addition to traditional functions, these nanofiber dressings were intended to reduce infection and inflammation and promote wound healing by creating a positive environment (Boateng et al. 2008). To prevent and treat wound infections, antimicrobial agents, antioxidants, growth factors, and enzymes have been incorporated into electrospun nanofibers (Chen et al. 2017). A hybrid composite of PLGA nanoparticles embedded in chitosan–poly(ethylene oxide) nanofibers was employed for the release of dual growth factor vascular endothelial growth factor (VEGF) and platelet-derived growth factor (PDGF). This nanoparticle-in-nanofiber system delivering both growth factors enhanced wound healing in vivo through VEGF-promoted angiogenesis and PDGF-mediated tissue regeneration and remodeling (Xie et al. 2013).

Naked and colloidal DNA have been delivered to wound sites by direct injection, gene gun, and electroporation. However, these techniques suffer from the need for repeated injections as well as inconsistent and short-term gene expression. These issues can be overcome by the use of electrospun nanofibrous meshes as matrices for gene encapsulation and wound dressing material. Nucleic acids have been impregnated into these nanofibers to enhance tissue regeneration and eventually decrease scar formation in normal and diabetic wounds (Choi et al. 2015).

12.3 3D Scaffolds for Wound Healing: Scope for Additive Manufacturing Techniques

Two main approaches which were used to replace or repair the damaged or lost tissue and organs are autografting or allografting. Limited availability and donor site morbidity of autografts and immune system rejections of allografts limit their medical applications (Rahmani Del Bakhshayesh et al. 2018). Further, they also suffer from a range of problems including wound contraction, scar formation, and poor integration with host tissue.

A paradigm shift is taking place in medical field from using synthetic implants and tissue grafts to a tissue-engineering approach that uses degradable porous material scaffolds integrated with biological cells or molecules to regenerate tissues. Scaffold structure is a novel carrier for cell and drug delivery that enhances wound healing through differentiation of endothelial and epithelial cells and production of angiogenic growth factors in cutaneous wounds (Chaudhary and Garg 2015). Both synthetic polymers and biodegradable polymeric biomaterials can be used in fabricating these 3D nanoscaffolds. These scaffolds have high surface area-to-volume ratio and mimic the ECM which assists in adhesion, proliferation, migration, and differentiation of the cells, all of which were deemed as the extremely desired features for tissue engineering. Its porous three-dimensional structure provides an excellent carrier for cell and drug and improves the wound healing through differentiation of endothelial and epithelial cells and production of angiogenic growth factors in cutaneous wounds.

Worldwide, approximately 230 million major surgical procedures are performed on a daily basis (Weiser et al. 2008). Most of these procedures involve reconstruction, repair, or replacement of one or more damaged tissues or organs. The primary objective of the current trends in tissue engineering is to provide patient-specific tailor-made substitutes that can help to restore, improve, or maintain tissue function (O'Brien 2011). Among the other methods, additive manufacturing has gained great interest in scaffold manufacturing (Mota et al. 2015). Additive manufacturing or 3D printing is a technologically sophisticated and advanced technique of manufacturing materials for different physical and biological applications. The conventional manufacturing techniques consist of molds and subtractive machining procedures that lack versatility to be modified into complex geometries and are labor-intensive with limited patient specific variability, limited compatible biomaterials, and lack the facility of in-process seeding of living cells due to long fabrication times (Ahangar et al. 2018). In addition, organic solvents are used to dissolve the synthetic polymers and the presence of their residues in fabricated scaffold can be toxic to cells.

The demand and application of the 3D printed products has witnessed a surprising increase in the healthcare industry, because of their high accuracy, precision, and reproducibility in designing therapeutic delivery systems and implants for surgical planning and tissue engineering (Ahangar et al. 2018). Further the process is environment friendlier as it offers reduced waste and minimal use of harmful chemicals (such as etching and cleaning solutions) as compared to traditional manufacturing techniques (Ivanova et al. 2013). 3D printing involves fabrication of complex structures by layer-by-layer processing of the material involving four steps, namely 3D modeling, data conversion and preprocessing, fabrication, and post-processing (Singh et al. 2016). Firstly, very precise information about the tissue defect is obtained for the material selection and the structure of the defect; secondly, the information is transferred to the computer system and a 3D model of the same is generated. The model is sliced in thousands of horizontal layers to get two-dimensional (2D) images. The connected printer uses this 2D data to fabricate a layer in X-Y plane. Layer-by-layer stacking gives the Z dimension to the product. Finer the thickness of the layer, smaller will be the stepping effect in the Z plane and a stable 3D structure is created to be incorporated onto the affected area (He et al. 2018; Gill et al. 2019).

There are numerous additive manufacturing techniques presently in use to fabricate range of products of complex geometry using various biopolymers. Broadly, they are grouped under four categories based on the material to be processed (i.e., liquid based, powder based, solid based, and bioink based). Figure 12.2 briefs some of the commonly employed additive manufacturing techniques used in bioprinting.

Extrusion bioprinting technique involves dispensing of viscous bioink (biomaterials, biomolecules, or cells) through a nozzle or syringe driven by mechanical or pneumatic forces according to the CAD (computer aided design) model (Bishop et al. 2017). It is a slow printing technique and capable of fabricating 3D pattern line by line and has a cell viability of maximum up to 90% (Jessop et al. 2017; Mandrycky et al. 2016). It can print with high cell densities for tissue reconstruction of skeletal muscle, skin, cardiac tissue, and liver (Vijayavenkataraman et al. 2018). Inkjet based bioprinting is a precise and high resolution printing technique which utilizes micro droplets of bioink (Jessop et al. 2017). It is an oncontact complex tissue printing technique, which uses thermal, electromagnetic, or piezoelectric based actuators to dispense bioink drops successively onto a CAD designed substrate (Bishop et al. 2017). Inkjet printers are conventional printers with a high cell viability (usually between 80 and 90%) and are commonly applied in the field of tissue engineering for blood vessels, bone, cartilage, and neurons (Mandrycky et al. 2016). Laser based

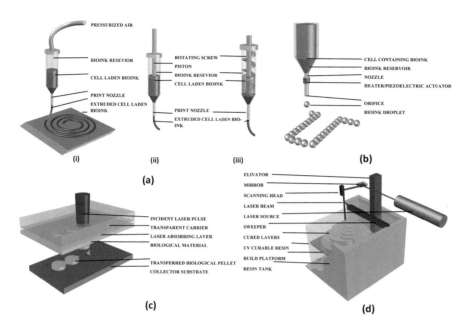

Fig. 12.2 Schematic representation of few selected additive manufacturing techniques. (**a**) Extrusion-based bioprinting (i) Pneumatic, (ii) Piston-driven, and (iii) Screw-driven; (**b**) Inkjet-based bioprinting; (**c**) Laser-assisted bioprinting; and (**d**) Stereolithography

bioprinting technique uses laser energy to pattern the cell loaded bioinks in a high resolution 2D and 3D arrangement (Vijayavenkataraman et al. 2018). It is a non-contact bioprinting method which does not provide any mechanical stress to the printed cells thus resulting in high cell viability (usually greater than 95%) (Mandrycky et al. 2016). Generally, it is used for regenerating tissues, which are damaged from burns, by the biofabrication of fibroblasts and keratinocytes (Singh et al. 2016; Vijayavenkataraman et al. 2018). Stereolithography technique is a fledging technique that utilizes photopolymerization in which UV light is directed in a pattern over a liquid polymer crosslinking it to a hardened structure (Bishop et al. 2017). It uses a photopolymerizable material with high fabrication accuracy than other techniques for manufacturing of complex 3D anatomical models (Bishop et al. 2017; Jessop et al. 2017). It consumes less time and offers higher cell viability (more than 90%). Steriolithography is generally used for the biofabrication of embryonic and dermal fibroblasts, mesenchymal progenitor cells, and ganglial cells (Vijayavenkataraman et al. 2018). Table 12.1 enlists various properties like compatible biomaterials, capabilities, advantages, limitations, and applications of a few selected biofabrication techniques commonly used in fabricating 3D scaffolds for tissue engineering.

Table 12.1 Comparative details of few selected biofabrication techniques

S. No	Process properties	Stereolithography	Laser direct write (LDW)	Inkjet printing	Extrusion printing
1	Compatible biomaterials	Alginate, polycaprolactone, polyethylene glycol, gelatin methacrylate, poly(ethylene glycol) diacrylate, poly(D,L-lactide)-based resin, ethyl lactate, polyurethane with hyaluronic acid, poly(trimethylene carbonate)-based resins, diethyl fumarate, bisacrylphosphrine oxide, poly(propylene fumarate), epoxy/hydroxyapatite, poly-4-hydroxybutyrate, polyhydroxyoctanoate, beta-tricalcium phosphate/collagen	Hydroxyapatite, polycaprolactone, alginate, poly (d-, l-lactide-coglycolide), zirconia, collagen, biotinylated bovine serum albumin	Alginate, polyethylene glycol, hydroxyapatite, polycaprolactone, bioactive glasses, poly(hydroxymethylglycolideco-ε-caprolactone), polylactic acid/polyethylene glycol, polystyrene, gelatin, methacrylic anhydride, collagen, agarose, fibrin	Cellulose, alginate, gelatin, polycaprolactone, gellan, collagen, carboxymethyl-chitosan, agarose, spider silk protein, hyaluronic acid, polyurethane, fibrinogen, polyethylene oxide, pluronic F127, gellan gum, sodium periodate, arginylglycylaspartic acid peptides, polylactic acid, decellularized extracellular matrix
2	Advantages	• Nozzle free technique • Can print complex designs • Growth factors, proteins and cell patterning is possible	• Can print both liquid and solid phase biomaterials • Suitable for organic and inorganic materials and cells because of mild conditions • Better quantitative control	• Both drug and biomolecules (proteins and living cells) can be plotted easily • Process is fast and suitable for low viscosity biomaterials	• Simple process • Vast range of biomaterials can be printed • Capable to print high cell densities

S. No	Process properties		Stereolithography	Laser direct write (LDW)	Inkjet printing	Extrusion printing
3	Limitations		• Limited for photopolymers only. • Multicells cannot be print. • The required photo curing can damage the cells. • UV light source toxicity to cells	• Chances of thermal damage due to nanosecond laser irritation • Requirement of homogeneous ribbon • Higher equipment cost	• Process suitable for certain range of viscosity • More suitable for drop on demand application and not unable to provide continuous flow • Poor functionality for vertical structures	• Only suitable for viscous liquids
4	Process capability	Resolution	100 μm	±5 μm	50 μm	100 μm
		Vertical printing ability	Good	Medium	Poor	Good
		Speed	Fast	Medium	Fast	Slow
		Cell density	Medium	Medium	Low	High
		Cell viability	>90%	>90%	80–95%	88–93%
5	Applications		Microscale cell patterning, tissue engineering, sacrificial molds for scaffold preparation, heart valve tissue engineering, cartilage tissue engineering, osteochondral tissue engineering, vascularized bone reconstruction	Tissue engineering, skin tissue like structures, fabricating biomimetic model for disease	Tissue engineering, soft tissue models, vascular tissue engineering	Wound dressing, bioprinting of tissue/ organ, tissue engineering (general), whole bone organ engineering, bioactive scaffolds, tissue regeneration, primary liver constructs

Adapted with permission from Gill et al. (2019)

12.4   Additive Manufacturing and Nanotherapeutics

Additive manufacturing or 3D printing technology will always be in the phase of "To be continued…" where new techniques keep emerging with each passing day. Various materials and processes are applied in conjugation to attain flexible, biologically stable and compatible treatment solutions. In recent times, researchers have tried to combine the positives of both 3D printing and nanotherapeutics for more effective action in different clinical implications by improving the drug performance and preparing a tailor-made product with better patient compliance. Lot of work has already been reported in the field of bone tissue regeneration. Nanomaterials like silicate nanoplatelets (Byambaa et al. 2017), calcium phosphate nanoparticles (Duan et al. 2010), and nanocrystalline hydroxyapatite (Holmes et al. 2016) were successfully printed using various additive manufacturing techniques to provide a biomimetic environment for osteogenesis. Nanostructures are incorporated into additive manufacturing printing media as an attempt to improve the properties of the final printed part. Ahangar and coworkers fabricated nanoporous scaffolds using Gel Lay, Lay FOMM 40, Lay FOMM 60 porous filaments and successfully evaluated them in spinal bone metastases. The developed nanoporous scaffolds not only assist in bone repair but also deliver the encapsulated chemotherapeutics locally for sustained drug release. This could reduce systemic negative effects and improve patient outcomes (Ahangar et al. 2018).

Additive manufacturing can provide the most efficient solution for both acute and chronic wounds by mimicking the ECM for better cell adherence, proliferation, and differentiation (Xu et al. 2018). The major factors contributing to these phenomena are the scaffold materials loaded with cells, drugs, and various other chemical and biological entities (Hamdan et al. 2017). Nanotherapeutics provides a high possibility of interaction with the biological target along with enhanced penetrating effect at the site of wound and results in controlled and sustained release of therapeutics for accelerated healing. Nanoengineered scaffolds loaded with cells, growth factors, and drugs can combine the benefits of both the technologies and revolutionize the research in the field of wound healing (Hamdan et al. 2017).

Rees et al. (2015) explored the application of carboxymethylated-periodate oxidized nanocellulose as a bioink to fabricate wound dressing using 3D bioprinting. The chemical oxidation of nanocellulose improves the rheological properties of the bioink. The fabricated 3D scaffolds were found to be highly porous and non-supportive to bacterial growth. Skardal et al. (2012) evaluated the ability of 3D printed amniotic fluid derived stem cells to augment wound healing in mouse model of skin regeneration. Results suggested that the wound close and re-epithelialization was significantly better than normal fibrin-collagen gel within 1 week of its application.

12.5   Conclusion and Future Perspective

Both nanotechnology and additive manufacturing have been explored individually to a great extent by numerous researchers to improve the drug performance and to prepare a tailor-made products for better patient compliance. The integration of nanotechnology with additive technology has the potential both to complement existing techniques and to create wholly new nanocomposites, alleviating some of the technologies limitations. Although lots of advancement in this field have taken place in bone tissue regeneration, still only few have worked for their application in wound healing. A lot remains unexplored.

References

Ahangar P, Akoury E, Ramirez Garcia Luna AS, Nour A, Weber MH, Rosenzweig DH (2018) Nanoporous 3D-printed scaffolds for local doxorubicin delivery in bone metastases secondary to prostate cancer. Materials (Basel) 11:1485

Archana D, Dutta J, Dutta PK (2013) Evaluation of chitosan nano dressing for wound healing: characterization, in vitro and in vivo studies. Int J Biol Macromol 57:193–203

Bishop ES, Mostafa S, Pakvasa M, Luu HH, Lee MJ, Wolf JM, Ameer GA, He TC, Reid RR (2017) 3-D bioprinting technologies in tissue engineering and regenerative medicine: current and future trends. Genes Dis 4:185–195

Boateng JS, Matthews KH, Stevens HNE, Eccleston GM (2008) Wound healing dressings and drug delivery systems: a review. J Pharm Sci 97:2892–2923

Byambaa B, Annabi N, Yue K, de Santiago GT, Alvarez MM, Jia W, Kazemzadeh-Narbat M, Shin SR, Tamayol A, Khademhosseini A (2017) Bioprinted osteogenic and vasculogenic patterns for engineering 3D bone tissue. Adv Healthc Mater 6:1700015–1700030

Chaudhary C, Garg T (2015) Scaffolds: a novel carrier and potential wound healer. Crit Rev Ther Drug Carrier Syst 32:277–321

Chen WY, Chang HY, Lu JK, Huang YC, Harroun SG, Tseng YT, Li YJ, Huang CC, Chang HT (2015) Self-assembly of antimicrobial peptides on gold nanodots: against multidrug-resistant bacteria and wound-healing application. Adv Funct Mater 25:7189–7199

Chen S, Liu B, Carlson MA, Gombart AF, Reilly DA, Xie J (2017) Recent advances in electrospun nanofibers for wound healing. Nanomedicine 12:1335–1352

Chigurupati S, Mughal MR, Okun E, Das S, Kumar A, McCaffery M, Seal S, Mattson MP (2013) Effects of cerium oxide nanoparticles on the growth of keratinocytes, fibroblasts and vascular endothelial cells in cutaneous wound healing. Biomaterials 34:2194–2201

Choi JS, Kim HS, Yoo HS (2015) Electrospinning strategies of drug-incorporated nanofibrous mats for wound recovery. Drug Deliv Transl Res 5:137–145

Chu Y, Yu D, Wang P, Xu J, Li D, Ding M (2010) Nanotechnology promotes the full-thickness diabetic wound healing effect of recombinant human epidermal growth factor in diabetic rats. Wound Repair Regen 18:499–505

Das S, Baker AB (2016) Biomaterials and nanotherapeutics for enhancing skin wound healing. Front Bioeng Biotechnol 4:82

Das S, Majid M, Baker AB (2016a) Syndecan-4 enhances PDGF-BB activity in diabetic wound healing. Acta Biomater 42:56–65

Das S, Monteforte AJ, Singh G, Majid M, Sherman MB, Dunn AK, Baker AB (2016b) Syndecan-4 enhances therapeutic angiogenesis after hind limb ischemia in mice with type 2 diabetes. Adv Healthc Mater 5:1008–1013

Dreifke MB, Jayasuriya AA, Jayasuriya AC (2015) Current wound healing procedures and potential care. Mater Sci Eng C 48:651–662

Duan B, Wang M, Zhou WY, Cheung WL, Yang Z, Lu WW (2010) Three-dimensional nanocomposite scaffolds fabricated via selective laser sintering for bone tissue engineering. Acta Biomater 6:4495–4505

Fife CE, Carter MJ (2012) Wound care outcomes and associated cost among patients treated in US outpatient wound centers: data from the US wound registry. Wounds 24:10–17

Fong J, Wood F (2006) Nanocrystalline silver dressings in wound management: a review. Int J Nanomedicine 1:441–449

Garay-Jimenez JC, Gergeres D, Young A, Lim DV, Turos E (2009) Physical properties and biological activity of poly(butyl acrylate-styrene) nanoparticle emulsions prepared with conventional and polymerizable surfactants. Nanomedicine 5:443–451

Gill AS, Deol PK, Kaur IP (2019) An update on the use of alginate in additive biofabrication techniques. Curr Pharm Des 25:1249–1264

Gokce EH, Korkmaz E, Dellera E, Sandri G, Bonferoni MC, Ozer O (2012) Resveratrol-loaded solid lipid nanoparticles versus nanostructured lipid carriers: evaluation of antioxidant potential for dermal applications. Int J Nanomedicine 7:1841–1850

Graham C (2005) The role of silver in wound healing. Br J Nurs 14:S22, S24, S26 passim

Gu H, Ho P, Tong E, Wang L, Xu B (2003) Presenting vancomycin on nanoparticles to enhance antimicrobial activities. Nano Lett 3:1261–1263

Guo SA, DiPietro LA (2010) Factors affecting wound healing. J Dent Res 89:219–229

Hafner A, Lovrić J, Lakoš GP, Pepić I (2014) Nanotherapeutics in the EU: an overview on current state and future directions. Int J Nanomedicine 9:1005

Hamdan S, Pastar I, Drakulich S, Dikici E, Tomic-Canic M, Deo S, Daunert S (2017) Nanotechnology-driven therapeutic interventions in wound healing: potential uses and applications. ACS Cent Sci 3:163–175

Han G, Ceilley R (2017) Chronic wound healing: a review of current management and treatments. Adv Ther 34:599–610

He P, Zhao J, Zhang J, Li B, Gou Z, Gou M, Li X (2018) Bioprinting of skin constructs for wound healing. Burns Trauma 6:5

Holmes B, Bulusu K, Plesniak M, Zhang LG (2016) A synergistic approach to the design, fabrication and evaluation of 3D printed micro and nano featured scaffolds for vascularized bone tissue repair. Nanotechnology 27:064001–064028

Ivanova O, Williams C, Campbell T (2013) Additive manufacturing (AM) and nanotechnology: promises and challenges. Rapid Prototyp J 19:353–364

Jacob DS, Bitton L, Grinblat J, Felner I, Koltypin Y, Gedanken A (2006) Are ionic liquids really a boon for the synthesis of inorganic materials? A general method for the fabrication of nano-sized metal fluorides. Chem Mater 18:3162–3168

Jessop ZM, Al-Sabah A, Gardiner MD, Combellack E, Hawkins K, Whitaker IS (2017) 3D bioprinting for reconstructive surgery: principles, applications and challenges. J Plast Reconstr Aesthet Surg 70:1155–1170

Ji HW, Sun HJ, Qu XG (2016) Antibacterial applications of graphene-based nanomaterials: recent achievements and challenges. Adv Drug Deliv Rev 105:176–189

Klasen HJ (2000) A historical review of the use of silver in the treatment of burns. II Renewed interest for silver. Burns 26:131–138

Kuchler S, Radowski MR, Blaschke T, Dathe M, Plendl J, Haag R, Schäfer-Korting M, Kramer KD (2009) Nanoparticles for skin penetration enhancement—a comparison of a dendritic core-multishell-nanotransporter and solid lipid nanoparticles. Eur J Pharm Biopharm 71:243–250

Kuchler S, Herrmann W, Panek-Minkin G, Blaschke T, Zoschke C, Kramer KD, Bittl R, Schäfer-Korting M (2010a) SLN for topical application in skin diseases—characterization of drug-carrier and carrier-target interactions. Int J Pharm 390:225–233

Kuchler S, Wolf NB, Heilmann S, Weindl G, Helfmann J, Yahya MM, Stein C, Schäfer-Korting M (2010b) 3D-wound healing model: influence of morphine and solid lipid nanoparticles. J Biotechnol 148:24–30

Lai HJ, Kuan CH, Wu HC, Tsai JC, Chen TM, Hsieh DJ, Wang TW (2014) Tailored design of electrospun composite nanofibers with staged release of multiple angiogenic growth factors for chronic wound healing. Acta Biomater 10:4156–4166

Lansdown AB (2002) Silver. I: its antibacterial properties and mechanism of action. J Wound Care 11:125–130

Leu JG, Chen SA, Chen HM, Wu WM, Hung CF, Yao YD (2012) The effects of gold nanoparticles in wound healing with antioxidant epigallocatechin gallate and alpha-lipoic acid. Nanomedicine 8:767–775

Liu SB, Zeng TH, Hofmann M, Burcombe E, Wei J, Jiang R, Kong J, Chen Y (2011) Antibacterial activity of graphite, graphite oxide, graphene oxide, and reduced graphene oxide: membrane and oxidative stress. ACS Nano 5:6971–6980

Maas M (2016) Carbon nanomaterials as antibacterial colloids. Mater Sci Eng C 9:617

Mandrycky C, Wang Z, Kim K, Kim DH (2016) 3D bioprinting for engineering complex tissues. Biotechnol Adv 34:422–434

Mele E (2016) Electrospinning of natural polymers for advanced wound care: towards responsive and adaptive dressings. J Mater Chem B 4:4801–4812

Mota C, Puppi D, Chiellini F, Chiellini E (2015) Additive manufacturing techniques for the production of tissue engineering constructs. J Tissue Eng Regen Med 9:174–190

Murphy PS, Evans GR (2012) Advances in wound healing: a review of current wound healing products. Plast Surg Int 2012:190436

O'Brien FJ (2011) Biomaterials & scaffolds for tissue engineering. Mater Today 14:88–95

Rahmani Del Bakhshayesh A, Annabi N, Khalilov R, Akbarzadeh A, Samiei M, Alizadeh E, Ghodsi MA, Davaran S, Montaseri A (2018) Recent advances on biomedical applications of scaffolds in wound healing and dermal tissue engineering. Artif Cells Nanomed Biotechnol 46:691–705

Rakhmetova AA, Alekseeva TP, Bogoslovskaya OA, Leipunskii IO, Ol'khovskaya IP, Zhigach AN (2010) Wound-healing properties of copper nanoparticles as a function of physicochemical parameters. Nanotechnol Russ 5:271–276

Randeria PS, Seeger MA, Wang XQ, Wilson H, Shipp D, Mirkin CA, Paller AS (2015) siRNA-based spherical nucleic acids reverse impaired wound healing in diabetic mice by ganglioside GM3 synthase knockdown. Proc Natl Acad Sci U S A 112:5573–5578

Rani S, Ritter T (2016) The exosome: a naturally secreted nanoparticle and its application to wound healing. Adv Mater 28:5542–5552

Rees A, Powell LC, Chinga-Carrasco G, Gethin DT, Syverud K, Hill KE Thomas DW (2015) 3D bioprinting of carboxymethylated-periodate oxidized nanocellulose constructs for wound dressing applications. Biomed Res Int 2015:925757

Sahoo SK, Parveen S, Panda JJ (2007) The present and future of nanotechnology in human health care. Nanomedicine 3:20–31

Sen CK, Gordillo GM, Roy S, Kirsner R, Lambert L, Hunt TK, Gottrup F, Gurtner GC Longaker MT (2009) Human skin wounds: a major and snowballing threat to public health and the economy. Wound Repair Regen 17:763–771

Singh D, Singh D, Han S (2016) 3D printing of scaffold for cells delivery: advances in skin tissue engineering. Polymers 8:19

Skardal A, Mack D, Kapetanovic E, Atala A, Jackson JD, Yoo J, Soker S (2012) Bioprinted amniotic fluid-derived stem cells accelerate healing of large skin wounds. Stem Cells Transl Med 1:792–802

Turos E, Shim JY, Wang Y, Greenhalgh K, Reddy GS, Dickey S, Lim DV (2007) Antibiotic-conjugated polyacrylate nanoparticles: new opportunities for development of anti-MRSA agents. Bioorg Med Chem Lett 17:53–56

Vijayavenkataraman S, Yan WC, Lu WF, Wang CH, Fuh JYH (2018) 3D bioprinting of tissues and organs for regenerative medicine. Adv Drug Deliv Rev 132:296–332

Wasiak J, Cleland H, Campbell F Spinks A (2013) Dressings for superficial and partial thickness burns. Cochrane Database Syst Rev (3):CD002106

Weiser TG, Regenbogen SE, Thompson KD, Haynes AB, Lipsitz SR, Berry WR, Gawande AA (2008) An estimation of the global volume of surgery: a modelling strategy based on available data. Lancet 372:139–144

Wong KK, Cheung SO, Huang L, Niu J, Tao C, Ho CM, Che CM, Tam PK (2009) Further evidence of the anti-inflammatory effects of silver nanoparticles. ChemMedChem 4:1129–1135

World Health Organization (2016) Golbal report on diabetes

Xie ZW, Paras CB, Weng H, Punnakitikashem P, Su LC, Vu K, Tang LP, Yang J, Nguyen KT (2013) Dual growth factor releasing multi-functional nanofibers for wound healing. Acta Biomater 9:9351–9359

Xu C, Molino BZ, Wang X, Cheng F, Xu W, Molino P, Bacher M, Su D, Rosenau T, Willfo S, Wallace G (2018) 3D printing of nanocellulose hydrogel scaffolds with tunable mechanical strength towards wound healing application. J Mater Chem B 6:7066–7075

Zhou EH, Watson C, Pizzo R, Cohen J, Dang Q, Ferreira de Barros PM, Park CY, Chen C, Brain JD, Butler JP, Ruberti JW et al (2014) Assessing the impact of engineered nanoparticles on wound healing using a novel in vitro bioassay. Nanomedicine 9:2803–2815

Ziv-Polat O, Topaz M, Brosh T, Margel S (2010) Enhancement of incisional wound healing by thrombin conjugated iron oxide nanoparticles. Biomaterials 31:741–747

Part III
Bone Infections and Toxicity

Chapter 13
The Bone Biology and the Nanotechnology for Bone Engineering and Bone Diseases

Fabio Franceschini Mitri and Avinash P. Ingle

Abstract The issues about the biology of bone tissue fascinate every researcher in the health area. Bone is a vital tissue and has a great mechanical strength and a remarkable resilience due to the compounds of its extracellular matrix. The bone matrix with organic and inorganic compounds is the starting point for the researchers who investigate the range of biomaterials applied in grafting procedures. Biomaterials are now produced at the nanoscale to work as a scaffold and facilitate bone repair, in an option to the autogenous graft. Different nanomaterials are being studied to apply in the treatment of various bone diseases including cancer. Nanomaterials as nanocarriers of drugs are being regarded as the safest system to treat cancer of bones, considering no side effects and tumor cells precision. Therefore, this chapter emphasizes all mechanisms of bone biology regarding healing and bone repair after application of nanomaterials, and also discusses the advancement of nanotechnology research in this area.

Keywords Bone biology · Bone engineering · Bone diseases · Nanotechnology · Nanomaterials · Implantology

13.1 Introduction

Bone is a mineralized connective tissue with an inert appearance macroscopically, but it is a highly dynamic organ with a continuous metabolism and active remodeling. It consists of calcified extracellular matrices and cells, such as the osteoprogenitor cells (OTCs) that give rise to osteoblasts, osteocytes, and osteoclasts

F. F. Mitri (✉)
Department of Human Anatomy, Biomedical Sciences Institute, Federal University of Uberlandia, Uberlandia, MG, Brazil
e-mail: fmitri@ufu.br

A. P. Ingle
Department of Biotechnology, Engineering School of Lorena, University of Sao Paulo, Lorena, SP, Brazil

(Buckwalter et al. 1996; Downey and Siegel 2006). Generally, the blast cells are responsible for producing new bone and the clastic cells resorb old bone. The bone matrix contains hydroxyapatite crystals formed due to the union of calcium and phosphate ions. In the skeletal system, bone supports and protects the soft tissue and organs, calcium and phosphate storage, and housing of bone marrow.

The mineral content of bone is the main feature to be considered in biomaterial production. The biomaterials had been investigated in the last decades to be an option in graft procedures and act as a scaffold. The development and application of the biomaterials have evolved over the past 50 years through a multidimensional interface among chemical engineering, the science of materials, mechanical engineering, biology, and medicine (Ratner and Bryant 2004).

The progress of the science has carried several studies about nanoscience and nanotechnology, which have increased the interest in manufacturing of nanosized biomaterials. Nanotechnology has been popularized in the 1980s and it is a multidisciplinary science that integrates engineering with biology, chemistry, and physics. The proposal of nanotechnology comes from the ability to control the material properties by the manufacturing of such biomaterials at the nanoscale. Nanomaterials are the materials with basic structural units, grains, particles, fibers, or other constituent components having size smaller than 100 nm in at least one dimension (Siegel and Fougere 1995) or structures at the grouped atom level up to 100 nm (Harvey et al. 2010), and it represents the pattern of manipulation of atoms and molecules over the scale of nanometer (Zhang et al. 2011).

Bone-forming osteoblasts are typically 25 nm in size (Harvey et al. 2010) and the inorganic content of the natural bone, nanocrystalline HA is 20–80 nm long and 2–5 nm wide (Zhang and Webster 2009). After decreasing material size into the nanoscale, the increased surface area, surface roughness, and surface area to volume ratios can consequently lead to ideal physicochemical properties favoring cell adherence and cell proliferation in an implanted nanomaterial. Nanomaterials are often used in combination with drugs to work as a delivery system in bone diseases, including bone infections, cancer, or tumor metastasis.

The aim of this chapter is to describe the bone biology and physiological mechanisms of bone tissue involved with the basic concepts of implantology, and the importance of these concepts to understanding of all mechanisms about the bionanomaterials implantation. In addition, to report in an overview of the application of nanotechnology and various types of nanomaterials in bone engineering and the most current systems of drug delivery in bone disease treatment.

13.2 The Bone Tissue

Bone is a highly vascularized mineralized connective tissue and it is constantly changing, with continuous and dynamic metabolism. The mechanical resistance, resilience, and high regeneration ability, including its organized response to injury, are the main characteristics of the bone. All these features are made possible by a set of tissue-specific cells embedded in a highly complex intercellular matrix, called osteoid matrix or osteoid, which is constituted by a mineralized and other non-mineralized component.

The bone matrix possesses organic material and inorganic mineral ions. The organic portion (non-mineralized) represents about 60–65% of the bone matrix and is mainly composed of type I collagen fibers, glycoproteins, and proteoglycans. On the other hand, about 35–40% is inorganic material with mineral ions, especially calcium and phosphate (ion originated from phosphor) composing the calcium phosphate, the main plentiful mineral constituent of bone. At the outset, these are the necessary minerals for the process of calcification, mechanism favored by alkaline phosphatase activity in osteoblasts, which raises the local concentrations of phosphate in the osteoid matrix. All this process starts the hydroxyapatite, which is the main crystalline unit in the bone tissue. This mineral content is composed of calcium, phosphate, and hydroxyl ions associated with other mineral ions. The union of both compounds, the organic and inorganic one, provides distinct mechanical properties to the bone. The organic compound assists in resilience, tensile and shear strength, and in contrast, the inorganic compound provides mechanical strength.

The main bone cells include stem cells (bone lining cell), osteoblasts (osteoprogenitor cells), osteocytes, and osteoclasts. Stem cells are the basis of bone-forming cells, and they are also called undifferentiated mesenchymal cells or simply mesenchymal cells (MSC) (Grigoriadis et al. 1988). Moreover, the MSC differentiates in osteoprogenitor cells, then this is known as osteoblasts. The osteoblast is a cuboid cell with a typical columnar form and uninucleate, and a larger and more developed nucleus (Capulli et al. 2014). These cells generally secrete a protein like osteoid which develops the bone extracellular matrix, undergoes calcification, and then the ossification of the bone tissue formation. During the secretion of osteoid, some osteoblasts can be surrounded and trapped by osteoid which makes these cells inactive and inert, thereby giving rise to osteocytes. The osteocytes are smaller cells than osteoblast, and it extends dendritic processes into the bone extracellular matrix. These dendritic extensions into the bone tissue will origin the vascular canaliculi. The osteoclast is a multinucleated cell from the union of monocytes, which are from a vascular origin. This cell has the small membrane flagella-like extensions to facilitate its adherence in the bone wall in which it secretes lacti and citric acid decreasing local pH to promote the mineral dissolution on bone surface, and then this cell promotes the resorption of old bone. Osteoclast remains inside the resorbed bone hole called Howship's lacuna (Everts et al. 2002), and then, the osteoid deposition by osteoclasts and new bone formation occurs simultaneously. This mechanism is related to the bone turnover, that is the constant substitution of old bone by new bone, and it is a part of bone remodeling. Bone remodeling is an active process in living bone during human life and it is responsible for formation of all complex architecture of bone.

The organic compound of the bone plays an essential role in the control of growth and differentiation of stem cells and osteoblasts, osteocytes and osteoclasts, and in the bone remodeling. Furthermore, bone development and bone regeneration are distinct processes and they are regulated by growth factors and transcription factors, which initialize and coordinate the cellular mechanisms and the cell interactions into the osteoid matrix.

13.3 Types of Bone

Macroscopically, bone is of clear coloring with a dense texture having cavities of varying sizes inside it. Depending on the presence or absence of these cavities, bone is classified into two types, i.e., compact bone or trabecular bone and cancellous bone or spongy bone. The term trabecular refers to the small bone spaces interspersed among small trabeculae, organized in a porous sponge-like pattern. The cancellous bone is filled by highly vascularized connective tissue consisting of a number of small blood vessels and capillaries, called bone marrow. Compact bone is located in the bone periphery of one bone piece, while the cancellous one is found inside and center of the bone. All bones of the human body are filled by red bone marrow at birth. During aging, the bone marrow is being infiltrated by adipose tissue giving rise to the yellow bone marrow. Red blood cells, platelets, leucocytes, and most white blood cells arise in red marrow, which is a source of blood cells. In adults, the red marrow is located in some flat bones such as ribs, sternal, base skull bones, and proximal epiphysis of long bones. Bone marrow is a source of stem cells, and these can give rise to any cell of any tissue of the human body.

The combination of architecture of the cancellous bone with that compact bone provides mechanical stability and strength to the skeleton (Seeman and Delmas 2006). These mechanical properties are very important to human skeleton since this acts as a base to the movement of the body, besides protecting the internal and vital organs. Furthermore, the bone is a mineral reservoir with the capacity to mobilize its mineral ions storage whenever the need for homeostasis of calcium blood level, under the action of parathyroid hormones. The thickness and the rate of compact bone regarding to cancellous one are variables according to the bone piece and to bony parts of skeleton.

13.4 Osteogenesis

Osteogenesis is the process of bone formation that follows after secretion of osteoid by bone-forming cells, the osteoblasts. It is a continuous process even after the skeleton growth because it also occurs during the bone remodeling.

There are two different types of bone development, the intramembranous and the endochondral ossification. In the first one, the ossification occurs directly in the mesenchyme or primitive connective tissue and it occurs in flat bones of the skull. In the second one, the bone develops into a preexisting cartilage template in most skeleton bones, such as long bones (extremities), vertebral column, and pelvis.

In the intramembranous ossification, the embryonic mesenchyme transformed into a vascularized connective tissue, then the fibroblast cells aggregate themselves in an extracellular matrix containing organized collagen fibers. This specific cell process is controlled by patterning signals from polypeptides of the fibroblast growth factor (FGF) and transforming growth factor-β families (TGF-β) (Linkhart et al. 1996), including the bone morphogenetic protein (BMP), which has an important role during the embryonic development in skeletal formation. The mesenchymal cells (MSCs) give rise to osteoblasts, which produce osteoid matrix. The calcification of the osteoid followed by its ossification is a well-orchestrated process that characterizes the primary ossification center of the bone. Calcium phosphate ions are deposited into the osteoid matrix, process known as mineralization front followed by the ossification. The various centers of ossifications develop and fuse, forming a network of anastomosing bone trabeculae, leading to the creation of cancellous bone. In the primary bone (or immature bone), the collagen fibers are randomly oriented; the lamellar bone (secondary bone or mature bone) is formed later through bone remodeling, a constant process supported by bone metabolism. At the birth, the bones of the calvaria are separated by membranous spaces denominated fonticulous or fontanelles. In addition, during the bone development, the internal and external connective tissue layers are condensed to form endosteum and periosteum, respectively. In endochondral ossification, the primary ossification center is derived from the chondrocytes proliferation and from the consequent deposition of type II collagen. The cells undergo hypertrophy and apoptosis giving spaces for the blood capillaries proliferation stimulated for the vascular endothelial growth factor (VEGF) (Kennedy et al. 2012; Wu et al. 2013); this event allows the appearance of OTCs and consequently calcification of the matrix, with the formation of a thin periosteal collar on the periphery of the bone. The primary ossification center is formed at the center of the bone, diaphysis, and the secondary ossification centers at the extremities of the bone, epiphysis. The growth cartilaginous plate, a structure of growth hyaline cartilage, remains at metaphysis (between diaphysis and epiphysis) while the bone grows in length. The bone growth in width is allowed for the periosteum, which is composed of a deep layer and a superficial mucosal layer. The deep one is a germinative layer that is made up of stem cells and osteoprogenitor cells; the superficial layer is a fibrous layer responsible for protection of the bone. In summary, in endochondral ossification, the bone replaces the bone cartilage template previously developed.

13.5   Structure and Micro-architecture of the Bone

The development of bone comes from an appositional growth of its tissue layers around a central vascular canal, therefore, these layers of new bone have been overlapping by osteoblasts forming lamellar bone. This pattern of bone tissue growth occurs both in cortical and cancellous bone. The bony lamellae may be arranged circumferentially and parallel to periosteal and endosteal surfaces, and they are

Fig. 13.1 Light microscopy (H/E) showing an osteon (Havers system), osteocytes, and bone canaliculi connecting neighboring vascular channels into bone tissue

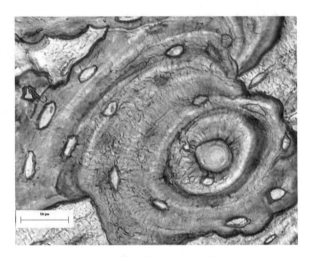

called primary or circumferential lamellae; when they are concentric around a vascular bone canal, they are known as osteon or secondary lamellae.

Inside the bone microstructure, the central vascular canal of each osteon (Haversian canal) is interconnected to the transversal canal (Volkmann's canal). Throughout bone tissue, there are bony canaliculi formed from osteoclast extensions. All this structural organization contributes to hemodynamic balance, bone nutrition, and consequently maintains basal metabolism of bone tissue. The lamellar structure is sited in both cortical and cancellous bone (Fig. 13.1) (Johnson 1966).

The lamellar bone around the central vascular canal is known as the osteon or Havers system in which each central vascular canal is the Haversian canal. So, first atypical osteons in immature bone are called primary osteons, no longer in mature bone with organized concentric lamellae around vascular canals are the secondary osteons representing typical Havers systems. For completion, the type of osteon observed in bone tissue as well as the collagen fibers organization represents the organization level of this tissue. There is an amorphous disposition of collagen fibers type I secreted by osteoblasts (Ducy et al. 1997) with varied sizes characterizing a primary tissue with primary osteons in reticulofibrous bone. The lamellar bone has an organized pattern of collagen fibers in its interstice, with these fibers being of the same size and morphologically more refined, including primary and secondary osteons in well-established bone tissue. The primary osteons are replaced by osteons and typical Havers systems as the bone matures.

13.6 Vascularization and Innervation of the Bone

The blood vascularization starts from one or more artery nutricia, either in a long bone (artery nutricia diaphyseal) or another morphological type, such as a face bone. The nutricia artery gives rise to wide capillaries network on the periosteum, a highly vascularized dense connective tissue. Artery nutricia from periosteum penetrates inside bone throughout nutricia foramina and canals. Consequently, the capillaries fill trabecular spaces of bones to constitute the bone marrow. The formation of venous structures from capillaries allows venous drainage, contributing for venous return. Small vessels converge at the level of nutricia veins, which return by nutricia foramina of cortical bone, taking the inverse path of arterial network. The sensorial nerves are widely distributed along periosteum making it highly sensitive. They are numerous near the joint ends of the bone. Thin myelinated fibers are around nutricia blood vessels on periosteum and in the perivascular spaces of osteons (Matsuo and Irie 2008; Elefteriou 2008).

13.7   Bone Repair: Stages of the Bone Healing

The bone is a dynamic and vascularized tissue with an effective and high capacity to heal and repair without leaving a scar. Bone regeneration is an organized process involving all the early-mentioned mechanisms of bone tissue, resulting in a truly continuous interplay between cells, growth, and transcription factors.

Generally, spontaneous bone regeneration starts as a response of an injury, in which primary reorganization and repairing of the bone morphological structure occurs. In the case of bone fracture, when there is not a large defect or a misalignment of the fractured osseous extremities, the bone heals very well under conservative surgical therapies.

Bone healing consists of four distinct and chronological sequential stages; they are the inflammatory stage, soft callus formation, hard callus (initial osseous union), and bone remodeling.

The initial inflammatory response of bone occurs immediately to an injury that remains for about 4 days. It is characterized by intraosseous bleeding, local edema with swelling and local pain. Damages in blood vessels lead to an intraosseous local hematoma causing the declining of oxygen ions and simultaneously decreasing of local pH making a consequently hypoxic and acidic microenvironment and thus releasing lysosomal enzymes, resulting in local tissue necrosis. Polymorphonuclear cells, mastocytes, and macrophages reach the injury site and they release chemical mediators, some of which stimulate the proliferation of stem cells and osteoprogenitor cells. Mastocytes cells are of local origin, and the other ones are hematogenous cells. Local hematoma helps in formation of an organized clot in a period of 6–8 h after injury, an important natural scaffold for cell proliferation and tissue development (Gerstenfeld et al. 2003).

During this initial stage, osteoclasts and phagocytic cells are responsible for the phagocytosis of the necrotic tissue. Blood clot acts as a scaffold for the vascular growth, which is unleashed by growth factors and mediators released from macrophages. In the sequence, fibroblasts proliferation and collagen fibers synthesis take place.

At the injury site, the MSCs are induced by growth factors secreted from bone morphogenetic proteins (BMPs) originating the osteoblasts. This mechanism is dependent on several biological factors, including the local oxygen level and the available BMPs (Kitaori et al. 2009). It is continued with the formation of soft callus stage within 4 weeks; that is a non-calcified wound tissue similar to an extracellular matrix with cellular proliferation, such as osteoblasts and fibroblasts, and it is rich in collagen fibers and glycoproteins. Osteoblasts in high proliferative activity leads to augment of osteoid with a fibrous tissue, not calcified overlaid at the injury site and onto the lesion margins giving union to osseous extremities. In local, the blood supply is re-established. From the clinical point of view, it is important to know that the local injury may be stable during all repairing bone processes. It means the osseous extremities of a fracture must be immobilized, without any movement, until the calcification of soft callus converts to the bone healing stage, called the hard callus stage (Gerstenfeld et al. 2006).

The hard callus is formed in the next 2 or 3 months. With the re-establishment of the local vascular, cellular and tissue patterns, combined with maintaining an ideal oxygen gradient, the pH is gradually increased to the neutral level. From this, the mineral ions deposition is started on the osteoid matrix, characterizing the matrix calcification followed by ossification, i.e., the primary bone formation. This mechanism provides a strong local osseous union. In this stage, the bone must be clinically activated or, in other words, any immobilizing device must be removed so that the bone is subjected to bone stress to receive loadings and other external stimulus in its surfaces, which are essential to activate bone remodeling, the last stage of healing bone (Gerstenfeld et al. 2006). This stage is started in 4 or 6 months after injury and can be continued for years.

The reticulofibrous bone from the hard callus is gradually matured in the lamellar bone. Osteoclasts remove the excess of the hard callus that is above the regular contour of bone and they remodel both endosteal and periosteal surfaces. Bone remodeling is substantially favored with vascular pattern re-establishment, the interstitial hemodynamic and the oxygen supply returned to normal. The damaged osteons have been precisely re-established by simultaneous and concomitant actions of the osteoblasts and osteoclasts. Then, as osteoclasts are reabsorbing the damaged tissue structure, at the same time that osteoblasts are acting to produce new bone. In the bone remodeling stage, the regular pattern of architecture and structure of the bone is repaired, revealing a complete and reliable healing bone, with no traces of scarring. This stage is essential also for bone adaptation, and consequently the skeleton adaptation during mechanical use.

13.8 Basic Concepts in Implantology

It is important to remember in implantology that natural or synthetic grafts act as a scaffold as well as the blood clot for bone repair. In majority, synthetic grafts are composed of calcium and phosphate as raw material, and then this graft mimics the mineral interstice of the bone matrix for the BMPs and other cells can stimulate stem cells to differentiate in osteoprogenitor cells from mediators releasing and start bone neoformation. The bone graft materials undergo action by macrophages and the smaller the granulation scale of the graft, the higher the resorption rate. The main goal in bone grafting is to achieve the total resorption of implanted biomaterial followed by bone neoformation, like this, the biomaterial will be totally replaced by new bone formation.

Some of the concepts widely applied in implantology are essentials for a good understanding of applying mechanisms of biomaterials. Osteoinduction involves bone neoformation from osteprogenitor cells derived from mesenchymal cells (stem cells); these are developed under the influence of osteoinductor biomaterial to stimulate cell differentiation. Osteoconduction is characterized by bone formation on biomaterial surface, thus biomaterial addresses bone formation for its own surface. Generally, an osteoconductor biomaterial is not totally resorbed in the biological microenvironment. Osseointegration means bone neoformation directly on the biomaterial surface with no interposition of dense connective tissue, in which there is the anchorage of the implant into the bone, it means the implant is osteointegrated. These three mechanisms occur during bone grafting procedures (Albrektsson and Johansson 2001).

A biomaterial implanted in a surgical site can be resorbed into microenvironment; however, this mechanism depends on the size of granules. If the size of granules is small, then the chances are more that the biomaterial will be completely resorbed into the biological environment. A low granulation biomaterial (nanomaterial) resorbed and replaced by newly formed bone is characteristic of osteoinduction. Otherwise, a high granulation biomaterial will not be resorbed into microenvironment and generally, the bone formation is addressed on its surface. This mechanism is well known by osteoconduction, in which new bone formation is conducted on a biomaterial surface. Calcium phosphate biomaterials can be osteoconductors or osteoinductors, the platelet concentrates tend to be osteoinductors, and the metallic biomaterials such as titanium implants are osteoconductors.

In general, biomaterials widely used in bone graft procedures are divided into four main types, according to its origin and/or raw material, such as autologous (autograft), allogenic, xenogenic, and synthetic (alloplastic). Bone autograft is the bone of the same patient, which is harvested from the donor site and transplanted or grafted in host surgical site, therefore, it is a straight transplant of living bone proteins of the same patient. An allogenic bone graft is bone of different living beings of the same species. A xenogenic graft is the specific harvested tissue of different living beings, and the bovine material is the most used, such as bone and collagen. And finally, the synthetic or alloplastic graft is the one fabricated in the laboratory from synthetic material generally the calcium phosphate, which is similar to the mineral base of human bone.

13.9   Biomaterials and Nanotechnology

The development of biomaterials and its application into bone graft procedures came from about the last 50 years. The majority of synthetic biomaterials are produced from calcium phosphate, such as the hydroxyapatite, which is similar to the mineral base of the bone.

Different types of biomaterials are produced and applied as a bone graft in reconstructive surgeries. The autogenous bone graft is well known, and the first choice or the gold standard to bone graft is because it helps in direct transplantation of the bone matrix and BMPs for the same patient. However, this graft depends on donor site, size, and morphology, quality of bone and requires initial stability. However, there is not always a suitable donor site to the host site, because the morbidity can increase with the higher quantity of bone graft harvested from the donor site. The bleeding or hematoma in a great area can lead to some complications, such as secondary infections and chronic pain.

When the autologous graft cannot indicate, the most commonly used bone graft are allogenic or xenogenic bone grafts or synthetic materials. There are the synthetic biomaterials or artificial bone grafts, which may help to overcome the problems related to morbidity or size limitations, as mentioned above. Considering tissue engineering as an interdisciplinary field, the application and indication of the biomaterials in the bone engineering and regenerative medicine is a main goal to restore, maintain, and improve the tissue morphology and function.

In the bone-engineering field, the reconstruction of small and moderate bone defects is technically feasible, including the application of autogenous and autologous bone graft; however, the large defects remain a challenge. In these cases, synthetic grafts can be used, but some aspects should be considered, such as the local vascularization, which is more suitable for small defects. The vascularization can be decreased in a large bone defect leading to tissue healing failure. Faced with the possibility of the choice of the kind of biomaterial, all the biological factors must be considered in the tissue engineering of bone. And it is for this reason that the prognostic of the reconstruction by bone graft procedure is unpredictable and difficult.

In general, nanotechnology is the field that refers to the study and management of matter in smaller scales, at the molecular level. The association of nanotechnology with biological sciences like biotechnology leads us to nanobiotechnology, which is referred to study and application of nanomaterials across all the other areas, such as chemistry, biology, materials science, and bioengineering. Since the half of last century, in 1959, the physicist Richard Feynman at the Annual American Physical Society Meeting at Caltech University in Pasadena, California, for the first time presented the concept of nanotechnology and introduced it to the scientific community as the manner to manipulation of atoms and molecules over the scale of nanometer, and then generates materials with at least one dimension in nanoscale. In 1974, that term was first used in a scientific publication (Webster 2017). Since then nanotechnology has emerged as the most advanced and highly promising approach to bioengineering. Therefore, nowadays, nanobiotechnology is widely applied in tissue reconstruction, bone engineering, and regenerative medicine, among other branches of health science.

As previously discussed, the nanomaterials possess specific characteristics when compared with the biomaterials, as the larger surface to volume ratio, which is suitable for its resorption in a biological environment. According to the specific raw material of the nanomaterial, it can mimic the biological tissue providing a scaffold to vascular and cell proliferation by favoring the formation of the biological matrix to tissue growth and development. Moreover, the application of these biocompatible nanomaterials implies in prospective approaches for bone engineering and regenerative medicine, including the treatment of several diseases.

Many areas of medicine have recognized the needs and application of proper nanomaterials, which mainly include orthopedics, oncology, and many others. Nanomaterials have been developed as nanoparticle-containing materials with enhanced mechanical properties. Nanomaterials and nanofibers scaffolds, or nanodelivery (nanocarrier) systems are used for delivery of the drugs into the affected area to promote bone repair or to heal a bone disease.

13.10   Nanotechnology in Bone Tissue Engineering

Tissue engineering was defined in 1993 as an "interdisciplinary area that applies the principles of engineering and the life sciences towards the development of biological substitutes to restore, maintain, or improve tissue function" (Webster 2017). Tissue engineering requires a deep understanding of embryology, tissue development and formation, and tissue regeneration (Langer and Vacanti 1993).

The bone tissue engineering procedures replace or reconstruct the lost bone tissue with the main purpose to bring the morphology and function of the determined part of the body to the patient, and then promoting a better quality of life and reintegration into society.

Vital tissue consists of matrix and cells (Kneser et al. 2006). The matrix acts as a biological tridimensional-scaffold for to host cells into tissues and provides to cells a tissue-specific environment and architecture (Huang and Ingber 1999). As explained previously, the nanomaterial possesses a dimension less than 100 nm and works like scaffolds providing the infiltration and cell proliferation to the defect site and assisting in the tissue development and bone growth. Therefore, any scaffold must be biocompatible and resorbable to be replaced for new bone.

In the last decades, the use of synthetic biomaterials has been promisingly increased in biomedical applications favoring the progress in nanotechnology and proving new approaches in bone repair. Nowadays, there are three types of nanomaterials, nanoparticles, nanofibers, and nanocomposites. Regarding the biomaterials, the nanomaterials have some advantages related to their size, one of that implies in an increased surface area demonstrating a suitable roughness and specific surface chemistries, wettability and surface energies (Griffin et al. 2016). All these characteristics of the nanomaterials are important for the formation of the extracellular matrix, the first step to the new tissue or new bone formation. The most common nanomaterials are nano-hydroxyapatite, because its mineral components are similar to bone mineral ions.

Protein adsorption onto the surface of nanomaterial is effective for cell adhesion and proliferation. This mechanism is allowed by those surface properties early cited, surface chemistry, wettability, and surface energy. Nanostructured surfaces promote protein adsorption and consequently, the cell adherence to the nanomaterial, since the proteins that govern cell attachment allow the signalizing to intracellular membrane proteins to control cell migration, proliferation, and differentiation and finally to determine tissue formation (Jell et al. 2009). However, to meet these requirements nanomaterials as scaffolds should mimic the architecture of native bone, and for this, it is essential that it should be produced with the raw material similar to mineral ions of bone, besides all the morphological characteristics and physical properties mentioned above.

Nanomaterials have a much larger surface as compared with biomaterials or to bulk materials (Zhang et al. 2011). The most important property already known for nanomaterials is the capacity to mimic the native tissue and provide the proper extracellular environment for cell growing and tissue development (Venugopal et al. 2008; Scheller et al. 2009; Khang et al. 2010). Nanomaterials can be implanted with cells, which could favor the tissue regeneration, and they can be applied as drug carrier implying prospective approaches for the treatment of bone diseases.

The surface of a nanomaterial provides better matrix for osteoblasts to grow and to function in osteogenesis (Webster et al. 2000). Metal biomaterials can also be manufactured at the nanoscale like other nanostructures, nanofibers, and nanotubes, and they present the same biological properties of ceramic biomaterial; for such reason, biomaterials are also applied in orthopedic surgeries. One of the first nanofiber scaffolds was manufactured from collagen due to its natural presence in the connective tissues (Laurencin et al. 2009; Prabbhakaran et al. 2009). Another great property of this type of nanomaterial is its high biodegradation rate, one of those requirements previously mentioned for the nanomaterial to be replaced for new formed bone. These scaffolds have an enhanced capacity of protein adsorption of osteoblasts (Wei and Ma 2004; Xiao et al. 2007), and improved mechanical strength (Jung et al. 2005). Approach and management of stem cells and osteogenic cells are one of the main parts of any tissue engineering area. In in vitro and in vivo study, Ti-Ag alloys with nanotubular coating presented a potential biomaterial for orthopedics, being able to achieve good osseointegration (Liu et al. 2019). Platelet-rich plasma were incorporated in polyvinyl-alcohol (PVA), chitosan, and HA nanofibers, and implanted in critical-sized rat calvarial defects which were almost filled, demonstrating a great potential for bone remodeling and tissue engineering (Abazari et al. 2019).

Synthetic nanomaterials such as polymers (PLA, a poly-lactide, and PLGA, a poly-lactide-co-glycolic) are highly biodegradable in a microenvironment without causing immunologic response, during a procedure of bone healing in bone graft. These materials present no risk of viral infection from the host, and the time of degradation depends on the general morphology, including density, nanoscale, and presence or absence of porosity, as well as their size and distribution. The biodegradation is an important process to target stem cells and then to activate signaling cascades for delivery of growth factors in human embryonic stem cells with large effect on cell differentiation (Ferreira et al. 2008).

Various methods to produce scaffolds with different materials have been developed with the common idea, to reach the perspectives in bone engineering. The incorporation of carbon nanotubes and micro-hydroxyapatite (HA) particles with PLA-based scaffolds to create nanocomposites increased the attachment of MSCs and their differentiation into osteoprogenitor cells (Ciapetti et al. 2012), besides stimulating the microenvironment of adherent osteoprogenitors and their viability and proliferation (Ciapetti et al. 2012). The potential of the nano-apatite to enhance the osteogenic capacity of MSCs explained for its constitution is similar and reflects the mineral structure of living bone. In fact, the apatite-coated PLGA promoted the differentiation of seeded OTCs (Chou et al. 2007), and porous nano HA-PLA scaffolds stimulated the expression of osteogenic proteins (BMP, osteopontin, collagen type I, osteocalcin) in rabbit bone marrow-derived MSCs promoting bone regeneration of critical size-defects of rabbit mandible (Guo et al. 2012). In addition, these osteogenic proteins act into cell signaling to osteoblastic differentiation. The addition of nano-HA into polymeric scaffolds alters its surface and is a great contribution for stimulation of cell adhesion and proliferation, continued by osteoblastic differentiation.

The integration of PLA, HA, and collagen into a single scaffold improved the MSC viability and increased the osteogenic gene expression through the elevated levels of osteogenic proteins, resulting in matrix mineralization and bone neoformation (Raghavendran et al. 2014). The benefits of different biomaterials into a scaffold may bring advantages of each material in order to give an ideal scaffold for stimulating bone heal combined with the importance of surface topography, which extends to the response of living cells to reconstruction grafting.

As a template for three-dimensional tissue growth, scaffolds must emulate the extracellular matrix, and then modifications of the nanomaterials into scaffolds may enhance the capacity to mimic the properties of the natural bone microenvironment and provide ideal conditions to cellular attachment, osteoblastic differentiation, and tissue formation for bone engineering (Wamsley et al. 2015). Multi-walled carbon nanotubes powder incorporated in poly-methyl methacrylate (PMMA) promoted the osteogenic differentiation, increased the integration between the bone cement and bone tissue, and revealed a large number of osteoblasts congregated and new bone formed in New Zealand rabbit bone defect model, revealing to be promising for use in orthopedic applications (Wang et al. 2019).

As far as the implantology is concerned, the use of nanocomposites of carbon nanotubes (CNT) is applied alone or with other polymers in regenerative therapies and to augment the process of osseointegration (Spin-Neto et al. 2013). During the loss of a tooth, the alveolar bone can be reabsorbed. To minimize this trouble, nano-composites can be grafted in the fresh dental socket to help the preservation in an alveolar ridge.

The guided tissue regeneration (GTR) is widely used in implantology to reconstruct or avoid the loss of bone in an alveolar ridge or to facilitate bone regeneration in periodontal disease. GTR is a technique, in which the collagen membrane is applied on the dental socket or alveolar bone defect to give it outline. Collagen membrane avoids the infiltration of dense connective tissue in a wound site. In this context, nanofibrous materials should be used in membranes for bone regeneration.

In addition, nanotechnology is very well employed in bone engineering, therefore, the reconstruction of large defects remains a challenge to the development of strategies improving the limited availability of nanomaterials.

Notwithstanding the foregoing, the nanotechnology for bone engineering requires an association of materials science and bone biology. Scaffolds must mimic the extracellular matrix to stimulate tridimensional tissue growth. The nanoparticles' modifications, including its surface, enhance this capacity to mimic the biological and physical properties of living bone tissue and provide favorable features for cell attachment and growth, osteprogenitor cells differentiation, increased osteoblast cells activity, and then the bone reconstruction.

13.11   Nanotechnology in Bone Diseases

Bone is one of the major organs of the human body, which consists of the human skeleton providing a basis for locomotion; it supports and protects various organs, including the vital ones; it is a font of blood cells and mineral ions. Therefore, some disorders in the bone can provoke serious morbidity, complications, or even the mortality of patients.

Tissue engineering and regenerative medicine are promising fields that have been developing intensely in the last decades due to the constant progress in organ transplantation and stem cell research, in concomitance with the advances of nano-material science.

There are many people in the world which suffers from bone cancer or other disorders and injuries (including infectious bone diseases), and some of these diseases progress to a degenerative stage, for instance, osteoporosis resulting in a deficient bone remodeling with risks of fracture to skeleton; some systemic diseases also negatively affect the bone metabolism leading to delay in healing bone. Bone metabolism and bone remodeling also can be decreased and/or altered for several stimuli like as radiotherapy, chemotherapy, and treatment with bisphosphonates, or others such as aging, malnutrition, hormonal disorders, and systemic diseases.

Nanomaterials associated with cellular therapy can be important tool to improve scaffolds doped with drugs and genes or cells, and then they act as a carrier in the delivery of these substances for the treatment of certain diseases. This kind of therapy is more effective and faster than conventional treatments.

Osteoarthritis is a very debilitating disease with limitation of movements consequently decreasing of life quality of the patient, and there is no effective treatment. The association of a growth factor to a cationic nanocarrier (PAMAM—Amine terminal polyamidoamine dendrimers with PEG—poly-ethylene glycol) conjugated to insulin-like growth factor 1 (IGF-1) for targeted delivery to chondrocytes (in deep within dense anionic cartilage tissue) and retention within cartilage through an intra-articular injection, which decreased the cartilage degeneration and the osteophyte volume in the model of rat osteoarthritis. The nanocarriers improved pharmacokinetics and efficacy of disease-modifying osteoarthritis drugs, a great prediction for clinical application (Geiger et al. 2018).

The development of antibacterial nanomaterials has a great potential for the management of infectious bone diseases. The synthetic nanomaterials mainly derived from calcium phosphate (CaP) are used as nanocarriers (drug delivery system) for treatment of bone infection (Eliaz and Metoki 2017). Silver nanoparticles (AgNPs) also act as an antimicrobial agent, being effective against both Gram-positive and

Gram-negative bacteria, and this nanomaterial effectively inhibited the growth of arthroplasty surgery-related infections caused by bacterial pathogens including *Staphylococcus aureus*, *Staphylococcus epidermidis*, and *Acinetobacter baumannii* (Kose et al. 2016). However, the fabrication of nanomaterials is concerned due to some limitations, such as specific morphology, mechanical properties, surface energy, and biomedical performance of living tissues. On the other hand, it is possible to create nanomaterials with specific porosities and mechanical strength similar to the complex architecture of bone-specific sites to optimize bone tissue regeneration (Harvey et al. 2010).

As discussed earlier, the use of nanomaterials as drug carriers can be an excellent tool for the prevention or treatment of various bone infections, and consequently reducing overall morbidity. The coating of implants with NPs doped with antimicrobial drugs found to inhibit the adhesion and colonization of bacteria such as *S. mutans*, *S. epidermidis*, and *Escherichia coli*, which are responsible for inflammation around implants (Della-Valle et al. 2012; Wang et al. 2017), and finally NPs with broad-spectrum antimicrobials have been found to be effective in the treatment of osteomyelitis (Qadri et al. 2017). In in vitro and in vivo study, nanosilver/poly (DL-lactic-co-glycolic acid) on titanium implant surface inhibited bacterial adhesion and accelerated the formation of new bone (Zeng et al. 2019). Type and cause of infection can be a challenge for conventional treatment of antimicrobial drug administration which may require weeks or months up to healing due to the vascular network and architecture of bone. Moreover, various NPs besides improving cell proliferation on its surface can be used for antimicrobial coatings of bone implants.

Several neoplastic conditions are the target in nanotechnology. The conventional treatment can affect other tissues and cells besides tumor cells. Nanocarriers can be perfect drug delivery vehicle agents as anticancer agents (Moore et al. 2017), then MSCs can be used as natural delivery drugs through their exosomes with a higher cell-target specific (Pascucci et al. 2014). A study review reported that the MSC-exosomes had revealed as a potential biological tool for cancer therapy with specificity for tumor cells and effective treatments with high safety (Zhou et al. 2018).

Keratin nanoparticles (KNPs) also are used as a carrier of anticancer drugs and are also useful for controlled release of doxorubicin (DOX), an effective chemotherapeutic agent for several neoplastic conditions such as leukemia, soft and bone sarcoma, breast cancer among others, but with limited application because of its cardiotoxicity. This method allowed a controlled release of doxorubicin which is efficient for antitumor activity and for decreasing drug toxicity (Aluigi et al. 2018). An in vitro study revealed that the combination between platinum NPs and doxorubicin could be a potent anticancer therapeutic strategy (Gurunathan et al. 2019). These reports represent a perspective for the future of nanotechnology in cancer treatment of several neoplastics, contributing for the progress of scientific investigation and clinical application of nanomaterials as carrier and delivery systems. However, a reduced number of studies about antitumor drug toxicity lead to a lack of understanding of the anticancer treatments and its relation to systemic toxicity, besides its real effect on the tumor.

To minimize the above, a new approach novel of integration between drug conjugates and nanocarriers based on a double sequential encrypted targeting system

(DSETS) capable to combine tissular and cellular targeting following an activatable cascade mechanism was presented on treatment of bone tumors. This technique provides the association of RGD tripeptide (Arg-Pr-Gly) with a bisphosphonate (BP), specific for exposed diseased bone (Villaverde et al. 2017). RGD becomes exposed only in presence of elevated concentrations of cathepsin-K (CK), a potent collagenase expressed in high osteoclast activity as in primary and secondary bone tumors (Husmann et al. 2008; Bonzi et al. 2015). RGD binds to specific receptors overexpressed in tumoral cells and provides selective responsivity to CK. The encrypted targeting system in a bone/culture in vitro model could avoid the reach of the drug in other non-diseased tissues reducing side effects and systemic toxicity, representing an ideal perspective in development of new approaches for the enhanced selectivity in antitumor drug delivery, which could be applied in loaded nanocarriers (Villaverde et al. 2017).

Nanocarriers loading with BPs have been projected to prevent primary bone cancer and cancer metastasis. Silica nanoparticles (SNPs) anchored by zoledronic acid (ZOL) and doped with DOX acted as a controlled delivery system in vitro, revealing a satisfactory ability for bone-targeting, increasing the efficacy of the anticancer drug (Sun et al. 2016); BPs present a high binding affinity in the surface of diseased bone sites and prevent the bone resorption, even used as surface ligands with nanoparticles (Tejinder et al. 2015).

Nanoparticles are very applied for bone repair and bone diseases treatment including nanocarriers (Mitri et al. 2018) (Fig. 13.2); the variety of nanomaterials designed for its application in bone engineering and regenerative medicine is wide (Mitri et al. 2018), then the following Table 13.1 presents some of the nanomaterials most investigated for applying in different bone diseases, according to the subject mentioned in this chapter.

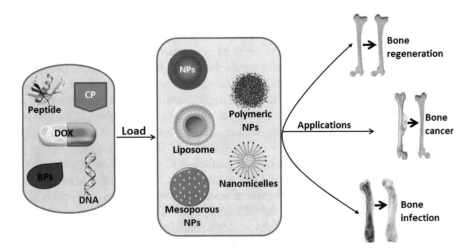

Fig. 13.2 Different biological molecules and nanomaterials used in management of different bone disorders (*CP* calcium phosphate, *DOX* doxorubicin, *BPs* bio-phosphates, *NPs* nanoparticles)

Table 13.1 Application of various nanomaterials or nanosystems in different bone diseases or bone engineering

Nanomaterials	Bone disease or bone engineering	Reference
AgNPs	To kill osteosarcoma cells	Kovács et al. (2016)
AgNP-loaded bone acrylic cement	To prevent the bacterial surface colonization in primary arthroplasty	Slane et al. (2015)
Nano-apatite/PCL membrane	For GTR/GBR applications. It is strong, enhances bioactivity, and supports osteoblast-like cell proliferation and differentiation	Yang et al. (2009)
TMC-Lip-DOX NPs	Periodontal and inflammatory diseases	Hu et al. (2019)
Nano/silver poly-coated titanium	Antibacterial activity (inhibited bacterial adhesion) and osteoinductive activities	Zeng et al. (2019)
Nanocarriers	(Levofloxacin-loaded mesoporous silica nanoparticles decorated with lectin concanavalin A) Antimicrobial efficacy for treatment for bone chronic infections	Martínez-Carmona et al. (2019)
Magnetic NPs-PEG-cisplatin	Increased anticancer effects compared with free cisplatin on the adhesion capacity of bone metastatic breast cancer	Mokhtari et al. (2017)
Nano-HA scaffolds	Bone regeneration	Elias et al. (2019)
Hydrophobic anticancer curcumin-loaded $(ASP)_8$-PEG-PCL NPs	Antitumorigenic ability in animal models with cancer metastasized to bone	Liu et al. (2017)
Nanosystem (nanomedicine)	To inhibit osteolysis and bone metastasis	Li et al. (2017)
KNPs	KNPs as DOX carriers for treatment of soft tissue and bone sarcomas, leukemia, neuroblastoma, breast and ovarian cancer, and others	Aluigi et al. (2018)
MSCs-exosome as natural nanocarrier	Natural nanocarrier as delivery therapy for several neoplastic conditions, including bone cancer	Zhou et al. (2018)
Nanomedicine (systemic RNA delivery)	Therapeutic gene silencing in cell malignances in bone	Weinstein et al. (2016)
NPs	Silica NPs doped with ZOL in bone cancer and bone cancer metastasis	Sun et al. (2016)
LDH NPs	Sheet-like layered double hydroxide NPs as efficient nanocarriers for drug and gene delivery to osteosarcoma cells (U2OS)	Li et al. (2018)
Chitosan NPs	Non-viral gene delivery for osteoarthritis	Lu et al. (2011)
Curcumin nanoparticles	Anti-inflammatory effects and anti-infective agent in treatment of periprosthetic joint infections	Peng et al. (2019)
PEGylated PAMAM	Delivery system with IGF-1 to reduce cartilage degeneration and osteophyte volume in osteoarthritis	Geiger et al. (2018)
ZnO-nanocrystals	Osteoinductive nanoantibiotic agent for bone tissue engineering	Garino et al. (2019)
SiO_2 nanocomposites	Nanocomposites with nanopores biomimicking native bone architecture to guide osteogenic differentiation of human stem cells	Greiner et al. (2019)

13.12 Conclusion and Future Perspectives

Nanotechnology is a promising field being applied in all branches of health, and it is progressing fast. Bone tissue engineering searches for an ideal scaffold that must have the strength and high rate of resorption, presence, and distribution of pores, proteins adhesion surface, and all these features to mimic living and native bone microenvironment and improve bone repair and bone remodeling. Even that fabricated from polymers trends to presenting needed mechanical strength, to allow protein adhesion, cellular proliferation and tissue growth, collaborating to the new bone tissue forming.

Some bone diseases, including infections and bone cancers, can be public health problems very common. Moreover, the unavailability of effective and precise treatment, at the cell level, is a challenge to be overcome by nanotechnology. A highlighted current trend is the ability of the nanocarriers to improve the drugs pharmacokinetic; nanocarriers doped or loaded with anticancer drugs and other associations are the very specific tools to directly attack the tumor cell with low or no side effects or systemic toxicity. This mechanism can prevent the growth of the tumor, avoid metastatic sites, and consequently preserve around organs and other tissues. Nanotechnology-based site-specific drug delivery is an important approach to direct the researches to the development of nanomaterials and provide better options for the clinicians about quality treatment strategies.

Current and future design concepts, and manufacturing techniques will order nanotechnology straightway to improve bone reconstruction and suitable forms of treatment for the different injuries of human bone.

References

Abazari MF, Nejati F, Nasiri N, Khazeni ZAS, Nazari B, Enderami SE, Mohajerani H (2019) Platelet-rich plasma incorporated electrospun PVA-chitosan-HA nanofibers accelerates osteogenic differentiation and bone reconstruction. Gene 720:144096–144102

Albrektsson T, Johansson C (2001) Osteoinduction, osteoconduction and osseointgration. Eur Spine J 10(2):S96–S101

Aluigi A, Ballestri M, Guerrini A, Sotgiu G, Ferroni C, Corticelli F, Gariboldi MB, Monti E, Varchi G (2018) Organic solvent-free preparation of keratin nanoparticles as doxorubicin carriers for antitumor activity. Mater Sci Eng C Mater Biol Appl 1(90):476–484

Bonzi G, Salmaso S, Scomparin A, Eldar-Boock A, Satchi-Fainaro R, Caliceti P (2015) Novel pullulan bioconjugate for selective breast cancer bone metastases treatment. Bioconjug Chem 26(3):489–501

Buckwalter A, Glimcher MJ, Cooper RR, Recker R (1996) Bone biology. I: structure, blood supply, cells, matrix, and mineralization. Instr Course Lect 5:371–386

Capulli M, Paone R, Rucci N (2014) Osteoblast and osteocyte: games without frontiers. Arch Biochem Biophys 561:3–12

Chou YF, Huang W, Dunn JC, Miller TA, Wu BM (2007) The effect of biomimetic apatite structure on osteoblast viability, proliferation, and gene expression. J Biomed Mater Res A 80(1):206–215

Ciapetti G, Granchi D, Devescovi V, Baglio SR, Leonardi E, Martini D, Jurado MJ, Olalde B, Armentano I, Kenny JM, Walboomers FX, Alava JI, Baldini N (2012) Enhancing osteoconduction of PLLA-based nanocomposite scaffolds for bone regeneration using different biomimetic signals to MSCs. Int J Mol Sci 13(2):2439–2458

Della-Valle C, Visai L, Santin M, Cigada A, Candiani G, Pezzoli D, Arciola CR, Imbriani M, Chiesa R (2012) A novel antibacterial modification treatment of titanium capable to improve osseointegration. Int J Artif Organs 35:864–875

Downey PA, Siegel MI (2006) Bone biology and the clinical implications for osteoporosis. Phys Ther 86(1):77–91

Ducy P, Zhang R, Geoffroy V, Ridall AL, Karsenty G (1997) Osf2/Cbfa1: a transcriptional activator of osteoblast differentiation. Cell 89(5):747–754

Elefteriou F (2008) Regulation of bone remodeling by the central and peripheral nervous system. Biophysics 473(2):231–236

Elias CMV, Maia-Filho ALM, Silva LR, Amaral FPM, Webster TJ, Marciano FR, Lobo AO (2019) In vivo evaluation of the genotoxic effects of poly (butylene adipate-co-terephthalate)/polypyrrole with nanohydroxyapatite scaffolds for bone regeneration. Materials 12:1330–1345

Eliaz N, Metoki N (2017) Calcium phosphate bioceramics: a review of their history, structure, properties, coating technologies and biomedical applications. Materials 10:334–438

Everts V, Delaissé JM, Korper W, Jansen DC, Tigchelaar-Gutter W, Saftig P, Beertsen W (2002) The bone lining cell: its role in cleaning Howship's lacunae and initiating bone formation. J Bone Miner Res 17(1):77–99

Ferreira L, Squier T, Park H, Choe H, Kohane DS, Langer R (2008) Human embryoid bodies containing nano- and microparticulate delivery vehicles. Adv Mater 20(12):2285–2291

Garino N, Sanvitale P, Dumontel B, Laurenti M, Colilla M, Izquierdo-Barba I, Cauda V, Vallet-Regi M (2019) Zinc oxide nanocrystals as a nanoantibiotic and osteoinductive agent. RSC Adv 9:11312–11321

Geiger BC, Wang S, Padera RF Jr, Grodzinsky AJ, Hammond PT (2018) Cartilage-penetrating nanocarriers improve delivery and efficacy of growth factor treatment of osteoarthritis. Sci Transl Med 28(10):469–488

Gerstenfeld LC, Culliname DM, Barnes GL, Graves DT, Einhorn TA (2003) Fracture healing as a post-natal developmental process: molecular, spatial, and temporal aspects of its regulation. J Cell Biochem 88(5):873–884

Gerstenfeld LC, Alkhiary YM, Krall EA, Nicholls FH, Stapleton SN, Fitch JL, Bauer M (2006) Three-dimensional reconstruction of fracture callus morphogenesis. J Histochem Cytochem 54(11):1215–1228

Greiner JFW, Gottschalk M, Fokin N, Büker B, Kaltschmidt C, Hütten A, Kaltschmidt B (2019) Natural and synthetic nanopores directing osteogenic differentiation of human stem cells. Nanomedicine 17:319–328

Griffin MF, Kalaskar DM, Seifalian A, Butler PE (2016) An update on the application of nanotechnology in bone tissue engineering. Open Orthop J 10(3):836–848

Grigoriadis AE, Heersche JNM, Aubin JE (1988) Differentiation of muscle, fat, cartilage, and bone from progenitor cells present in a bone-derived clonal cell population: effect of dexamethasone. J Cell Biol 106(6):2139–2151

Guo J, Meng Z, Chen G, Xie D, Wang H, Liu L, Jing W, Long J, Guo W, Tian W (2012) Restoration of critical-size defects in rabbit mandible using porous nanohydroxyapatite-polyamide scaffolds. Tissue Eng A 18(11–12):1239–1252

Gurunathan S, Jeyaraj M, Kang MH, Kim JH (2019) Tangeretin-assisted platinum nanoparticles enhance the apoptotic properties of doxorubicin: combination therapy for osteosarcoma treatment. Nanomaterials 9:1089–1119

Harvey EJ, Henderson JE, Vengallatore ST (2010) Nanotechnology and bone healing. J Orthop Trauma 24:25–30

Hu F, Zhou Z, Xu Q, Fan C, Wang L, Ren H, Xu S, Ji Q, Chen X (2019) A novel pH-responsive quaternary ammonium chitosan-liposome nanoparticles for periodontal treatment. Int J Biol Macromol 129(15):1113–1119

Huang S, Ingber DE (1999) The structural and mechanical complexity of cell-growth control. Nat Cell Biol 1:131–138

Husmann K, Muff R, Bolander ME, Sarkar G, Born W, Fuchs B (2008) Cathepsins and osteosarcoma: expression analysis identifies cathepsin K as an indicator of metastasis. Mol Carcinog 47:66–73

Jell G, Minelli C, Stevens M (2009) Biomaterial-related approaches: surface structuring. In: Fundamentals of tissue engineering and regenerative medicine. Springer, New York, pp 469–484

Johnson LC (1966) The kinetics of skeletal remodeling. Birth Defects Orig Artic Ser 2(1):66–142

Jung Y, Kim SS, Kim YH, Kim SH, Kim BS, Kim S, Choi CY (2005) A poly(lactic acid)/calcium metaphosphate composite for bone tissue engineering. Biomaterials 26:6314–6322

Kennedy OD, Herman DM, Laudier DM, Majeska RJ, Sun HB, Schaffler MB (2012) Activation of resorption in fastigue-loaded bone involves both apoptosis and active pro-osteoclastogenic signaling by distinct osteocyte populations. Bone 50(5):1115–1122

Khang D, Carpenter J, Chun YW, Pareta R, Webster TJ (2010) Nanotechnology for regenerative medicine. Biomed Microdevices 12:575–587

Kitaori T, Ito H, Schwarz EM, Tsutsumi R, Yoshitomi H, Oishi S, Nakano M, Fujii N (2009) Stromal cell-derived factor 1/CXCR4 signaling is critical for the recruitment of mesenchymal stem cells to the fracture site during skeletal repair in a mouse model. Arthritis Rheum 60(3):813–823

Kneser U, Schaefer DG, Polykandriotis E, Horch RE (2006) Tissue engineering of bone: the reconstructive surgeon's point of view. J Cell Mol Med 10(1):7–19

Kose N, Çalak R, Pekşen C, Kiremitçi A, Burukoglu D, Koparal S, Doğan A (2016) Silver ion doped ceramic nano-powder coated nails prevent infection in open fractures: *in vivo* study. Injury 47:320–324

Kovács D, Igaz N, Keskeny C, Bélteky P, Tóth T, Gáspar R, Madarász D, Rázga Z, Kónya Z, Boros IM, Kiricsi M (2016) Silver nanoparticles defeat p53-positive and p53-negative osteosarcoma cells by triggering mitochondrial stress and apoptosis. Sci Rep 13(6):27902–27914

Langer R, Vacanti JP (1993) Tissue engineering. Science 260:920–926

Laurencin CT, Kumbar SG, Nukavarapu SP (2009) Nanotechnology and orthopedics: a personal perspective. Wiley Interdiscip Rev Nanomed Nanobiotechnol 1:6–10

Li C, Zhang Y, Chen G, Hu F, Zhao K, Wang Q (2017) Engineering multifunctional nanomedicine for simultaneous stereotactic chemotherapy and inhibited osteolysis in an orthotopic model of bone metastasis. Adv Mater 29:1605754–1605760

Li L, Zhang R, Gu W, Xu ZP (2018) Mannose-conjugated layered double hydroxide nanocomposite for targeted siRNA delivery to enhance cancer therapy. Nanomedicine 14(7):2355–2364

Linkhart TA, Mohan S, Baylink DJ (1996) Growth factors for bone growth and repair: IGF, TGF beta and BMP. Bone 19(1):1–19

Liu J, Zeng Y, Shi S, Xu L, Zhang H, Pathak JL, Pan Y (2017) Design of polyaspartic acid peptide-poly (ethylene glycol)-poly (ε-caprolactone) nanoparticles as a carrier of hydrophobic drugs targeting cancer metastasized to bone. Int J Nanomedicine 12:3561–3575

Liu X, Chen C, Zhang H, Tian A, You J, Wu L, Lei Z, Li X, Bai X, Chen S (2019) Biocompatibility evaluation of antibacterial Ti-Ag alloys with nanotubular coatings. Int J Nanomedicine 14:457–468

Lu HD, Zhao HQ, Wang K, Liv LL (2011) Novel hyaluronic acid-chitosan nanoparticles as non-viral gene delivery vectors targeting osteoarthritis. Int J Pharmacol 420:358–365

Martínez-Carmona M, Izquierdo-Barba I, Colilla M, Vallet-Regí M (2019) Concanavalin A-targeted mesoporous silica nanoparticles for infection treatment. Acta Biomater 96:547–556

Matsuo K, Irie N (2008) Osteoclast-osteoblast communication. Arch Biochem Biophys 473(2):201–209

Mitri FF, Ingle AP, Rai M (2018) Nanotechnology in the management of bone diseases and as regenerative medicine. Curr Nanosci 14:95–103

Mokhtari MJ, Koohpeima F, Mohammadi H (2017) A comparison inhibitory effects of cisplatin and MNPs-PEG-cisplatin on the adhesion capacity of bone metastatic breast cancer. Chem Biol Drug Des 90(4):618–628

Moore C, Kosgodage U, Lange S, Inal J (2017) The emerging role of exosome and microvesicle- (EMV-) based cancer therapeutics and immunotherapy. Int J Cancer 141:428–436

Pascucci L, Coccè V, Bonomi A, Ami D, Ceccarelli P, Ciusani E, Viganò L, Locatelli A, Sisto F, Doglia SM, Parati E, Bernardo ME, Muraca M, Alessandri G, Bondiolotti G, Pessina A (2014) Paclitaxel is incorporated by mesenchymal stromal cells and release in exosomes that inhibit in vitro tumor growth: a new approach for drug delivery. J Control Release 192:262–270

Peng KT, Chiang YC, Huang TY, Chen PC, Chang PJ, Lee CW (2019) Curcumin nanoparticles are a promising anti-bacterial and anti-inflammatory agent for treating periprosthetic joint infections. Int J Nanomedicine 14:469–481

Prabbhakaran MP, Venugal J, Ramakrishna S (2009) Electrospun nanostructured sacaffolds for bone tissue engineering. Acta Biomater 5:2884–2893

Qadri S, Haik Y, Mensah-Brown E, Bashir G, Fernandez-Cabezudo MJ, Al-Ramadi BK (2017) Metallic nanoparticles to eradicate bacterial bone infection. Nanomedicine 13:2241–2250

Raghavendran HRB, Puvaneswary S, Talebian S, Murali MR, Naveen SV, Krishnamurithy G, McKean R, Kamarul T (2014) A comparative study on in vivo osteogenic priming potential for electron spun scaffold PLLA/HA/Col, PLLA/Col for tissue engineering application. PLoS One 9(8):e104389

Ratner BD, Bryant SJ (2004) Biomaterials: where we have been and where we are going. Annu Rev Biomed Eng 6:41–75

Scheller EL, Krebsbach PH, Kohn DH (2009) Tissue engineering: state of the art in oral rehabilitation. J Oral Rehabil 36:368–389

Seeman E, Delmas PD (2006) Bone quality-the material and structural basis of bone strength and fragility. N Engl J Med 354(21):2250–2261

Siegel RW, Fougere GE (1995) Mechanical properties of nanophase metals. Nanostruct Mater 6(1–4):205–216

Slane J, Vivanco J, Rose W, Ploeg HL, Squire M (2015) Mechanical, material, and antimicrobial properties of acrylic bone cement impregnated with silver particles. Mater Sci Eng C 48:188–196

Spin-Neto R, Stravopoulos A, Dias-Pereira LA, Marcantonio-Junior E, Wenzel A (2013) Fate of autologous and fresh-frozen allogenic block bone grafts used for ridge augmentation. A CBCT-based analysis. Clin Oral Implants Res 24:167–173

Sun W, Han Y, Li Z, Ge K, Zhang J (2016) Bone-targeted mesoporous silica nanocarrier anchored by zoledronate for cancer bone metastasis. Langmuir 32(36):9237–9244

Tejinder S, Veerpal K, Manish K, Prabhjot K, Murthy RSR, Rawal RK (2015) The critical role of bisphosphonates to target bone cancer metastasis: an overview. J Drug Target 23:1–15

Venugopal J, Low S, Choon AT, Ramakrishna S (2008) Interaction of cells and nanofiber scaffolds in tissue engineering. J Biomed Mater Res B Appl Biomater 84:34–48

Villaverde G, Nairi V, Baeza A, Vallet-Regi M (2017) Double sequential encrypted targeting sequence: a new concept for bone cancer treatment. Chemistry 23(30):7174–7179

Wamsley GG, McArdle A, Tevlin R, Momeni A, Atashroo D, Hu MS, Feroze AH, Wong VW, Lorenz PH, Longaker MT, Wan DC (2015) Nanotechnology in bone tissue engineering. Nanomedicine 11(5):1253–1263

Wang L, Hu C, Shao L (2017) The antimicrobial activity of nanoparticles: present situation and prospects for the future. Int J Nanomedicine 12:1227–1249

Wang C, Yu B, Fan Y, Ormsby RW, McCarthy H, Dunne N, Li X (2019) Incorporation of multi-walled carbon nanotubes to PMMA bone cement improves cytocompatibility and osseointegration. Mater Sci Eng C Mater Biol Appl 103:109823–109835

Webster TJ (2017) IJN's second year is now a part of nanomedicine history. Neuropsychiatr Dis Treat 2:1–2

Webster TJ, Ergun C, Doremus RH, Siegel RW, Bizios R (2000) Enhanced functions of osteoblasts on nanophase ceramics. Biomaterials 21:1803–1810

Wei G, Ma PX (2004) Structure and properties of nanohydroxyapatite/polymer composite scaffolds for bone tissue engineering. Biomaterials 25:4749–4757

Weinstein S, Toker IA, Emmanuel R, Ramishetti S, Hazan-Halevy I, Rosenblum D, Goldsmith M, Abraham A, Benjamini O, Bairey O, Raanani P, Nagler A, Lieberman J, Peer D (2016) Harnessing RNAi-based nanomedicines for therapeutic gene silencing I B-cells malignancies. Proc Natl Acad Sci U S A 113:16–22

Wu AC, Morrison NA, Kelly WL, Forwood MR (2013) MCP-1 expression is specifically regulated during activation on skeletal repair and remodeling. Calcif Tissue Int 92(6):566–575

Xiao X, Liu R, Huang Q (2007) Preparation and characterization of nano-hydroxyapatite/polymers increase osteoblast attachment. Int J Nanomedicine 2:487–492

Yang F, Both SK, Yang X, Walboomers F, Jansen JA (2009) Development of an electrospun nanoapatite/PCL composite membrane for GTR/GBR application. Acta Biomater 5:3295–3304

Zeng X, Xiong S, Zhuo S, Liu C, Miao J, Liu D, Wang H, Zhang Y, Zheng Z, Ting K, Wang C, Liu Y (2019) Nanosilver/poly (DL-lactic-co-glycolic acid) on titanium implant surfaces for the enhancement of antibacterial properties and osteoconductivity. Int J Nanomedicine 14:1849–1863

Zhang H, Webster TJ (2009) Nanotechnology and nanomaterials: promises for improved tissue regeneration. Nano Today 4(1):66–80

Zhang ZG, Li ZH, Mao XZ (2011) Advances in bone repair with nanobiomaterials: mini-review. Cytotechnology 63:439–443

Zhou J, Tan X, Tan Y, Li Q, Ma J, Wang G (2018) Mesemchymal stem cell derived exosomes in cancer progression, metastasis and drug delivery: a comprehensive review. J Cancer 9(17):3129–3137

Chapter 14
Diabetic Foot Osteomyelitis: Control and Therapy Through Nanotechnology

Vandita Kakkar, Parina Kumari, Priyanka Narula, and Mohd Yaseen

Abstract Osteomyelitis (OM) also known as bone infection is a subtle but a severe condition. OM in diabetic foot is a complication of a foregoing foot infection. The conventional remedies for osteomyelitis include prolonged and aggressive use of antibiotics and surgical intervention in case of severe infections. The treatment of bone infections through antibiotics often fails due to a widespread range of drug-resistant bacteria, poor accessibility of many antimicrobials to the deeper parts of the bones, facile formation of biofilm on the bone surface, and elevated hazards associated with drug toxicity. Nanotechnology-based interventions provide the possible solutions owing to their high targeting potential and efficient delivery, thus leading to the development of novel anti-infective formulations. The nanodelivery systems can be devised with precise functional moieties capable of selective transport of drugs to the specific site in a controlled manner, thus overcoming the most significant milestone in formulating anti-infectives. This chapter aims to explore the application of nanotechnology for the treatment of OM. Further, the pathogenic events along with the available therapeutic remedies, their disadvantages, and the role of nanosizing in OM have been discussed at length.

Keywords Osteomyelitis · Diabetes · Nanotechnology · Infections · Anti-infectives

Abbreviations

AG	Antibiotic group
AgNPs	Silver nanoparticles
CAPs	Calcium phosphates
CI	Confidence interval

V. Kakkar (✉) · P. Kumari · P. Narula · M. Yaseen
Department of Pharmaceutical Sciences, University Institute of Pharmaceutical Sciences, Panjab University, Chandigarh, India
e-mail: vanditakakkar@pu.ac.in

© Springer Nature Switzerland AG 2020
M. Rai (ed.), *Nanotechnology in Skin, Soft Tissue, and Bone Infections*,
https://doi.org/10.1007/978-3-030-35147-2_14

CNS	Coagulase-negative staphylococci
CT	Computed tomography
DDS	Drug delivery system
DFO	Diabetic foot osteomyelitis
DFUs	Diabetic foot ulcers
DO	Diabetic osteomyelitis
ESR	Erythrocyte sedimentation rate
FDG-PET	Fluorodeoxyglucose positron emission tomography
HA	Hydroxyapatite
LR	Likelihood ratio
MBIC	Minimal biofilm inhibitory concentration
MDR	Multidrug resistance
MIC	Minimal inhibitory concentrations
MRI	Magnetic resonance imaging
OM	Osteomyelitis
PEG	Poly (ethylene glycol)
PLGA	Poly (lactic-*co*-glycolic acid)
PTB	Probe-to-bone test
SG	Surgical group
TCP	Tricalcium phosphate
TMP-SMX	Trimethoprim/sulfamethoxazole
WBC	White blood cell

14.1   Introduction

"Osteomyelitis" (OM) draws its origin from the Greek words *osteon*, *myelos*, and *itis*. It is an inflammatory and infectious disease of bone, usually caused by bacteria (Malhotra et al. 2014). Osteomyelitis is present in ~20% of patients suffering from foot infections with diabetes referred to as diabetic foot osteomyelitis (DFO) (Lipsky 2014). DFO can be either acute or chronic and results from diabetic complications, especially peripheral neuropathy. This disorder is a unique clinical and pathologic problem which usually occurs after a soft tissue infection in the diabetic foot ulcer (DFU) area and spreads into the bone, involving the cortex first and then the marrow (Berendt et al. 2008). OM normally occurs in the forefoot (90%), followed by the midfoot (5%) and the hindfoot (5%). Diagnosis of OM can be done easily in the forefoot than the midfoot and hindfoot (Giurato et al. 2017). Amputation risk is significantly higher for hindfoot (50%) than midfoot (18.5%) and forefoot (0.33%) (Faglia et al. 2013). Since undiagnosed and untreated DO often leads to major risk factors for minor or major lower-extremity amputation, a high index of clinical suspicion is required to make a diagnosis (Malhotra et al. 2014). Both the neuropathic and ischemic ulcers can be complicated in DFUs by the underlying infections (Margolis and Jeffcoate 2013; Giurato et al. 2017).

With an increase in the prevalence of diabetes, a sequential rise in cases of foot complications have been reported. Diabetes is the fundamental cause for up to 8–10 nontraumatic amputations, of which 85% follow a foot ulcer (Siitonen et al. 1993; Bader 2008). About 15–25% of diabetic patients develop a foot ulcer at some time during their life, and 40–80% of these ulcers become infected (Singh 2005). Limb amputation is the most costly and feared consequence of a foot ulcer and occurs 10–30 times more often in diabetic persons than in the general population (Armstrong et al. 1997). The advancement of a foot infection due to the occurring foot ulcer leads to considerable morbidity, including discomfort and physical psychosomatic issues leading to a poor quality of life (Yazdanpanah et al. 2015).

Nanotechnology has emerged as a new field in producing biomedicine and biotechnology-based applications through the synthesis of nanomaterials. It has been applied successfully to enhance drug delivery for the treatment of many diseases such as cancers (Tiwari et al. 2012), inflammation, and hypertension (McLendon et al. 2015). Nanotechnology can be used for solving the limitations of antimicrobial therapy such as antimicrobial resistance by delivering new platforms for effective drug delivery by means of new antimicrobial nanomaterials which pathogens may not be able to develop resistance (Huh and Kwon 2011). Also, drug delivery through nanosystems improves cellular internalization, thereby decreasing the side effects by uniform distribution in the target tissue and improving the pharmacokinetic profiles and patient compliance to antibiotics (Walmsley et al. 2015). The preparation of nanoparticles is cost-effective as compared to antibiotic synthesis, thus giving stable formulations for long-term storage. Nanoparticles can withstand high temperature and sterilization unlike antibiotics that can be degraded easily in harsh conditions (Ranghar et al. 2014).

14.2   Pathophysiology

DFO involves a complex pathophysiology and is a consequence of soft tissue infections (usually an infected diabetic foot ulcer) that spreads to the underlying osteoarticular structures. It also results from either penetrating injury or ischemic soft tissue loss or contiguous spread of pathogens from infection, complicating a diabetic foot ulcer to the bones underlying these ulcers. Recent observations have ruled out any neuropathic event to be an important factor (Hobizal and Wukich 2012). Occurrence of neuropathy due to metabolic imbalances in diabetes has been reported in 80% of patients with foot disease. Patients with decreased sensation can suffer from thermal or mechanical injuries unknowingly leading to skin ulcerations. Motor neuropathy affects intrinsic muscles of the foot leading to gait disorders. This anatomic alteration leads to maldistribution of weight with increased focal pressure resulting in skin ulceration (Pendsey 2010). The autonomic neuropathy acts by interfering with sweating and causing dry, cracked skin. It makes a way for entry of microorganisms through the skin, leading to soft tissue infections that acts as a focus for bone infection. Moreover, as fungal infections are common in diabetic

Fig. 14.1 Pathophysiology
of DFO

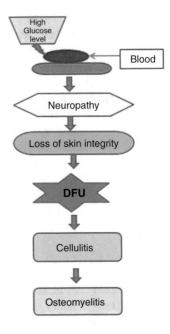

patients, there are chances that it may enter into blood to causes further infection. Diabetic patients have impaired wound healing due to poorly characterized defects in host immunity, leading to a delay in the onset of ulceration resulting in the spread of the infection to other parts (Mayfield et al. 1998; Zinman et al. 2004) as shown in Fig. 14.1. OM is accompanied by osseous changes, biofilm formation, and major defects caused by neutrophils throughout its natural course (Garwood and Kim 2015).

14.3 Microbiology

The most common pathogenic agent of OM is *Staphylococcus aureus* which is cultured from bone samples. *Staphylococcus epidermidis* is also known to be one of the causative agents for OM. Other pathogenic species include *Enterobacteriaceae*, *Escherichia coli*, *Klebsiella pneumoniae*, and *Proteus* sp. followed by *Pseudomonas aeruginosa* (Hartemann and Senneville 2008). A study showed the occurrence of obligate anaerobes in only 5% of patients in which all bone samples were directly vaccinated with Rosenow's broth (Senneville et al. 2006). The most predominant bacteria among the obligate anaerobes included *Finegoldia magna* (formerly *Peptostreptococcus magnus*) and other anaerobic streptococci as shown in Fig. 14.2. Bacteria such as coagulase-negative staphylococci (CNS) and *Corynebacterium* sp. are also highly pathogenic to cause OM of the diabetic foot (Bessman et al. 1991).

Fig. 14.2 Illustration of causative agents

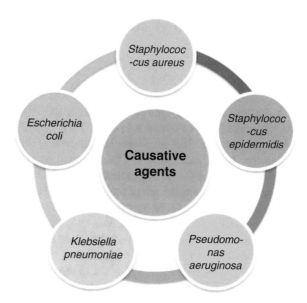

14.4   Classification of Diabetic Foot Osteomyelitis

OM can be classified into two main categories as proposed by Waldvogel and colleagues (Waldvogel et al. 1970; Lipsky 1997). First, the one that is caused due to hematogenous infection of the bone. Second, the one that spreads to the bone from a contiguous center (Waldvogel et al. 1970). It can be subdivided into those with and without vascular insufficiency, which could lead to acute or chronic OM. Chronic infections typically proceed in a gradual way but with very harmful effects and involve necrotic or ischemic bones. Almost all diabetic patients with lower extremity OM have chronic contiguous infections, usually associated with vasculopathy (Lipsky 1997).

An alternative classification of OM which combines anatomic disease types and physiological host categories (local and systemic factors) has been proposed. It clearly defines the 12 clinical stages of OM (Cierny et al. 1985).

14.5   Diagnosis

This involves mainly the histopathological examination and growth on culture of an aseptically obtained bone specimen. Bone biopsy is an incursive procedure, and histology and culture are relatively expensive and time-consuming (Kaleta et al. 2001). Thus, it is important to evaluate the suitability of an appropriate diagnostic test for DFO in selected patients.

14.5.1   Inflammatory Markers and Blood Tests

Erythrocyte sedimentation rate (ESR) is the most useful laboratory test for the diagnosis of diabetic foot OM at present (Kaleta et al. 2001). An increase in ESR level > 70 mm/h raises the chances of OM in a diabetic foot with a pooled +LR (likelihood ratio) of 11 (confidence interval, 1.6–79) and −LR of 0.34 (Butalia et al. 2008). Another recent study was carried out in patients with OM, and it revealed increased levels of ESR for 3 months, and hence, ESR was suggested to be used for the follow-up of patients with OM (Michail et al. 2013). Another study showed increased levels of C-reactive protein (CRP) value >3.2 mg/dL, thus differentiating bone infection from infection of the soft tissue (Fleischer et al. 2009). Another study revealed increased levels of both the neutrophils and CRP in patients with soft tissue infection without OM compared with those with OM (Eneroth et al. 1999). The usefulness of CRP (compared with ESR) or procalcitonin in the diagnosis of diabetic foot OM is not sufficiently established in the published literature (Mutluoğlu et al. 2011). However, increased white blood cells (WBCs) and swab cultures confirm the diagnosis of diabetic foot OM in an effective manner (Newman et al. 1991).

14.5.2   Bone Exposure and Probe-to-Bone Tests

The exposed bone shows a likelihood ratio (+LR) of 9.2 (Newman et al. 1991). The chances of OM are increased on striking the bone with a blunt, sterile metal probe as per the pretest probability of OM. As per the reports, the +LR for a positive probe-to-bone (PTB) test ranges between 4.3 and 9.4 in case of high pretest probability of bone infection, i.e. >50% (Grayson 1995; Shone et al. 2006; Dinh et al. 2008). Therefore, a positive PTB in case of an infected wound has a strong indication of OM, but a negative PTB test does not deny the likelihood of the disease. A negative PTB test in case of uninfected ulcers shows unlikeliness of OM, and in such cases, the positive PTB test exhibits a low relevance (Lavery et al. 2007; Markanday 2014).

14.5.3   Plain Radiographs

Radiographs play an important role during the initial stages of patient evaluation and can be used for diagnosis when cortical bone abnormalities, i.e., cortical erosion, periosteal reaction, and osteolysis, have been reported. However, it has been reported that the sensitivity and specificity of the initial X-ray examinations are low as these abnormalities are detected only after 7–15 days of the onset of the acute clinical OM. It has been evidenced that early precise changes are not easily differentiated due to charcot osteoarthropathy (Miller 2006; Pineda et al. 2009). As a result, a follow-up examination should be performed 2–4 weeks later, if the initial X-ray examination of a diabetic patient with suspected OM is negative. In case the imaging findings remain unchanged, it confirms that the infection is confined to the soft tissue. The characteristic cortical abnormalities depict a positive diagnosis of OM. Further imaging examinations can be considered if the radiographic findings are consistent with the diagnosis of OM (Miller 2006). A study by Dinh et al. (2008) revealed a pooled sensitivity and specificity of 0.54 and 0.68 and a diagnostic odds ratio of 2.84, with a Q statistic of 0.60 for plain radiography in the diagnosis of OM (Dinh et al. 2008). Further, a +LR of 2.3 and a –LR of 0.63 were revealed in another review (Shult et al. 1989; Kapoor et al. 2007; Butalia et al. 2008). Thus it was concluded that variations in the plain radiography after a particular time interval may lead to accurate results for diagnosing OM (Markanday 2014).

14.5.4   Radiolabeled White Blood Cell Scanning

It is purported that the leukocyte scans provide a more accurate diagnosis than the triple-phase bone scan. Indium-111-labeled or technetium-99-labeled leukocytes do not usually aggregate at the site of new bone formation without infection as they are not taken up by healthy bone. However, the dimensional resolution is reported to be a drawback in this technique. Technetium-99 labeling allegedly provides a better spatial resolution than indium-111-labeled scans. A ^{99m}Technetium-phosphate bone scan demonstrates the activity at unsuspected sites, which cannot be detected during scintigraphy, and it can detect lesions at sites which may be difficult to examine radiographically, e.g., in the spine or in the pelvic bones (Markanday 2014). A study by Dinh et al. (2008) showed a pooled sensitivity of 0.74 and a specificity of 0.68 for leukocyte scans. The pooled diagnostic odds ratio was found to be 10 with a Q statistic of 0.59 (Dinh et al. 2008). Another study showed positive prognostic values of 70–90% and negative predictive values of 81–83% for technetium- and indium-labeled scans, respectively (Capriotti et al. 2006). The diagnosis and evaluation of the extent of OM can be better performed with white blood cell scans than the bone scans. They were reported to be more useful even during the follow-up of medical treatment (Capriotti et al. 2006). WBC scans have been recommended by the United Kingdom National Institute for Health and Care Excellence guidelines as the next test to be performed when OM is suspected and in case of nonavailability or contra-indication of (magnetic resonance imaging) MRI (Markanday 2014).

14.5.5   Computed Tomography (CT)

CT scan can be used as the first step to distinguish between inflammatory mechanisms and a malignant one. However, the radiation associated with it limits its application (Power et al. 2016). Fluorodeoxyglucose positron emission tomography

(FDG-PET) shows a high sensitivity value between 0.94 and 1.00 and a specificity value between 0.87 and 1.00 (Lipsky et al. 2012). It has been reported that the combination of FDG-PET and CT scan can provide a better diagnostic accuracy. However, the result to the present date is preliminary, and additional research is still warranted in this area (Kagna et al. 2012).

14.5.6 Magnetic Resonance Imaging (MRI)

MRI has been recognized as the most accurate imaging technique for detecting DFO and for evaluating soft tissue involvement (Kapoor et al. 2007; Markanday 2014). Leukocyte or anti-granulocyte bone scans may be performed when MRI is unavailable or contraindicated. It is a noninvasive imaging technique and highly sensitive to active and remitted inflammatory lesions in bone and soft tissues (Jurik and Egund 1997; Jurik 2004). MRI can detect abnormal bone marrow edema before changes are revealed in X-ray of bone scintigraphy (Girschick et al. 1998). MRI has the best indicative potential to distinguish active medullary OM as an area of abnormal marrow with decreased signal intensity on T1-weighted images that correspond to an area of high intensity on T2-weighted images. MRI can very well detect the level and morphology of deep soft tissue infections. A pooled sensitivity of around 0.90 (CI, 0.82–0.95) and specificity value of around 0.85, with a diagnostic odds ratio of 24.4, have been reported by various studies showing excellent discriminant power of MRI (Markanday 2014; Lee et al. 2016). Table 14.1 shows the comparison between different diagnostic techniques.

14.6 Medical Management

Foot infections are among the most recurring causes for hospitalization linked to diabetes leading to lower extremity amputation in these patients (Lipsky et al. 2012). Infection generally starts in ulcerated soft tissues, but can spread promptly to underlying bone (Lipsky 1997). It has been reported that about 20% of patients with

Table 14.1 Comparison of different imaging techniques

Test modality	Approximate mean sensitivity, % (range)	References
MRI	90 (very high)	Jurik and Egund (1997), Jurik (2004)
Indium bone scan	89 (high)	Dinh et al. (2008), Markanday (2014)
Technetium bone scan	86 (high)	Capriotti et al. (2006), Dinh et al. (2008), Markanday (2014)
Plain radiography	60 (moderate)	Miller (2006), Pineda et al. (2009)
CT scan	45 (low)	Kagna et al. (2012), Power et al. (2016)

Less than 50 = low, 50–70 = moderate, 71–90 = high, above 90 = very high a diabetic foot infection and over 60% of those with severe infection suffer from OM, which conclusively increases the risk of lower extremity amputation (Eneroth et al. 1999; Jeffcoate and Lipsky 2004). The treatment of DFO remains a hot topic in the field of diabetic foot. The most deliberated theories have been surgical or antibiotic therapy as first approach (Barwell et al. 2017).

14.6.1 Antimicrobial Treatment

The conventional therapy of OM involves surgical debridement, segregation of implants, necrotic tissues, restoration of blood stream, soft tissue, and systemic distribution of antibiotics (Insall et al. 2002; Hanssen and Spangehl 2004). Active antimicrobial therapy is the foundation for efficacious management of OM. However, clinical response to antimicrobials always remains elusive because of deprived permeability of the drugs due to biofilm formation in case of necrotic bone, thereby inhibiting the drug to achieve the required minimum inhibitory concentration (MIC) level in bone tissue and extended course of therapy (Kim et al. 2013). Drugs such as β-lactams, i.e. penicillin, cephalosporins, and carbapenems, cannot effectively permeate the bone tissue, and bone level of drugs only attains 5–20% of the serum level (Fraimow 2009). Thus, the specific surgical process employed to treat chronic OM involves surgical amputation of infected and necrotic bone (Williams et al. 1983). Diabetic foot OM treatment involves administration of fluoroquinolones, clindamycin, and rifampicin which attain the highest concentrations in bone and prevent the action of infection-causing microorganisms (Hartemann and Senneville 2008). These antimicrobial moieties should only be administered in effective combinations to avoid the development of resistant bacteria (specifically in case of rifampicin) as they have the dominant menace of resistant-mutant selection. The choice of agents should be done on the basis of bone culture results in order to ensure that the combination of drugs is effective against pathogen(s) engaged in causing bone infection (Diamantopoulos et al. 1998).

14.6.1.1 Duration

The duration of antibiotic therapy depends on the cause and level of infection and the clinical course. The usual duration ranges from 3 to 6 weeks and is based on the severity of illness and clinical response. Rifampicin, fusidic acid, and fluoroquinolones should not be used as first-line therapy in patients with acute soft tissue infections as they tend to develop resistance with high inoculums and thus should be reserved for foot OM when it has been conferred via bone specimens (Liu et al. 2011). It has been endorsed that patients with chronic bone infection be treated by antimicrobial therapy for at least 4 weeks except where antimicrobial agents such as fusidic acid, levofloxacin, and rifampicin have complete oral bioavailability (Kim et al. 2013). Currently, the suggested period of treatment is 2–5 days in case of absence of residual infection of tissue (postamputation), 2–4 weeks in case of residual infection of soft tissue alone, 4–6 weeks for residual infection in viable bone, and 3 months or more if persistent bone necrosis is present (Hartemann and Senneville 2008).

Mader et al. (1999) reported that the use of trimethoprim/sulfamethoxazole (TMP-SMX) oral therapy alone for a period above 6 months with appropriate surgical debridement could treat approximately 98% of chronic OM (Mader et al. 1999). Likewise, using TMP-SMX alone or in combination with linezolid was successful in curing almost 80% of the patients with chronic OM as reported by Nguyen et al. (2009). Oral therapy of TMP-SMX demonstrated effective management of chronic OM when used alone or in combination with rifampin and rifampin plus ciprofloxacin for a duration of more than 10 weeks (Nguyen et al. 2009). Table 14.2 shows the antimicrobial therapy involved in the course of DFO.

Orthopedic surgical management by employing antibiotic impregnated bone cement was introduced in 1970 in Europe for the treatment of OM. The antibiotic impregnated bone cements are advantageous over parenteral or oral application of drugs as the concentration of antibiotic is much higher in the drug-coated beads, and it can be maintained for a long time, favoring the healing process in a more appropriate way (Henry and Galloway 1995; Wininger and Fass 1996). The use of drug-coated beads also reduced the probability of systemic toxicity which is common after the subsequent parenteral administration of the drugs. Studies have shown that the occurrence of ototoxicity, nephrotoxicity, and other adverse hypersensitivity reactions is lowered by the use of antibiotic-coated cement beads (Wininger and Fass 1996), which aid in the elevation of the local concentration of the drug,

Table 14.2 Antibiotics used for diabetic foot osteomyelitis

Antibiotics	Infection severity	Comments	References
Flucloxacillin, dicloxacillin, cephalexin, amoxicillin clavulanate	Mild	Methicillin-sensitive S. aureus (MSSA)	Barwell et al. (2017)
Doxycycline, trimethoprim sulfamethoxazole	Mild	Methicillin-resistant S. aureus (MRSA)	Lipsky et al. (2012), Barwell et al. (2017)
Flucloxacillin 1 g QDS (oral) or 2 g QDS (IV) ± metronidazole 400 mg TDS (oral)	Moderate	Combination of two or more antibiotics (oral plus IV)	Barwell et al. (2017)
Ceftriaxone 2 g OD (IV) or teicoplanin (IV) or daptomycin or linezolid	Moderate	Outpatient intravenous antibiotic therapy (OPAT)	Barwell et al. (2017)
Flucloxacillin + clindamycin ± gentamicin (max 4 days) or aztreonam ± metronidazole	Severe	Combination therapy	Barwell et al. (2017)
Piperacillin TAZO, gentamicin, cefepime, meropenem	Severe	Used in case of multidrug-resistant organism	Lipsky et al. (2012), Barwell et al. (2017)

maintaining their systemic concentration at minimum level. Besides, they can plug the post-surgical debridement dead spaces (Belt et al. 2001).

14.6.2 Traditional Surgical Management

Surgery is the ultimate curative approach for the treatment of diabetic foot OM. It is indicated for OM when the patient fails to respond to a specific antimicrobial treatment (Aragón-Sánchez 2010). In some cases, debridement of necrotic tissues, removal of foreign materials, and skin closure of chronic unhealed wounds become necessary, as surgery alone is not enough which requires additional antibiotic treatment. Empirical therapy starts after microbiological analysis of deep tissue samples and is directed against the expected pathogen spectrum. Beta-lactam antibiotics are well tolerated and can attain high enough effective serum concentrations (Walter et al. 2012). Alternatively, lincosamides and gyrase inhibitors can be administered. Usefulness of combination therapy has also been reported in patients with implant-related and periprosthetic infections (Perlroth et al. 2008; Euba et al. 2009) and in treating infections with problem pathogens.

The surgical procedure which involves resectioning of the affected bone can be preceded with patients having an ability to bear weight on the foot. Studies have shown that about a quarter of patients treated for OM requires surgical intervention in cases where traditional surgery was initially performed or if necrosis or ischemia was involved (Hannan and Attinger 2009). The risk of amputation was reportedly increased with hindfoot OM (50%), compared to forefoot OM (0.33%) and midfoot OM (18.5%) (Faglia et al. 2013). The change of foot dynamics and anatomy is one of the main drawbacks of surgery. Partial amputations and even conventional surgery can cause biomechanical changes in the feet which may incite re-ulceration at a new position (Molines-Barroso et al. 2013). Murdoch et al. (1997) reported a second amputation in 60% of patients within a year subsequent to a great toe or first ray amputation (Murdoch et al. 1997).

This conventional approach of treatment involves a great risk as it often removes healthy bone segments along with infected bone. For example, treatment of metatarsal head or even digit infection is done by total ray amputation. A transmetatarsal amputation is implemented when multiple digits are involved even when the infection in the metatarsal heads is lacking (van Baal 2004). In this regard, the technique cannot be clearly defined as "conservative" surgery. Nehler et al. reported a success ratio of 34% through healing without amputation in a group of 97 patients with forefoot infections, 56% of which were OM (Nehler et al. 1999; Jeffcoate and Lipsky 2004).

Tan et al. (1996) showed that an aggressive surgical approach with minor amputation reduces not only the risk of major amputation but also long-time hospitalization and associated costs. The authors report that forefoot amputation reduces the risk of major amputation in comparison to medical therapy performed (Tan et al. 1996).

14.6.3   Conservative Surgery or Medicosurgical Management

Medicosurgical treatment involves antibiotic therapy with conservative surgery. Conservative surgery signifies the restricted resectioning of the infected digit or metatarsal bone, without resection of noninfected bone (Qin et al. 2019). It does not involve amputation of any ray rather involves removing a single metatarsal head, or one or two phalanges. Four to 6 weeks of antibiotic treatment has been recommended after surgery. A medicosurgical approach is reported to elevate the rate of healing as compared to medical treatment alone; however, this assumption requires further investigation (Qin et al. 2019). Nonetheless, the conservative surgical approach possibly increases the risk of re-ulceration due to changed foot biomechanics, even though the risk is less than that with traditional surgery, where more bone segments are removed. The published studies however do not include prolonged clinical and radiological follow-ups that appraise the rates of recurrence of OM and of foot ulcers. This limitation towards medicosurgical approach to OM thus requires a further investigation. To prove the fact, Ha Van et al. (1996) have made a comparison with the conservative surgical treatment involving resection of the phalanx and/or metatarsal head, associated with antibiotic therapy against antibiotic therapy alone. The conservative approach was found to be more efficient in terms of rapid healing times (Ha Van et al. 1996).

14.7   Clinical Evaluation

Several recent reports on diabetic foot OM have been published. In one study, a survey on patients with diabetic foot ulceration and OM was carried out by Niazi et al. (2019), who were treated by using an adjuvant local antibiotic carrier. The survey comprised of 70 patients (average mean age of 68 years) with Texas Grade 3B and 3D lesions. In this study, an antibiotic-loaded absorbable calcium sulfate/hydroxyapatite bio-composite Cerament G was used along with intraoperative multiple bone sampling and culture-specific systemic antibiotics. A follow-up of patients was taken until the complete eradication of infection or the ulcer healing was evidenced. The mean follow-up was 10 months (4–28 months). Charcot foot deformity was found to be present in nine patients; peripheral vascular disease was reported in 14 patients. About 62% of patients had forefoot, 5% midfoot, and 33% hind foot involvement. Fifty-three patients (87%) suffered from polymicrobial infection. The main causative agent isolated was *Staphylococcus aureus*. Ulcer healing was achieved in about 90% of the patients within 12 weeks. Seven patients however were reportedly not cured. Five patients had to undergo leg amputation. Hence, it was concluded that adjuvant, local antibiotic therapy with an absorbable bio-composite can help achieve up to 90% cure rates in diabetic foot ulceration with OM. Cerament G was thus reported to be an effective void filler allowing dead space management after excision and could also prevent reinfection and requirement for multiple surgical procedures (Niazi et al. 2019).

In August 2019, ClinicalTrials.gov (identifier number: NCT03012529) investigation of rifampin to reduce pedal amputations for OM in diabetic patients was reported in VA Office of Research and Development (U.S. National Library of Medicine). The total number of participants was 880, who were randomly assigned to adjunctive rifampin and received a 600 mg oral daily dose for a period of 6 weeks. In case of gastrointestinal intolerance, the patients were advised for once daily dosing and were observed.

In another study conducted by Tone et al. (2015), a comparative randomized trial on therapeutic effectiveness of 6 versus 12 weeks of antibiotic therapy in patients with DFO without any surgical treatment was performed. A total of 40 patients were involved in the clinical trial. Of these 50% (20 individuals) were given the treatment for 6 weeks and the rest 20 for 12 weeks with antibiotics. The two groups were comparable for all variables recorded at the start of the study. Remission was obtained in 26 (65%) patients, with no significant differences between patients treated for 6 versus 12 weeks (12/20 vs. 14/20, respectively; $P = 0.50$). The authors of the multicenter prospective randomized study concluded that 6-week duration of antibiotic therapy may be sufficient in patients with DFO who were treated without surgical removal of the infected bone and is linked to better gastrointestinal tolerance (Tone et al. 2015).

In 2014, a team of Lazaro team conducted a clinical trial involving comparative studies of the treatment of diabetic foot OM in patients treated exclusively with antibiotics versus patients who underwent conservative surgery. The patients were randomly divided into two groups: antibiotic group (AG) and surgical group (SG). Antibiotic therapy was carried out for a period of 90 days in the AG. A conservative surgery with postoperative antibiotic treatment was carried out for 10 days in patients in the SG. Primary healing was achieved in 18 patients (75%) in the AG and 19 (86.3%) in the SG ($P = 0.33$). The average time involved in healing was 7 weeks in the AG and 6 weeks in the SG ($P = 0.72$). Four patients (16.6%) from the AG underwent surgery because of the worsened condition. Three patients from the SG needed reoperation. No variation was found between the two groups regarding minor amputations ($P = 0.336$). Thus it was reported that similar outcomes could be derived from both the antibiotic therapy and the surgical treatment with regard to the healing rates, healing time, and short-term complications in case of patients with complex neuropathic forefoot ulcers due to OM without ischemia or necrotizing soft tissue infections (Lázaro-Martínez et al. 2014).

14.8 Nanotechnology in OM

Nanotechnology opens new avenues for biomedicine and biotechnology through the principles of particle size. Their nanometric scale (between 1 and 100 nm) endows them their unique physicochemical properties (Heiligtag and Niederberger

Fig. 14.3 Classification of nanoparticles

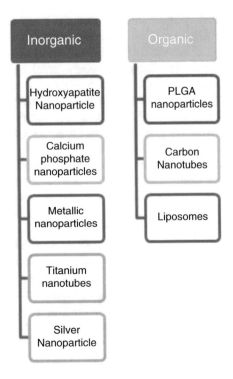

2013). Thus, nanotechnology can be an alternative approach to overcome infectious diseases through the use of antimicrobial nanomaterials (Huh and Kwon 2011). Various types of nanoparticles used for bone-targeted drug delivery are shown in Fig. 14.3.

14.8.1   Hydroxyapatite Nanoparticles

Bone loss due to OM can significantly affect the quality of life of patients. Recently, tissue engineering has emerged as a possible alternative approach for bone tissue repair/regeneration (Walmsley et al. 2015). Many efforts have been made for the regeneration of bone tissue and have led to the development of composite scaffolds with nanoparticles, and fibers as bones is a nanocomposite of collagen and hydroxyapatite (Visakh and José 2016; Zhang et al. 2018). The development of nanobiomaterials and nanocomposites has been achieved using a variety of materials and methods to recapitulate the content and architecture of native bones (McMahon et al. 2013). The composition of bone tissue includes protein materials, i.e., nanoscale molecules and fibrils including collagen, laminin, fibronectin, vitronectin, etc., and hard inorganic components, i.e., nanocrystalline hydroxyapatite (HA) (Lu et al. 2018). Ceramics, such as HA, tricalcium phosphate (TCP), and silicate and phosphate bioglasses hold potential applications in orthopedics owing to their high compressive strength and hardness along with good biocompatibility. These materials can be considered as bioinert, active, and resorbable (Baino et al. 2015). TCP is broadly used as a bioresorbable bone graft for low-weight-bearing orthopedic applications (Wang and Yeung 2017). Hydroxyapatite (HA) is the most popular material to be used as a bone graft substitute due to its structural resemblance with the minerals found in natural bone, thus leading to the formation of tight bonds with surrounding native tissues and osteoconductive properties (Walmsley et al. 2015). Nanophase HA (nanoscale grain size) has been shown to have enhanced cytocompatibility and promote bone formation as compared to conservative, micronstructured HA (Rumpel et al. 2006; Gong et al. 2015). However, low fracture toughness leading to brittleness and low strength of HA restrict its use for load-bearing applications, so composite materials are being explored (Zhou and Lee 2011). Nanomaterials and nanocomposites have emerged as promising constructs with improved reformative abilities, when compared with conservative materials as frameworks for bone repair and rejuvenation.

This has been illustrated by both in vitro and in vivo experiments with nano-featured materials. Nanomaterials, irrespective of their composition or manufacturing process, have been shown to endorse new bone formation in both small and large animal models (Bramhill et al. 2017). A recent study has illustrated the use of calcium sulfate nanoparticles for both antibiotic release and bone regeneration. The study involved a total of 51 patients of which 25 patients required infection irrigation and bone grafting, 16 patients required fracture reparation, 23 of the 25 entirely recovered from infection, and 14 of 16 recovered from infection as well as fracture repair upon use of calcium sulfate nanoparticles. These results confirmed that the in vitro results can be applied to a clinical setting. However, the absence of control group was one drawback to this study even though the graft used was biodegradable in nature. The study also showed that few participants required a second surgery owing to the use of stabilizers for repairing of the fracture. Various mechanisms are being tried in this field comprising scaffolds and injectable materials. The increased surface area, porosity, and bone compatibility of nanomaterials leads to an increased concentration of antibiotics along with the duration for release. Thus, it can be predicted that antibiotics can be confined to a site of infection for treatment through fabrication of biodegradable nanoparticles and compounds. This mechanism of action would endorse bone regeneration without the need for a second surgery (Snoddy and Jayasuriya 2016).

14.8.2 Calcium Phosphate Nanoparticles

Apart from HA, nanosized calcium phosphate (CAP) is one of the most widely accepted choices for antibiotic delivery platforms in bone therapy (Desai and Uskokovic 2013). Nano-CAP is one of the natural mineral components of bone. CAP crystals in bone have the potential to impart sufficient compressive strength to innately tough collagen fibers and can yield a composite material that is both strong and tough. CAPs are bioactive, bioresorptive, and osteo-conductive, hence promote bone growth. They have been evaluated to be nontoxic and most biocompatible nanomaterials and can be prepared in nanoform in a variety of configurations by simple and green precipitation methods (Uskokovic and Desai 2013). The control of stoichiometry of CAP makes it possible to tune its degradation rate, and therefore, the drug releases kinetics. This effect has been employed to vary the in vitro drug release time scale from hours to months. Literature reports on the antibiotic-loaded nanoparticle-loaded scaffolds as an emerging drug delivery system (DDS) for bone regeneration. Such combination hints at the improved antibiotic efficiency even against bacterial biofilms. Nanoparticles are sub-micron sized, hence are capable of crossing the biological barriers, thus improving drug bioavailability and drug permeation at the infected site. Moreover, nanoparticles prevent degradation of the drug and thus achieve a gradual drug release pattern with improved antibiotic effect (Dorati et al. 1999).

14.8.3 Poly (Lactic-co-Glycolic Acid) (PLGA) Nanoparticles

Peng et al. (2010) have reported teicoplanin-loaded biodegradable thermosensitive hydrogel nanoparticles composed of poly(ethylene glycol) monomethyl ether (mPEG) and poly(lactic-co-glycolic acid) (PLGA) copolymer in an injectable form as a sol-gel drug delivery system for treating bone infection (Peng et al. 2010). The injectable thermogelling polymers possess several additional advantages, including easy preparation, high encapsulation efficiency of drugs or bioactive molecules, and above all, they are free of the harmful organic solvents involved in the formulation process (Yu and Ding 2008). A study carried out by Abdelghany and coworkers showed gentamicin-loaded PLGA nanoparticles and tested them against *Pseudomonas aeruginosa* PA01 in both planktonic and biofilm cultures as well as in peritoneal murine infection model. The nanoparticles demonstrated significant improvement of antimicrobial effect by the reduction of inflammatory indicators interleukin-6 and myeloperoxidase in the murine model (Peng et al. 2010; Abdelghany et al. 2012).

14.8.4 Metallic Nanoparticles

Another approach for the treatment of OM is by way of metallic nanoparticles with inherent antimicrobial activity where treatment through conventional antibiotics has proven to be challenging owing to the limited accessibility to the site of infection. Inorganic routes against bacterial infection have been reported for external and topical applications. However, application of these antimicrobials in vivo has not been fully analyzed. Targeted delivery of metallic nanoparticles has been reported by Qadri et al. (2017), demonstrating antimicrobial function of Ag-Cu-B in vivo as a therapeutic agent for bone infection. This strategy represents an alternative means of overcoming the challenges posed by multidrug-resistant bacteria and may potentially reduce the overall morbidity (Stewart et al. 2012; Qadri et al. 2017).

14.8.5 Silver Nanoparticles

As reported in the literature, silver nanoparticles (AgNPs) possess excellent microbicidal activity against wild and nosocomial strains of multidrug resistance (MDR) microorganisms. They have emerged as the most useful nanomaterials in medical products in the form of bandages, wound dressings, catheters, and textiles (Barros et al. 2018). The infections presented in DFU are polymicrobial in nature, and in many cases, this increases the risk for a chronic infection, limb amputation, and morbidity (Marambio-Jones and Hoek 2010). Almonaci Hernandez et al. (2017) have reported disappearance or significant reduction in the area of DFU without developing infection by using silver nanoparticles in the treatment of DFU in two cases of patients with DFU classified as Wagner ulcers II and III. The ulcers were treated with AgNP solution at 1.8 mg/mL of metallic silver topically administered, and the progress of wound healing during treatment was documented by photography (Gonzalez-Sanchez et al. 2015; Hernández et al. 2017).

14.8.6 Titanium Nanoparticles

Juan et al. (2010) illustrated the use of silver nanoparticles by grafting them on the surface of titanium devices such as joint replacements. The efficacy of the nanoparticles was tested with *S. aureus*, and the results confirmed efficient antibacterial properties. The drawback of the study was that the nanoparticles aggregated on the surface of titanium instead of distributing themselves uniformly (Juan et al. 2010). This could lead to challenging antibacterial properties in the future. DeGiglio et al. carried out a similar study except that the nanoparticles were produced through a "green" method of synthesis and showed that silver nanoparticles could be applied to the surface of titanium implants by using a hydrogel method (De Giglio et al. 2013).

14.8.7 Carbon Nanotubes

Nanotubes can be used by modifying their surfaces with different materials to form a more composite assembly and to deliver the antibacterial properties to an optimum level. The cylindrical structure of CNTs enables designing of effective scaffolds loaded with antibiotic and materials in an alignment similar to osteocytes and osteons of the bone. This allows a strong biocompatibility and promotes bone regeneration (Afzal et al. 2013). An increase in the mobilization and bacterial interaction leads to elevated efficiency of isolated single-walled CNTs to exhibit antibacterial properties with greater efficiency (Liu et al. 2009). CNTs possess a stable configuration, are biocompatible, and uphold a high drug-loading ability, making them future candidates for medical applications (Zhang et al. 2010).

14.8.8 Lipid Nanoparticles

Biofilm formation plays a vital role in the progression of diabetic foot ulcer due to antibiotic resistance to the pathogen found in foot infections. The treatment of biofilm infections is one of the biggest challenges to overcome the resistance and tolerance against antimicrobial agents. Several mechanisms have been proposed to overcome the antimicrobial resistance and tolerance such as limited diffusion of antimicrobial agents in the biofilm matrix, deactivation of the antimicrobial agent in the outer layers of the biofilm via binding to matrix components, or enzymatic modification (Banu et al. 2015). Development of innovative strategies to overcome these mechanisms of resistance is the need of the hour. One possible approach to achieve the goal is via lipid nanoparticles for antimicrobial drug delivery. Liposomes are spherical vesicles consisting of one or more phospholipid double layers. Lipophilic drugs can be assimilated into the phospholipid double layers while hydrophilic drugs can be encapsulated into the aqueous core. Several authors have reported that the encapsulation of antibiotics in liposomes resulted in lower minimal inhibitory concentration (MIC) for clinically relevant biofilm-forming organisms and/or lower minimal biofilm inhibitory concentration (MBIC) compared to the free antibiotic in vitro (Kadry et al. 2004).

14.9 Conclusions

The treatment of diabetic foot OM remains challenging, thus opening several avenues for the upcoming nano-based technologies. Nanoparticle modifications of scaffolds boost the capacity to mimic the multifaceted properties of the natural bone environment and provide a more favorable atmosphere for cellular attachment, ingrowth, and bone formation. Despite the appalling advances within this field of nanointerventions, one needs to understand the mechanistic approach involving molecular interactions among the nanoscale surface topography and the biological system. Changes at nanostructural level to polymer surfaces may offer a more favorable milieu for bone regenerative strategies by means of promotion of cellular survival, osteoblastic differentiation, or variation of immunological response. Surface characteristics such as wettability, surface energy and roughness, surface curvature and nanoscale features, proliferation, integration, and viability require a further in-depth investigation. It seems that nano-based interventions behold a great potential for the treatment of diabetes foot osteomyelitis once the mechanisms have been established.

References

Abdelghany SM, Quinn DJ, Ingram RJ, Gilmore BF, Donnelly RF, Taggart C, Scott CJ (2012) Gentamicin-loaded nanoparticles show improved antimicrobial effects towards Pseudomonas aeruginosa infection. Int J Nanomedicine 7:40–53

Afzal MAF, Kalmodia S, Kesarwani P, Basu B, Balani K (2013) Bactericidal effect of silver-reinforced carbon nanotube and hydroxyapatite composites. J Biomater Appl 27:967–978

Almonaci Hernandez CA, Juarez-Moreno K, Castañeda-Juarez ME, Almanza-Reyes H, Pestryakov A (2017) Silver nanoparticles for the rapid healing of diabetic foot ulcers. Int J Med Nano Res 4:1–6

Aragón-Sánchez J (2010) Treatment of diabetic foot osteomyelitis: a surgical critique. Int J Low Extrem Wounds 9:37–59

Armstrong DG, Lavery LA, Quebedeaux TL, Walker SC (1997) Surgical morbidity and the risk of amputation due to infected puncture wounds in diabetic versus nondiabetic adults. J Am Podiatr Med Assoc 87:321–326

Bader MS (2008) Diabetic foot infection. Am Fam Physician 78:71–79

Baino F, Novajra G, Vitale-Brovarone C (2015) Bioceramics and scaffolds: a winning combination for tissue engineering. Front Bioeng Biotechnol 3:202–225

Banu A, Hassan MMN, Rajkumar J, Srinivasa S (2015) Spectrum of bacteria associated with diabetic foot ulcer and biofilm formation: a prospective study. Australas Med J 8:280–285

Barros C, Fulaz S, Stanisic D, Tasic L (2018) Biogenic nanosilver against multidrug-resistant bacteria (MDRB). Antibiotics 4:1–24

Barwell ND, Devers MC, Kennon B, Hopkinson HE, McDougall C, Young MJ, Leese GP (2017) Diabetic foot infection: antibiotic therapy and good practice recommendations. Int J Clin Pract 71:1–10

Belt HVD, Neut D, Schenk W, Horn JRV, Mei HCVD, Busscher HJ (2001) Infection of orthopedic implants and the use of antibiotic-loaded bone cements: a review. Acta Orthop Scand 72:557–571

Berendt A, Peters E, Bakker K, Embil J, Eneroth M, Hinchliffe R, Jeffcoate W, Lipsky B, Senneville E, Teh J, Valk G (2008) Diabetic foot osteomyelitis: a progress report on diagnosis and a systematic review of treatment. Diabetes Metab Res Rev 24:S145–S161

Bessman A, Geiger P, Page J, Sapico F, Canawati H (1991) Prevalence of corynebacterium in diabetic foot infections. Diabetes Care 15:1531–1533

Bramhill J, Ross S, cry Ross G (2017) Bioactive nanocomposites for tissue repair and regeneration: a review. Int J Environ Res Public Health 14:1–21

Butalia S, Palda VA, Sargeant RJ, Detsky AS, Mourad O (2008) Does this patient with diabetes have osteomyelitis of the lower extremity. J Am Med Assoc 299:806–813

Capriotti G, Chianelli M, Signore A (2006) Nuclear medicine imaging of diabetic foot infection: results of meta-analysis. Nucl Med Commun 27(10):757–764

Cierny G, Jon TM, Johan JP (1985) A clinical staging system for adult osteomyelitis. Contemp Orthop 10:17–37

De Giglio E, Cafagna D, Cometa S et al (2013) An innovative, easily fabricated, silver nanoparticle based titanium implant coating: development and analytical characterization. Anal Bioanal Chem 405:805–816

Diamantopoulos EJ, Haritos D, fandi GY, Grigoriadou M, Margariti G, Paniara O, A RS (1998) Management and outcome of severe diabetic foot infections. Exp Clin Endocrinol Diabetes 106:346–352

Dinh MT, Abad CL, Safdar N (2008) Diagnostic accuracy of the physical examination and imaging tests for osteomyelitis underlying diabetic foot ulcers: meta-analysis. Clin Infect Dis 47:519–527

Dorati R, De Trizio A, Genta I, Merelli A, ModeMader JT, Shirtliff ME, Bergquist SC, Calhoun J (1999) Antimicrobial treatment of chronic osteomyelitis. Clin Orthop Relat Res 360:47–65

Eneroth M, Larsson J, Apelqvist J (1999) Deep foot infections in patients with diabetes and foot ulcer: an entity with different characteristics, treatments, and prognosis. J Diabetes Complications 13:254–263

Euba G, Murillo O, Fernandez-Sabe N, Mascaro J, Cabo J, Perez A, Tubau F, Verdaguer R, Gudiol F, Ariza J (2009) Long-term follow-up trial of oral rifampin-cotrimoxazole combination versus intravenous cloxacillin in treatment of chronic staphylococcal osteomyelitis. Antimicrob Agents Chemother 53:2672–2676

Faglia E, Clerici G, Caminiti M, Curci V, Somalvico F (2013) Influence of osteomyelitis location in the foot of diabetic patients with transtibial amputation. Foot Ankle Int 34:222–227

Fleischer AE, Didyk AA, Woods JB, Burns SE, Wrobel JS, Armstrong DG (2009) Combined clinical and laboratory testing improves diagnostic accuracy for osteomyelitis in the diabetic foot. J Foot Ankle Surg 48:39–46

Fraimow HS (2009) Systemic antimicrobial therapy in osteomyelitis. Semin Plast Surg 23:90–99

Garwood CS, Kim PJ (2015) Relevance of osteomyelitis to clinical practice. In: Boffeli TJ (ed) Osteomyelitis of the foot and ankle. Springer, Cham, pp 1–11

Girschick HJ, Krauspe R, Tschammler A, Huppertz HI (1998) Chronic recurrent osteomyelitis with clavicular involvement in children: diagnostic value of different imaging techniques and therapy with non-steroidal anti-inflammatory drugs. Eur J Pediatr 157:28–33

Giurato L, Meloni M, Izzo V, Uccioli L (2017) Osteomyelitis in diabetic foot: a comprehensive overview. World J Diabetes 8:135–142

Gong T, Xie J, Liao J, Zhang T, Lin S, Lin Y (2015) Nanomaterials and bone regeneration. Bone Res 3:1–7

Gonzalez-Sanchez MI, Perni S, Tommasi G, Morris NG, Hawkins K, Lopez-Cabarcos E, Prokopovich P (2015) Silver nanoparticle based antibacterial methacrylate hydrogels potential for bone graft applications. Mater Sci Eng C 50:332–340

Grayson ML (1995) Probing to bone in infected pedal ulcers. A clinical sign of underlying osteomyelitis in diabetic patients. 273(9):721–723

Hannan CM, Attinger CE (2009) Special considerations in the management of osteomyelitis defects (diabetes, the ischemic or dysvascular bed, and irradiation). Semin Plast Surg 23:132–140

Hanssen AD, Spangehl MJ (2004) Treatment of the infected hip replacement. Clin Orthop Relat Res 420:63–71

Hartemann HA, Senneville E (2008) Diabetic foot osteomyelitis. Diabetes Metab 34:87–95

Heiligtag FJ, Niederberger M (2013) The fascinating world of nanoparticle research. Mater Today 16:262–271

Henry SL, Galloway KP (1995) Local antibacterial therapy for the management of orthopaedic infections. Clin Pharmacokinet 29:36–45

Hernández CAA, Juarez-Moreno K, Castañeda-Juarez ME, Almanza-Reyes H, Pestryakov A, Bogdanchikova N (2017) Silver nanoparticles for the rapid healing of diabetic foot ulcers. Int J Med Nano Res 4:1–6

Hobizal KB, Wukich DK (2012) Diabetic foot infections: current concept review. Diabetic Foot Ankle 3:1–18

Huh AJ, Kwon YY (2011) "Nanoantibiotics": a new paradigm for treating infectious diseases using nanomaterials in the antibiotic resistant era. J Control Release 156:128–145

Insall JN, Thompson FM, Brause BD (2002) Two-stage reimplantation for the salvage of infected total knee arthroplasty. J Bone Joint Surg Am 84(3):490

Jeffcoate WJ, Lipsky BA (2004) Controversies in diagnosing and managing osteomyelitis of the foot in diabetes. Clin Infect Dis 39:S115–S122

Juan L, Zhimin Z, Anchun M, Lei L, Jingchao Z (2010) Deposition of silver nanoparticles on titanium surface for antibacterial effect. Int J Nanomedicine 5:261–267

Jurik AG (2004) Chronic recurrent multifocal osteomyelitis. Semin musculoskelet Radiol 8:243–253

Jurik AG, Egund N (1997) MRI in chronic recurrent multifocal osteomyelitis. Skelet Radiol 26:230–238

Kadry AA, Al-Suwayeh SA, Abd-Allah AR, Bayomi MA (2004) Treatment of experimental osteomyelitis by liposomal antibiotics. J Antimicrob Chemother 54:1103–1108

Kagna O, Srour S, Melamed E, Militianu D, Keidar Z (2012) FDG PET/CT imaging in the diagnosis of osteomyelitis in the diabetic foot. Eur J Nucl Med Mol Imaging 39:1545–1550

Kaleta JL, Fleischli JW, Reilly CH (2001) The diagnosis of osteomyelitis in diabetes using erythrocyte sedimentation rate: a pilot study. J Am Podiat Med Assn 91:445–450

Kapoor A, Page S, LaValley M, Gale DR, Felson DT (2007) Magnetic resonance imaging for foot osteomyelitis: a meta-analysis. Arch Intern Med 167:125–132

Kim BN, Kim ES, Oh MD (2013) Oral antibiotic treatment of staphylococcal bone and joint infections in adults. J Antimicrob Chemother 69:309–322

Lavery LA, Armstrong DG, Peters EJ, Lipsky BA (2007) Probe-to-bone test for diagnosing diabetic foot osteomyelitis: reliable or relic. Diabetes Care 30:270–274

Lázaro-Martínez JL, Aragón-Sánchez J, García-Morales E (2014) Antibiotics versus conservative surgery for treating diabetic foot osteomyelitis: a randomized comparative trial. Diabetes Care 37:789–795

Lee YJ, Sadigh S, Mankad K, Kapse N, Rajeswaran G (2016) The imaging of osteomyelitis. Quant Imaging Med Surg 6:184

Lipsky BA (1997) Osteomyelitis of the foot in diabetic patients. Clin Infect Dis 25(6):1318–1326

Lipsky BA (2014) Treating diabetic foot osteomyelitis primarily with surgery or antibiotics: have we answered the question? Diabetes Care 37:593–595

Lipsky BA, Berendt AR, Cornia PB, Pile JC, Peters EJ, Armstrong DG, Pinzur MS (2012) Infectious Diseases Society of America clinical practice guideline for the diagnosis and treatment of diabetic foot infections. Clin Infect Dis 54:132–173

Liu S, Wei L, Hao L, Fang N, Chang MW, Xu R, Chen Y (2009) Sharper and faster "nano darts" kill more bacteria: a study of antibacterial activity of individually dispersed pristine single-walled carbon nanotube. ACS Nano 3:3891–3902

Liu C, Bayer A, Cosgrove SE, Daum RS, Fridkin SK, Gorwitz RJ, Rybak MJ (2011) Clinical practice guidelines by the Infectious Diseases Society of America for the treatment of methicillin-resistant Staphylococcus aureus infections in adults and children. Clin Infect Dis 52:e18–e55

Lu J, Yu H, Chen C (2018) Biological properties of calcium phosphate biomaterials for bone repair: a review. RSC Adv 8:2015–2033

Mader JT, Shirtliff ME, Bergquist SC, Calhoun J (1999) Antimicrobial treatment of chronic osteomyelitis. Clin Orthop Relat Res 360:47–65

Malhotra R, Chan CSY, Nather A (2014) Osteomyelitis in the diabetic foot. Diabetic Foot Ankle 5:24445

Marambio-Jones C, Hoek EMV (2010) A review of the antibacterial effects of silver nanomaterials and potential implications for human health and the environment. J Nanopart Res 12:1531–1551

Margolis DJ, Jeffcoate W (2013) Epidemiology of foot ulceration and amputation: can global variation be explained. Med Clin 97:791–805

Markanday A (2014) Diagnosing diabetic foot osteomyelitis: narrative review and a suggested 2-step score-based diagnostic pathway for clinicians. Open Forum Infect Dis 1(2):ofu060

Mayfield JA, Reiber GE, Sanders LJ, Janisse D, Pogach LM (1998) Preventive foot care in people with diabetes. Diabetes Care 21:2161–2177

McLendon JM, Joshi SR, Sparks J, Matar M, Fewell JG, Abe K, Oka M, McMurtry IF, Gerthoffer WT (2015) Lipid nanoparticle delivery of a microRNA-145 inhibitor improves experimental pulmonary hypertension. J Control Release 210:67–75

McMahon RE, Wang L, Skoracki R, Mathur AB (2013) Development of nanomaterials for bone repair and regeneration. J Biomed Mater Res B Appl Biomater 101:387–397

Michail M, Jude E, Liaskos C, Karamagiolis S, Makrilakis K, Dimitroulis D, Tentolouris N (2013) The performance of serum inflammatory markers for the diagnosis and follow-up of patients with osteomyelitis. Int J Low Extrem Wounds 12:94–99

Miller (2006) Osteomyelitis and the diabetic foot. Radiol Rounds 4:1–4

Molines-Barroso RJ, Lázaro-Martínez JL, Aragón-Sánchez J, García-Morales E, Beneit-Montesinos JV, Álvaro-Afonso FJ (2013) Analysis of transfer lesions in patients who underwent surgery for diabetic foot ulcers located on the plantar aspect of the metatarsal heads. Diabet Med 30:973–976

Murdoch DP, Armstrong DG, Dacus JB, Laughlin TJ, Morgan CB, Lavery LA (1997) The natural history of great toe amputations. J Foot Ankle Surg 36:204–208

Mutluoğlu M, Uzun G, İpcioğlu OM, Sildiroglu O, Özcan Ö, Turhan V, Yildiz S (2011) Can procalcitonin predict bone infection in people with diabetes with infected foot ulcers. A pilot study. Diabetes Res Clin Pract 94:53–56

Nehler MR, Whitehill TA, Bowers SP, Jones DN, Hiatt WR, Rutherford RB, Krupski WC (1999) Intermediate-term outcome of primary digit amputations in patients with diabetes mellitus who have forefoot sepsis requiring hospitalization and presumed adequate circulatory status. J Vasc Surg 30:509–518

Newman LG, Waller J, Palestro CJ, Schwartz M, Klein MJ, Hermann G, Stagnaro-Green A (1991) Unsuspected osteomyelitis in diabetic foot ulcers: diagnosis and monitoring by leukocyte scanning with indium in 111 oxyquinoline. J Am Med Assoc 266:1246–1251

Nguyen S, Pasquet A, Legout L, Beltrand E, Dubreuil L, Migaud H, Senneville E (2009) Efficacy and tolerance of rifampicin-linezolid compared with rifampicin-co-trimoxazole combinations in prolonged oral therapy for bone and joint infections. Clin Microbiol Infect 15:1163–1169

Niazi NS, Drampalos E, Morrissey N, Jahangir N, Wee A, Pillai A (2019) Adjuvant antibiotic loaded bio composite in the management of diabetic foot osteomyelitis—a multicentre study. Foot 39:22–27

Pendsey SP (2010) Understanding diabetic foot. Int J Diabetes Dev Ctries 30:75

Peng KT, Chen CF, Chu IM, Li YM, Hsu WH, Hsu RWW, Chang PJ (2010) Treatment of osteomyelitis with teicoplanin-encapsulated biodegradable thermosensitive hydrogel nanoparticles. Biomaterials 31:5227–5236

Perlroth J, Kuo M, Tan J, Bayer AS, Miller LG (2008) Adjunctive use of rifampin for the treatment of Staphylococcus aureus infections: a systematic review of the literature. Arch Intern Med 168:805–819

Pineda C, Espinosa R, Pena A (2009) Radiographic imaging in osteomyelitis: the role of plain radiography, computed tomography, ultrasonography, magnetic resonance imaging, and scintigraphy. Semin Plast Surg 23:80–89

Power SP, Moloney F, Twomey M, James K, O'Connor OJ, Maher MM (2016) Computed tomography and patient risk: facts, perceptions and uncertainties. World J Radiol 8:902

Qadri S, Haik Y, Mensah-Brown E, Bashir G, Fernandez-Cabezudo MJ, Ramadi BK (2017) Metallic nanoparticles to eradicate bacterial bone infection. Nanomedicine 13:2241–2250

Qin CH, Zhou CH, Song HJ, Cheng GY, Zhang HA, Fang J, Tao R (2019) Infected bone resection plus adjuvant antibiotic-impregnated calcium sulfate versus infected bone resection alone in the treatment of diabetic forefoot osteomyelitis. BMC Musculoskelet Disord 20:246–252

Ranghar S, Sirohi P, Verma P, Agarwal V (2014) Nanoparticle-based drug delivery systems: promising approaches against infections. Braz Arch Biol Technol 57:209–222

Rumpel E, Wolf E, Kauschke E, Bienengräber V, Bayerlein T, Gedrange T, Proff P (2006) The biodegradation of hydroxyapatite bone graft substitutes in vivo. Folia Morphol (Warsz) 65:43–48

Senneville E, Melliez H, Beltrand E, Legout L, Valette M, Cazaubie M, Mouton Y (2006) Culture of percutaneous bone biopsy specimens for diagnosis of diabetic foot osteomyelitis: concordance with ulcer swab cultures. Clin Infect Dis 42:57–62

Shone A, Burnside J, Chipchase S, Game F, Jeffcoate W (2006) Probing the validity of the probe-to-bone test in the diagnosis of osteomyelitis of the foot in diabetes. Diabetes Care 29:945–945

Shults DW, Hunter GC, McIntyre KE, Parent FN, Piotrowski JJ, Bernahd VM (1989) Value of radiographs and bone scans in determining the need for therapy in diabetic patients with foot ulcers. Am J Surg 158:525–530

Singh N (2005) Preventing foot ulcers in patients with diabetes. JAMA 293(2):217

Siitonen OI, Niskanen LK, Laakso M, Siitonen JT, Pyörälä K (1993) Lower-extremity amputations in diabetic and nondiabetic patients: a population-based study in eastern Finland. Diabetes Care 16:16–20

Snoddy B, Jayasuriya AC (2016) The use of nanomaterials to treat bone infections. Mater Sci Eng C 67:822–833

Stewart SB, Engiles J, Hickok NH, Shapiro IM, Richardson DW (2012) Vancomycin-modified implant surface inhibits biofilm formation and supports bone-healing in an infected osteotomy model in sheep: a proof-of-concept study. J Bone Joint Surg 94:1406–1415

Tan JS, Friedman NM, Hazelton-Miller C, Flanagan JP, File TM Jr (1996) Can aggressive treatment of diabetic foot infections reduce the need for above-ankle amputation? Clin Infect Dis 23:286–291

Tiwari G, Tiwari R, Sriwastawa B, Bhati L, Pandey S, Pandey P, Bannerjee SK (2012) Drug delivery systems: an updated review. Int J Pharm Investig 2:2–20

Tone A, Nguyen S, Devemy F, Topolinski H, Valette M, Cazaubiel M, Senneville E (2015) Six-week versus twelve-week antibiotic therapy for nonsurgically treated diabetic foot osteomyelitis: a multicenter open-label controlled randomized study. Diabetes Care 38:302–307

Uskoković V, Desai TA (2013) Phase composition control of calcium phosphate nanoparticles for tunable drug delivery kinetics and treatment of osteomyelitis. I. Preparation and drug release. J Biomed Mater Res Part A 101A (5):1416–1426

van Baal JG (2004) Surgical treatment of the infected diabetic foot. Clin Infect Dis 39:S123–S128

Van GH, Siney H, Danan JP, Sachon C, Grimaldi A (1996) Treatment of osteomyelitis in the diabetic foot: contribution of conservative surgery. Diabetes Care 19:1257–1260

Visakh PM, José M (2016) Introduction for nanomaterials and nanocomposites: state of art, new challenges, and opportunities, Chapter 1. In: Nanomaterials and nanocomposites: zero- to three-dimensional materials and their composites. Wiley, New York

Waldvogel FA, Medoff G, Swart MN (1970) Osteomyelitis: a review of clinical features, therapeutic considerations and unusual aspects. N Engl J Med 282:260–266

Walmsley GG, McArdle A, Tevlin R, Momeni A, Atashroo D, Hu MS, Wan DC (2015) Nanotechnology in bone tissue engineering. Nanomedicine 11:1253–1263

Walter G, Kemmerer M, Kappler C, Hoffmann R (2012) Treatment algorithms for chronic osteomyelitis. Dtsch Arztebl Int 109:257

Wang W, Yeung KW (2017) Bone grafts and biomaterials substitutes for bone defect repair: a review. Bioactive Mater 2:224–247

Williams DN, Gustilo RB, Beverly R, Kind AC (1983) Bone and serum concentrations of five cephalosporin drugs. Relevance to prophylaxis and treatment in orthopedic surgery. Clin Orthop Relat Res 179:253–265

Wininger DA, Fass RJ (1996) Antibiotic-impregnated cement and beads for orthopedic infections. Antimicrob Agents Chemother 40:2675

Yazdanpanah L, Nasiri M, Adarvishi S (2015) Literature review on the management of diabetic foot ulcer. World J Diabetes 6:37

Yu L, Ding J (2008) Injectable hydrogels as unique biomedical materials. Chem Soc Rev 37:1473–1481

Zhang Y, Bai Y, Yan B (2010) Functionalized carbon nanotubes for potential medicinal applications. Drug Discov Today 15:428–435

Zhang D, Wu X, Chen J, Lin K (2018) The development of collagen based composite scaffolds for bone regeneration. Bioactive Mater 3:129–138

Zhou H, Lee J (2011) Nanoscale hydroxyapatite particles for bone tissue engineering. Acta Biomater 7:2769–2781

Zinman LH, Bril V, Perkins BA (2004) Cooling detection thresholds in the assessment of diabetic sensory polyneuropathy: comparison of case IV and Medoc instruments. Diabetes Care 27:1674–1679

Chapter 15
Genotoxicity of Silver Nanoparticles (Ag-NPs) in In Vitro and In Vivo Models

Anita K. Patlolla and Paul B. Tchounwou

Abstract Genotoxicity represents impairment to a cell's DNA or RNA by geno-toxic vehicle. Materials with at least one dimension of 100 nm or less are called nanomaterials. They vary greatly in size, composition, and structure. A phenomenal rapid growth in the use of metal nanomaterials (NPs) in various consumer products and biomedical applications resulted in increased exposure to humans and the environment. Many of the metal NPs used widely (Ag, Au, Ni, Cu, Co, Ti, Zn, and their corresponding oxides) have shown cytotoxicity and genotoxicity in various animal (mammalian/cell) models. Due to their antimicrobial activity silver nanoparticles (Ag-NPs) are one of the most commonly used metal nanoparticles in consumer, medical, and industrial products. Interactions of metal nanomaterials with cells have shown to cause alterations in the expression of several cellular macromole-cules. Overall the major adverse effects include reactive oxygen species (ROS) mediated biomolecular damage to DNA, lipids, and proteins. Although it is likely that the impairment in genotoxicity and oxidative stress biomarkers is associated with Ag-NPs toxicity, it may be from the smaller particles' proclivity to release silver ions from the surface compared to larger particles. This chapter emphasizes on genotoxicity of Ag-NPs in in vitro and in vivo models.

Keywords Silver nanoparticles · Genotoxicity · DNA · Chromosome aberrations · In vitro · In vivo · Reactive oxygen species

A. K. Patlolla (✉) · P. B. Tchounwou
CSET, Department of Biology, Jackson State University, Jackson, MS, USA
e-mail: anita.k.patlolla@jsums.edu

© Springer Nature Switzerland AG 2020
M. Rai (ed.), *Nanotechnology in Skin, Soft Tissue, and Bone Infections*,
https://doi.org/10.1007/978-3-030-35147-2_15

269

15.1   Introduction

The antimicrobial properties of silver nanoparticles (Ag-NPs) have emerged in their large-scale implementation in consumer and healthcare commodities. They are among the most commercialized metal nanomaterial worldwide. Ag-NPs can be found in many consumer commodities including textiles, contraceptive, sports items, cosmetics, cleaning solutions, and food products and packing (Song et al. 2012). In the treatment of a range of diseases including malaria, lupus, tuberculosis, typhoid, tetanus, and cancer, Ag-NPs have been used extensively (FDA 1999). The general populations have a greater chance to be exposed to it in daily life through occupational, environmental, and consumer products (Stebounova et al. 2011). Additionally, the adverse effects of Ag-NPs on human health and the environment are of increasing concern (Fig. 15.1). To date the reports on toxicological effects of Ag-NPs either in vitro (Ahamed et al. 2008; Hsin et al. 2008; Gliga et al. 2014) or in vivo (Asharani et al. 2009; Song et al. 2012; Magdolenova et al. 2014; Patlolla et al. 2015) further provides data indicating adverse effects on cells exposed to Ag-NPs. Exposure to nanoparticles (NPs) takes place through different routes via dermal, inhalation, and ingestion which might lead to a wide range of toxicological effects. From the site of deposition, the NPs are translocated to different parts of the body through circulatory system. Due to their stability, nanomaterials are expected to remain in the body and the environment for long period of time (Karn et al. 2009).

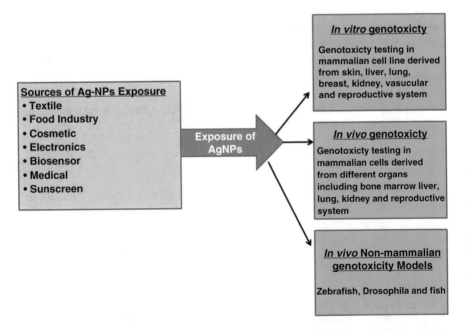

Fig. 15.1 Schematic representation of applications and exposure of Ag-NPs leading to genotoxicity studies in mammalian and non-mammalian cells

Different types of DNA damage (DNA adduct, alkali labile sites, strand breaks) and mutations ranging from gene to structural or numerical chromosome changes are considered as genotoxic effects. Studies on genotoxicity and cellular interactions of metal nanomaterials manufactured on the low nanometer scale have been limited. The reports on genotoxicity of Ag-NPs especially regarding in vivo effects are limited. Although Ag-NPs have great potential benefits, their side effects are unknown and seem inevitable due to their ability to reach the nucleus and damage genetic material.

15.2   Mechanisms of Nanoparticle-Induced Genotoxicity

The exact mechanism through which NPs interact with genetic material is not well established however, insight into factors that affect the physio-chemical properties of a NP would prove helpful in understanding the phenomenon of genotoxicity. Several aspects of NPs specifically size, surface area, particle shape, aspect ratio, surface charge, composition and crystalline structure, aggregation, and concentration have been extensively studied, which may contribute to their reactivity with biomolecules. Such properties on the one hand confer beneficial characteristics on the NPs but on the other hand impart exclusive mechanisms of toxicity, as toxicity has been linked to the aforementioned properties of NPs (Gatoo et al. 2014). The distribution and elimination of NPs by biological systems is almost determined by the particle size (Powers et al. 2007). NPs smaller than 50 nm have been reported to result in toxic manifestations in different tissues while positively charged NPs of greater size (100–120 nm) are readily phagocytosed by mononuclear phagocyte system (De Jong et al. 2008). The rationale behind small size NPs being more reactive is their high surface area to volume ratio, therefore, enhancing their ability to generate ROS-mediated oxidative damage of biomolecules (Risom et al. 2005) and also causing epithelial inflammatory responses (Holgate 2010). Shape and aspect ratio of NPs influence the process of cellular uptake. Spherical NPs are easily and speedily engulfed by cells as compared to rod shaped or fiber-like NPs (Champion and Mitragotri 2006). Aspect ratio is the average ratio of the highest to the lowest dimension of a NP. Higher aspect ratio results in higher toxicity. There are evidences that imply NPs larger in length are more toxic (Lippmann 1990; Hamilton et al. 2009) as macrophages are unable to phagocytose them and thus they are not effectively cleared from the biological system. It has been recorded that uptake of nanorods reaches maximum when aspect ratio is equal to unity (Chen et al. 2009). Surface charge largely affects the behavior of NPs with their surrounding environment. The ability of NPs to get across membranes, binding with biomolecules is mainly regulated by surface charge (Pietroiusti et al. 2011). Positively charged NPs exhibit significant cellular uptake due to the presence of correspondent negatively charged plasma proteins as compared to the negatively charged and neutral NPs (Goodman et al. 2004). Structural differences existing among NPs of the same size and chemical composition have found to be detrimental. Soluble and crystalline forms of some NPs are more toxic than those of the same dimensions (Gurr et al. 2005; Griffitt et al. 2008). Aggregation is the accumulative effect of size, shape, surface charge, structure, and composition of NPs. Agglomerated NPs show more toxicity than well dispersed NPs (Wick et al. 2007). Furthermore, it has been observed that with increase in the concentration of NPs, the toxicity decreases at higher concentration.

A common hypothesis suggests that genotoxicity may be triggered in two different ways: primary direct contact between NPs and the genetic material or primary indirect damage from NPs induced ROS, and by hyperreactive ions generated from soluble NPs (Kisin et al. 2007) while secondary genotoxicity is also caused by ROS but through activated phagocytes (neutrophils, macrophages) at the time of NPs-triggered inflammation (Stone et al. 2009). Schemes of different types of potential NPs induced genotoxicity are well explained diagrammatically by Magdolenova et al. (2014). NPs that reach across cellular membranes may infiltrate the nucleus through diffusion across the nuclear membrane or transiting through the nuclear pore complexes and mesh directly with DNA. The overall nuclear pore complex size varies among eukaryotic species, however the diameter measures 100–150 nm on average (Wente and Rout 2010), therefore, it is most convenient to get across through the nuclear pore complexes easily as NPs used generally well fall within this size range. As considered by Barillet et al. (2010), studies conducted in vitro showed that smaller size NPs might enter the nucleus through nuclear pores (diameter 8–10 nm), while bigger NPs such as SiCNPs (15–60 nm) might only interfere with the DNA in mitotic cells while the nuclear membrane disappears during mitosis (Singh et al. 2009). For example, TiO_2 NPs (Shukla et al. 2011), ZnO-NPs (Hackenberg et al. 2011b), and Ag-NPs (Hackenberg et al. 2011a) are reported to accumulate in the nucleus after in vitro exposure. Larger intranuclear aggregates of TiO_2-NPs have also been located in the nucleus (the mean size of studied TiO_2NPs was 285±52 nm and in particular cases aggregates could reach diameters up to 2000 nm, thus corroborating higher toxicity of agglomerates as mentioned before (Hackenberg et al. 2010)). In vitro genotoxicity of TiO_2-NPs on human nasal mucosa cells was not observed by the same authors (Hackenberg et al. 2010) but in another study an efficacious effect of ZnO was observed with the comet assay (Hackenberg et al. 2011c) and also of Ag-NPs, observed with the chromosome aberration assay (Hackenberg et al. 2011a). According to the study of Di Virgilio et al. (2010) nucleus can even be deformed by large lumps of NPs as demonstrated by in vitro transmission electron microscopy (TEM) examinations in the Chinese hamster ovary cells CHO-KI. Clusters of TiO_2-NPs wreaked the formation of cellular vesicles which had impressed and modified the form of the nucleus, which may afterwards adversely affect the mitotic process, substantially not allowing the proper isolation of chromosomes and the actual working of the mitotic apparatus. The NP clusters could also unreasoningly damage the chromosomes. Di Virgilio et al. (2010) observed an enhanced recurrence of MN formation and sister chromatid swap after TiO_2NPs exposure. However, NPs presence in the nuclei could not be manifested.

15.3 Methods for Genotoxicity Testing

Several methods have been adapted to assess genotoxicity of NPs. Principal mechanisms may vary but focus of the method being utilized remains the same i.e., NPs induced genetic damage.

15.3.1 Ames Test

The Ames test exploits the principal of reverse mutation, which utilizes several strains of the mutated bacteria Salmonella *typhimurium* lacking the means to synthesize the amino acid histidine, so they need exogenous supply of histidine as a growth additive. The bacteria accompanied with the test compound are cultured on a minimal media and only those bacteria will be able to grow into colonies that have regained their histidine synthesis genes function (hist) through reverse mutation. The density of colonies formed is equivalent to the mutation recurrence instigated by the test compound at a specific dose (Ames et al. 1972).

15.3.2 Chromosome Aberration Test

Using this assay chromosomal alteration can be determined by blocking cell cycles of cultured mammalian cells exposed to the test agent at metaphase stage just before formation of two daughter nuclei by the replicated chromosomes. The chromosome samples collected at metaphase stage are then mounted on slides, followed with Giemsa staining to distinguish the banding patterns on the chromosomes. Microscopic study of the cells is then performed to analyze the presence of chromosomal anomalies subjected to their respective structures and number (Galloway et al. 1987).

15.3.3 Comet Assay

The comet assay, also known as the single-cell gel electrophoresis (SCGE) assay is used for measuring DNA single- and double-strand breaks at the level of individual cells. DNA released as a result of individual cell's lysis in a thin layer of agarose gel (having low melting point) on a microscope slide is electrophoreses. The applied electric charge causes minimal movement of unbroken DNA owing to its large size, but small broken/damaged DNA fragments extend much further forming a comet body(with an elongated tail outstretched) toward the anode. The extent of DNA damage can be correlated to the length and fluorescence intensity of the comet tail as observed with either ethidium bromide or propidium iodide staining (Collins et al. 2008).

15.3.4 Cytokinesis-Blocked Micronucleus Assay

Cell cycle at cytokinesis can be blocked by the use of cytochalasin B, which is an actin polymerization inhibitor, forming binucleated cells. Cells are subjected to divide in the presence of test substance, if the test substance inflicts chromosomal breakdown or loss, as a result the affected genetic material does not contribute to chromosomal disjunction and is absent in either of the two daughter nuclei. Rather they are isolated in the form of a MN and their number in resultant binucleated cells can provide an estimate of genotoxicity caused by the test substance at a given amount (Fenech and Morley 1986). The nature of genetic damages either is chromosome fragmentation (clastogenic) or whole chromosome loss (aneugenic) can be determined by coupling MN assays with kinetochore staining. Kinetochores are basically protein bodies that appear at the centromere of all chromosomes throughout nuclear division, thus positively stained kinetochore MN carry a whole chromosome and characterize an aneugenic case. Whereas the negatively stained kinetochore MN are a result of a clastogenic event as they carry chromosome fragments (Fenech 2000).

15.3.5 HPRT Forward Mutation Assay

The HPRT (hypoxanthine–guanine phosphoribosyltransferase) primarily functions to regain purines from degraded DNA and reintroduce them into the purine synthetic pathways. When cells are cultured along with 6-thioguanine, a poisonous purine base pair analogue, HPRT enzyme will also integrate this counterpart into DNA at the time of replication, resulting in mortality of normal cells. However, if a mutation appears in this gene following treatment with the test substance, the nucleotide salvage will no more be able to integrate the toxic counterpart during DNA replication hence viable cell clusters will be observed. The cell's viability frequency shows the extent of damaging point mutations at a given dose of the test substance (DeMarini et al. 1989).

15.3.6 g-H2AX Staining

g-H2AX is formed by modification of histone H2A variant in higher eukaryotes at DNA double strand breaks (DSB), which acts as a precursor signaling for recruitment of DNA repair proteins to DSB region. Adapting immunofluorescence microscopy that employ fluorescently labeled antibodies targeting g-H2AX can report DNA damage and can locate the damaged sites (Petrini and Stracker 2003).

15.3.7 8-Hydroxydeoxyguanosine DNA Adducts

8-hydroxydeoxyguanosine (8-OHdG), also known as DNA adduct is formed due to modification of guanine base as a result of attack on DNA by ROS induced by oxidative stress. Such DNA adduct can cause potent alterations while DNA replication occurs as DNA polymerases are incapable of recognizing it as guanine base. Oxidative stress DNA damage can, therefore, be considered if there is presence of this DNA adduct. Numerous methods particularly HPLC and mass spectrometry (GC-MS) based analytical techniques are being used for the detection of 8-OHdG. Alternative practices include antibody involving procedures such as immunofluorescence, immunohistochemistry, and DNA dot blots (Halliwell and Gutteridge 2015).

15.4 Genotoxicity of Silver NPs (Ag-NPs)

Among the nano-sized materials available in the market Ag-NPs are noticeably the most used nanocompounds (Ahamed et al. 2008). In a most recent genotoxicity study of Ag-NPs synthesized from Adeniumobesum leaf extracts conducted on MCF-7 breast cancer cells which were exposed to three different concentrations (50, 100, and 150 µg/mL) for 24 h, alkaline comet assay determined the DNA damage (Farah et al. 2016). Microscopic imaging showed dose dependent increase in DNA fragmentation (significantly longer comet tail lengths) as well decrease in cell survival was also observed for treated cells. A notable increase of 2.5-folds in ROS generation at the highest concentration of 150 µg/mL was confirmed by both qualitative and quantitative tests suggesting ROS-mediated DNA damage and apoptosis of MCF-7 cells. Dose dependent increase in various comet parameters such as tail length, intensity, and movement was also observed in mice orally instilled with Ag-NPs and carbon nanotubes, respectively (Awasthi et al. 2015). Results obtained from DNA damage study after photodynamic therapy (PDT) of lung cancer cells (A549 cell line) also showed the presence of DNA fragmentation through the generation of ROS detected via mitochondrial membrane potential changes and comet assay (El-Hussein 2016). In another study dose and time-dependent genotoxic effects of Ag-NPs were observed on human lung epithelial cells (Suliman et al. 2015). Oral exposure of Ag-NPs to mice showed induction of large DNA deletions in developing embryos, uncorrectable chromosomal damage in bone marrow, DSB and oxidative DNA damage along with modulation of DNA repair gene expression system particularly the downregulation of base excision repair (BER) genes enhancing susceptibility to cancer (Kovvuru et al. 2015). A concentration dependent but low level genotoxic effect of Ag-NPs has been reported in Ntera2 (NT2, human testicular embryonic carcinoma cell line), (Asare et al. 2012). Comparison of cytotoxicity and genotoxicity results of different studies conducted separately for uncapped Ag-NPs having size of 20–50 nm and concentrations less than 10 mg/mL in different experimental models inferred proclivity of lethal dose (LD_{50}) to be ranging from 1 to 7 mg/mL for both in vitro and in vivo studies as evaluated for various aquatic organisms (Griffitt et al. 2008; Griffitt et al. 2009), cell culture (Wise et al. 2010), crustaceans (Park and Choi 2010), or larvae (Nair et al. 2011). Zebra fish, Daphnia, and *Pseudokirchneriella subcapitata* were treated with commercial Ag-NPs nanopowder (size 20–30 nm) and the response was recorded. The toxicity response was developmental stage dependent, whether the treatment was done to an adult or juvenile fish, after 48 h treatment LD_{50} of 7.0–7.2 mg/mL in Zebra fish and 0.040–0.067 mg/mL in Daphnia was obtained. In *P. subcapitata* LD_{50} was recorded to be 0.19 mg/mL. For soluble metal treatment, LD_{50} of 0.022 mg/mL and 0.008–0.16 mg/mL was recorded for Zebra fish and *Daphnia*, respectively. These results showed that soluble metal was more toxic compared with Ag-NPs (Griffitt et al. 2008). Microarray test revealed induction of gene expression changes by nanosilver (1 mg/mL) after 24 and 48 h of exposure. These results showed that 82 genes were downregulated and 66 genes were upregulated during 24 h, whereas 126 genes observed upregulated and 336 genes observed downregulated during 48 h. Furthermore, among the observed genes some of them represented similarities to human genes, most of them found connected to cell death, mitosis initiation, and proliferation signaling (Griffitt et al. 2009). 100% fatality occurred for *Daphnia magna* at 1 mg/mL of Ag-NPs (35 nm) at 96 h, and 43.33% for 0.1 mg/mL treatment. Long-term experiments in which *Daphnia magna* was exposed to Ag-NPs showed significant toxicity at lower concentrations of Ag-NPs 0.001 mg/mL (Gaiser et al. 2011). In another work, Gaiser et al. (2012) compared the potential effects of micro (600–1.600) and nano-sized (35 nm) particles in a range of cells including fish hepatocyte, intestinal and human hepatocyte and two animal models, *Daphnia magna* and *Cyprinus carpio*. A comparable biological response was obtained from different models in this study. The authors noted that Ag-NPs were found to be comparatively more harmful than greater micro-sized Ag-NPs. Observing shared toxic attributes in these different models as a result of the same Ag-NPs, they concluded that it would be suitable to extend the application of these results over a range of living systems for future test development and planning. Freshwater crustacean *Daphnia magna* was tested for comparative genotoxicity and ecotoxicity analysis of less than 50 nm Ag-NPs (Sigma, pre-filtered) and Ag ions [aqueous silver nitrate, ($AgNO_3$)]. 100% mortality was recorded for up to 2 mg/mL concentration (24 h; LD50 ~1.2 mg/mL) in case of acute toxicity but 0% mortality occurred at 1 mg/mL. Repetitively, increasing mortality was observed in connection with DNA damage in the Ag-NPs, which suggests that Ag-NPs induced DNA damage might incite higher-level complications. The results of the comparative toxicological study of Ag-NPs and Ag ions advocated that the aforementioned were meagerly more toxic and it was considered that Ag ions contributed to the damaging effects of Ag-NPs (Park and Choi 2010). It was established that mice are comparatively more susceptible than fish to capped Ag-NPs. For example, capping Ag-NPs with starch (sizes 8–15 nm), capping with bovine serum albumin (sizes 10–20 nm (Asharani et al. 2008)), and capping with polyvinyl alcohol (sizes 5–35 nm) (Asharani et al. 2011), none of these complexes caused genotoxicity on zebra fish embryos up to concentrations of 25 mg/mL. However, a significant raise in the concentration to >100 mg/mL produced genotoxicity as well a relative increase in apoptosis and abnormalities in the embryos, these effects were noticed to be more prominent for albumin-capped Ag-NPs than for other complexes. In a similar study, comparative genotoxicity evaluation was performed for Ag-NPs, anionic surfactant (AOT) used as dispersant of the particles and Ag ions (silver nitrate; $AgNO_3$), size ranged from 3 to 15 nm. Results showed LD_{50} value of 3 mg/mL, prevalence of abnormal sperm heads, and DNA damage after the addition of Ag-NPs in concentrations of half of the $LD_{50/30}$ values (Ordzhonikidze et al. 2009). It was concluded that mortality was caused in the decreasing order of Ag-NPs > AOT >> AgNO3.AOT had more DNA damaging effects than uncapped Ag-NPs; however, abnormal sperm morphology as a result of either chromosomal aberrations or somatic DNA damage in the reproductive cells received almost same damaging effects from both Ag-NPs and AOT at same concentrations. Ag ions were least toxic. Various in vivo studies report genotoxicity due to Ag-NPs at significantly elevated dose exposure. Patlolla et al. (2015) reported an increase in micronuclei formation, as well as structural chromosome aberrations, damage to DNA as seen via the comet assay, and a decrease in the mitotic index in bone marrow cells of male Sprague Dawley rats administered orally with 10 nm Ag-NPs (5, 25, 50, 100 mg/kg) once a day for five days. The highest two doses (50 and 100 mg/kg) induced a remarkable increase in all tested biomarkers, and caused an increase in ROS as measured by H_2DCFDA. Li et al. (2017) explored the differential genotoxicity mechanisms of Ag-NPs and silver ions in Human TK6 cells. To evaluate genotoxicity and induction of oxidative stress TK6 cells were treated with 5 nM Ag-NP or $AgNO_3$ (silver nitrate). The results of this study demonstrated that both Ag-NPs and AgNOs induced genotoxicity via oxidative stress, although the mechanisms and nanoparticles are different not the released ions that contributed to the genotoxicity of Ag-NPs. The effects of size and coating on the cytotoxicity and genotoxicity of Ag-NPs were reported by Guo et al. (2016). Six different types of Ag-NPs having three different sizes and two different coatings were examined using the Ames test, mouse lymphoma assay (MLA) and in vitro micronucleus (MN) assay. All types of silver compounds in Ames test generated inconclusive outcomes. Size-dependent cytotoxicity and genotoxicity were observed in both MLA and MN assays. The effects of coating was relatively less in inducing genotoxicity by Ag-NPs. Comparative genotoxic effects of Ag-NPs with/without coating in human liver HepG2 cells and in mice were reported by Wang et al. (2019). The study examined DNA damage and chromosomal aberrations in $HepG_2$ cell line and micronucleus test in bone marrow of mice. Polyvinylpyrrolidone (PVP)-coated and uncoated Ag-NPs were used for exposure to HepG2 cell line and mice. Uncoated Ag-NPs caused more DNA-damage than PVP-coated, while it was vice-versa in chromosomal aberrations (CA). In the micronucleus test on mouse bone marrow cells, the highest dose 250 mg/kg body weight showed chromosomal aberrations. The outcome of this study was that Ag-NPs have genotoxic effects in HepG2 cells and limited effects on bone marrow in mice.

15.5   Conclusion and Future Perspectives

The presence of DNA damage, structural and numerical chromosomal aberrations and mutations are the fundamental outcomes that need to be assessed in order to confirm genotoxicity. Predominantly the studies, both in vitro and in vivo, demonstrate that silver nanoparticles has genotoxic effects, nonetheless, other studies do not report any genotoxicity. Numerous in vitro genotoxicity assays may be assessed, these in vitro assays expressed to be greatly fragile but not very precise. Therefore, in vivo testing is necessary for validation. However, the available data seems equivocal to arrive at a final conclusion about the safety issues of NPs related with living systems as most of the NPs exhibit a time and dose (increasing order) dependent manner of genotoxicity, also many NPs such as gold NPs are considered the future elements of theranostics applications specifically cancer therapy so there is a need for research that could provide a powerful insight into mechanisms underlying these risks thus would clearly demarcate associated risks and benefits.

Acknowledgments Authors are thankful to National Institutes of Health (Grant # G12MD007581) through the RCMI Center for Environmental Health at Jackson State University for support.
   Conflict of Interest Statement: The authors declare no conflict of interest.

References

Ahamed M, Karns M, Goodson M, Rowe J, Hussain SM, Schlager JJ, Hong Y (2008) DNA damage response to different surface chemistry of silver nanoparticles in mammalian cells. Toxicol Appl Pharmacol 233(3):404–410

Ames BN, Gurney E, Miller JA, Bartsch H (1972) Carcinogens as frameshift mutagens: metabolites and derivatives of 2-acetylaminofluorene and other aromatic amine carcinogens. Proc Natl Acad Sci U S A 69(11):3128–3132

Asare N, Instanes C, Sandberg WJ, Refsnes M, Schwarze P, Kruszewski M, Brunborg G (2012) Cytotoxic and genotoxic effects of silver nanoparticles in testicular cells. Toxicology 291(1):65–72

Asharani P, Wu YL, Gong Z, Valiyaveettil S (2008) Toxicity of silver nanoparticles in zebrafish models. Nanotechnology 19(25):255102

Asharani PV, Hande MP, Valiyaveettil S (2009) Anti-proliferative activity of silver nanoparticles. BMC Cell Biol. 10:65

Asharani P, Lianwu Y, Gong Z, Valiyaveettil S (2011) Comparison of the toxicity of silver, gold and platinum nanoparticles in developing zebrafish embryos. Nanotoxicology 5(1):43–54

Awasthi KK, Awasthi A, Verma R, Soni I, Awasthi K, John P (2015) Silver nanoparticles and carbon nanotubes induced DNA damage in mice evaluated by single cell gel electrophoresis. Wiley Online Library, Hoboken, NJ, pp 210–217

Barillet S, Jugan M-L, Laye M, Leconte Y, Herlin-Boime N, Reynaud C, Carriere M (2010) In vitro evaluation of SiC nanoparticles impact on A549 pulmonary cells: cyto-, genotoxicity and oxidative stress. Toxicol Lett 198(3):324–330

Champion JA, Mitragotri S (2006) Role of target geometry in phagocytosis. Proc Natl Acad Sci U S A 103(13):4930–4934

Chen Y-S, Hung Y-C, Liau I, Huang GS (2009) Assessment of the in vivo toxicity of gold nanoparticles. Nanoscale Res Lett 4(8):858

Collins AR, Oscoz AA, Brunborg G, Gaivao I, Giovannelli L, Kruszewski M, Smith CC, Štětina R (2008) The comet assay: topical issues. Mutagenesis 23(3):143–151

De Jong WH, Hagens WI, Krystek P, Burger MC, Sips AJ, Geertsma RE (2008) Particle size dependent organ distribution of gold nanoparticles after intravenous administration. Biomaterials 29(12):1912–1919

DeMarini DM, Brockman HE, de Serres FJ, Evans HH, Stankowski LF, Hsie AW (1989) Specific-locus mutations induced in eukaryotes (especially mammalian cells) by radiation and chemicals: a perspective. Mutat Res Rev Genet Toxicol 220(1):11–29

Di Virgilio A, Reigosa M, Arnal P, De Mele MFL (2010) Comparative study of the cytotoxic and genotoxic effects of titanium oxide and aluminium oxide nanoparticles in Chinese hamster ovary (CHO-K1) cells. J Hazard Mater 177(1):711–718

El-Hussein A (2016) Study DNA damage after photodynamic therapy using silver nanoparticles with A549 cell line. J Nanomed Nanotechnol 7(1):1000346

Farah MA, Ali MA, Chen S-M, Li Y, Al-Hemaid FM, Abou-Tarboush FM, Al-Anazi KM, Lee J (2016) Silver nanoparticles synthesized from Adenium obesum leaf extract induced DNA damage, apoptosis and autophagy via generation of reactive oxygen species. Colloids Surf B 141:158–169

FDA (1999) Food and Drug Administration issues final ruling on OTC products containing colloidal silver. http://www.fda.gov/bbs/topics/ANSWERS/ANS00971.html

Fenech M (2000) The in vitro micronucleus technique. Mutat Res Fund Mol Mech 455(1):81–95

Fenech M, Morley AA (1986) Cytokinesis-block micronucleus method in human lymphocytes: effect of in vivo ageing and low dose X-irradiation. Mutat Res Fund Mol Mech 161(2):193–198

Gaiser BK, Biswas A, Rosenkranz P, Jepson MA, Lead JR, Stone V, Tyler CR, Fernandes TF (2011) Effects of silver and cerium dioxide micro-and nano-sized particles on Daphnia magna. J Environ Monitor 13(5):1227–1235

Gaiser BK, Fernandes TF, Jepson MA, Lead JR, Tyler CR, Baalousha M, Biswas A, Britton GJ, Cole PA, Johnston BD (2012) Interspecies comparisons on the uptake and toxicity of silver and cerium dioxide nanoparticles. Environ Toxicol Chem 31(1):144–154

Galloway S, Armstrong M, Reuben C, Colman S, Brown B, Cannon C, Bloom A, Nakamura F, Ahmed M, Duk S (1987) Chromosome aberrations and sister chromatid exchanges in Chinese hamster ovary cells: evaluations of 108 chemicals. Environ Mol Mutagen 10(S10):1–35

Gatoo MA, Naseem S, Arfat MY, Mahmood Dar A, Qasim K, Zubair S (2014) Physico-chemical properties of nanomaterials: implication in associated toxic manifestations. Bio Med Res Int 2014:498420

Gliga AR, Skoglund S, Wallinder IO, Fadeel B, Karlsson HL (2014) Size-dependent cytotoxicity of silver nanoparticles in human lung cells: the role of cellular uptake, agglomeration and Ag release. Part Fibre Toxicol 11:11

Goodman CM, McCusker CD, Yilmaz T, Rotello VM (2004) Toxicity of gold nanoparticles functionalized with cationic and anionic side chains. Bioconjugate Chem 15(4):897–900

Griffitt RJ, Luo J, Gao J, Bonzongo JC, Barber DS (2008) Effects of particle composition and species on toxicity of metallic nanomaterials in aquatic organisms. Environ Toxicol Chem 27(9):1972–1978

Griffitt RJ, Hyndman K, Denslow ND, Barber DS (2009) Comparison of molecular and histological changes in zebrafish gills exposed to metallic nanoparticles. Toxicol Sci 107(2):404–415

Guo X, Li Y, Yan J, Ingle T, Jones MY, Mei N, Boudreau MD, Cunningham CK, Abbas M, Paredes AM, Zhou T, Moore MM, Howard PC, Chen T (2016) Size- and coating-dependent cytotoxicity and genotoxicity of silver nanoparticles evaluated using in vitro standard assays. Nanotoxicology 10(9):1373–1384

Gurr J-R, Wang AS, Chen C-H, Jan K-Y (2005) Ultrafine titanium dioxide particles in the absence of photoactivation can induce oxidative damage to human bronchial epithelial cells. Toxicology 213(1):66–73

Hackenberg S, Friehs G, Froelich K, Ginzkey C, Koehler C, Scherzed A, Burghartz M, Hagen R, Kleinsasser N (2010) Intracellular distribution, geno-and cytotoxic effects of nanosized titanium dioxide particles in the anatase crystal phase on human nasal mucosa cells. Toxicol Lett 195(1):9–14

Hackenberg S, Scherzed A, Kessler M, Hummel S, Technau A, Froelich K, Ginzkey C, Koehler C, Hagen R, Kleinsasser N (2011a) Silver nanoparticles: evaluation of DNA damage, toxicity and functional impairment in human mesenchymal stem cells. Toxicol Lett 201(1):27–33

Hackenberg S, Scherzed A, Technau A, Kessler M, Froelich K, Ginzkey C, Koehler C, Burghartz M, Hagen R, Kleinsasser N (2011b) Cytotoxic, genotoxic and proinflammatory effects of zinc oxide nanoparticles in human nasal mucosa cells in vitro. Toxicol In Vitro 25(3):657–663

Hackenberg S, Zimmermann FZ, Scherzed A, Friehs G, Froelich K, Ginzkey C, Koehler C, Burghartz M, Hagen R, Kleinsasser N (2011c) Repetitive exposure to zinc oxide nanoparticles induces DNA damage in human nasal mucosa mini organ cultures. Environ Mol Mutagen 52(7):582–589

Halliwell B, Gutteridge JM (2015) Free radicals in biology and medicine. Oxford University Press, New York

Hamilton RF, Wu N, Porter D, Buford M, Wolfarth M, Holian A (2009) Particle length dependent titanium dioxide nanomaterials toxicity and bioactivity. Part Fibre Toxicol 6(1):1

Holgate ST (2010) Exposure, uptake, distribution and toxicity of nanomaterials in humans. J Biomed Nanotechnol 6(1):1–19

Hsin Y, Chen C, Huang S, Shih T, Lai P, Chueh PJ (2008) The apoptotic effect of nanosilver is mediated by a ROS- and JNK-dependent mechanism involving the mitochondrial pathway in NIH3T3 cells. Toxicol Lett 179:130–139

Karn B, Kuiken T, Otto M (2009) Nanotechnology and in situ remediation: a review of the benefits and potential risks. Environ Health Perspect 117(12):1813–1831

Kisin ER, Murray AR, Keane MJ, Shi X-C, Schwegler-Berry D, Gorelik O, Arepalli S, Castranova V, Wallace WE, Kagan VE (2007) Single-walled carbon nanotubes: geno-and cytotoxic effects in lung fibroblast V79 cells. J Toxicol Environ Health A 70(24):2071–2073

Kovvuru P, Mancilla PE, Shirode AB, Murray TM, Begley TJ, Reliene R (2015) Oral ingestion of silver nanoparticles induces genomic instability and DNA damage in multiple tissues. Nanotoxicology 9(2):162–171

Li Y, Qin T, Ingle T, Yan J, He W, Yin JJ, Chen T (2017) Differential genotoxicity mechanisms of silver nanoparticles and silver ions. Arch Toxicol 91(1):509–519

Lippmann M (1990) Effects of fiber characteristics on lung deposition, retention, and disease. Environ Health Perspect 88:311

Magdolenova Z, Collins A, Kumar A, Dhawan A, Stone V, Dusinska M (2014) Mechanisms of genotoxicity. A review of in vitro and in vivo studies with engineered nanoparticles. Nanotoxicology 8(3):233–278

Nair PMG, Park SY, Lee SW, Choi J (2011) Differential expression of ribosomal protein gene, gonadotrophin releasing hormone gene and Balbiani ring protein gene in silver nanoparticles exposed Chironomus riparius. Aquat Toxicol 101(1):31–37

Ordzhonikidze C, Ramaiyya L, Egorova E, Rubanovich A (2009) Genotoxic effects of silver nanoparticles on mice in vivo. Acta Naturae 1(3):99–101

Park SY, Choi JH (2010) Geno-and ecotoxicity evaluation of silver nanoparticles in Fresh water crustacean Daphnia magna. Environ Eng Res 15(1):23–27

Patlolla AK, Hackett D, Tchounwou PB (2015) Silver nanoparticle-induced oxidative stress-dependent toxicity in Sprague-Dawley rats. Mol Cell Biochem 399(1–2):257–268

Petrini JH, Stracker TH (2003) The cellular response to DNA double-strand breaks: defining the sensors and mediators. Trends Cell Biol 13(9):458–462

Pietroiusti A, Massimiani M, Fenoglio I, Colonna M, Valentini F, Palleschi G, Camaioni A, Magrini A, Siracusa G, Bergamaschi A (2011) Low doses of pristine and oxidized singlewall carbon nanotubes affect mammalian embryonic development. ACS Nano 5(6):4624–4633

Powers KW, Palazuelos M, Moudgil BM, Roberts SM (2007) Characterization of the size, shape, and state of dispersion of nanoparticles for toxicological studies. Nanotoxicology 1(1):42–51

Risom L, Moller P, Loft S (2005) Oxidative stress-induced DNA damage by particulate air pollution. Mutat Res Fund Mol Mech 592(1):119–137

Shukla RK, Sharma V, Pandey AK, Singh S, Sultana S, Dhawan A (2011) ROS-mediated genotoxicity induced by titanium dioxide nanoparticles in human epidermal cells. Toxicol In Vitro 25(1):231–241

Singh N, Manshian B, Jenkins GJ, Griffiths SM, Williams PM, Maffeis TG, Wright CJ, Doak SH (2009) NanoGenotoxicology: the DNA damaging potential of engineered nanomaterials. Biomaterials 30(23):3891–3914

Song MF, Li YS, Kasai H, Kawai K (2012) Metal nanoparticle-induced micronuclei and oxidative DNA damage in mice. J Clin Biochem Nutr 50(3):211–216

Stebounova LV, Adamcakova-Dodd A, Kim JS, Park H, O'Shaughnessy PT, Grassain VH, Thorne PS (2011) Nanosilver induces minimal lung toxicity or inflammation in a subacute murine inhalation model. Part Fibre Toxicol 8:5

Stone V, Johnston H, Schins RP (2009) Development of in vitro systems for nanotoxicology: methodological considerations. Crit Rev Toxicol 39(7):613–626

Suliman Y, Omar A, Ali D, Alarifi S, Harrath AH, Mansour L, Alwasel SH (2015) Evaluation of cytotoxic, oxidative stress, proinflammatory and genotoxic effect of silver nanoparticles in human lung epithelial cells. Environ Toxicol 30(2):149–160

Wang X, Li T, Su X, Li J, Li W, Gan J, Wu T, Kong L, Zhang T, Tang M, Xue Y (2019) Genotoxic effects of silver nanoparticles with/without coating in human liver HepG2 cells and in mice. J Appl Toxicol 39(6):908–918

Wente SR, Rout MP (2010) The nuclear pore complex and nuclear transport. Cold Spring Harbor Perspect Biol 2(10):a000562

Wick P, Manser P, Limbach LK, Dettlaff-Weglikowska U, Krumeich F, Roth S, Stark WJ, Bruinink A (2007) The degree and kind of agglomeration affect carbon nanotube cytotoxicity. Toxicol Lett 168(2):121–131

Wise JP, Goodale BC, Wise SS, Craig GA, Pongan AF, Walter RB, Thompson WD, Ng AK, Aboueissa A-M, Mitani H (2010) Silver nanospheres are cytotoxic and genotoxic to fish cells. Aquat Toxicol 97(1):34–41

Index

Printed in the United States
By Bookmasters